Handbook of
Mental Illness in
the Mentally Retarded

Handbook of Mental Illness in the Mentally Retarded

Edited by

Frank J. Menolascino, M.D.

Nebraska Psychiatric Institute
University of Nebraska Medical Center
Omaha, Nebraska

and

Jack A. Stark, Ph.D.

Departments of Pediatrics and Psychiatry
University of Nebraska Medical Center
Omaha, Nebraska

Plenum Press • New York and London

Library of Congress Cataloging in Publication Data

Main entry under title:

Handbook of mental illness in the mentally retarded.

Includes bibliographies and indexes.
1. Mentally handicapped—Mental health services—Handbooks, manuals, etc. I.
Menolascino, Frank J., 1930–   . II. Stark, Jack A., 1946–   . [DNLM: 1.
Mental Disorders. 2. Mental Retardation—complications. WM 307.M5 H236]
RC451.4.M47H36   1984   362.3   84-13263
ISBN 0-306-41648-4

©1984 Plenum Press, New York
A Division of Plenum Publishing Corporation
233 Spring Street, New York, N.Y. 10013

Printed in the United States of America

Contributors

Diana W. Allin, M.A., Chesterfield Mental Health and Mental Retardation Services, Lucy Corr Court, Chesterfield, Virginia

Robert B. Allin, M.A., Chesterfield Mental Health and Mental Retardation Services, Lucy Corr Court, Chesterfield, Virginia

Daniel H. Baker, Ph.D., Department of Psychiatry, Meyer Children's Rehabilitation Institute, University of Nebraska Medical Center, Omaha, Nebraska

William J. Bates, M.D., Department of Psychiatry, Ohio State University, Columbus, Ohio

Frederic B. Chanteau, B.A., Executive Director, the Rock Creek Foundation, Silver Spring, Maryland

Christine L. Cole, M.S.S.W., Waisman Center on Mental Retardation and Human Development, University of Wisconsin, Madison, Wisconsin

John Y. Donaldson, M.D., Department of Psychiatry, Nebraska Psychiatric Institute, University of Nebraska Medical Center, Omaha, Nebraska

Ellen S. Fabian, M.A., Director of Research and Training, the Rock Creek Foundation, Silver Spring, Maryland

Robert J. Fletcher, M.S.W., C.S.W., A.C.S.W., Founder and Executive Director, National Association for the Dually Diagnosed and Director, Dual Diagnosed Day Treatment Program, Beacon House, Ulster County Mental Health Services, Kingston, New York

Larry Folk, B.A., Mental Health Coordinator, Dual Diagnosis Service, Nebraska Psychiatric Institute, University of Nebraska Medical Center, Omaha, Nebraska

William I. Gardner, Ph.D., Waisman Center on Mental Retardation and Human Development, University of Wisconsin, Madison, Wisconsin

Bruce Gutnik, Ph.D., Department of Psychiatry, Nebraska Psychiatric Institute, University of Nebraska Medical Center, Omaha, Nebraska

Helen Houston, C.S.W., Chief Executive Officer, Middletown Psychiatric Center, New York State Office of Mental Health, Middletown, New York

Jack G. May, Jr., Ph.D., Department of Psychology, Florida State University, Tallahassee, Florida

John J. McGee, Ph.D., Department of Psychiatry, Nebraska Psychiatric Institute and Meyer Children's Rehabilitation Institute, University of Nebraska Medical Center, Omaha, Nebraska

Frank J. Menolascino, M.D., Departments of Psychiatry and Pediatrics, Nebraska Psychiatric Institute, University of Nebraska Medical Center, Omaha, Nebraska

Paul E. Menousek, Ph.D., Department of Psychiatry, Meyer Children's Rehabilitation Institute, University of Nebraska Medical Center, Omaha, Nebraska

Michael J. Monfils, M.S.W., Department of Psychiatry, Nebraska Psychiatric Institute, University of Nebraska Medical Center, Omaha, Nebraska

Ruth Parkhurst, M.D., North Dorchester Health Services, Hurlock, Maryland

Julie A. Parsons, Ph.D., Palo Alto Center for Stress Related Disorders, 675 Forest Avenue, Palo Alto, California

Stephen Ruedrich, M.D., Department of Psychiatry, Nebraska Psychiatric Institute, University of Nebraska Medical Center, Omaha, Nebraska

Michael W. Smull, B.A., Deputy Director, Mental Retardation Program, University of Maryland School of Medicine, Baltimore, Maryland

Jack A. Stark, Ph.D., Departments of Psychiatry and Pediatrics, Meyer Children's Rehabilitation Institute, University of Nebraska Medical Center, Omaha, Nebraska

Donald A. Swanson, M.D., Department of Psychiatry, Nebraska Psychiatric Institute, University of Nebraska Medical Center, Omaha, Nebraska

Ludwik S. Szymanski, M.D., Department of Psychiatry, Children's Hospital, 300 Longwood Avenue, Boston, Massachusetts

Peter E. Tanguay, M.D., Department of Psychiatry, University of California at Los Angeles, Los Angeles, California

Luke S. Watson, Jr., Ph.D., Therapeutic Homes, Inc., 6214 Presidential Court, S.W., Suite C, Fort Myers, Florida

Preface

This volume aims to provide the reader with a contemporary account of historical, diagnostic, treatment–management (including the individual and the service systems perspectives), and training dimensions of mentally ill/mentally retarded individuals from interdisciplinary perspectives. Emphasis is placed on current and evolving aspects of this topic. The broad scope of our approach is consistent with the concepts and practices that currently typify this topical area of clinical and research activity.

This volume is divided into five sections. Part I deals with the definitional aspects: the nature and incidence, the historical aspects, and a view of assessing the types of needs of mentally ill/mentally retarded individuals. Part II addresses the key issues in treatment intervention: from an individual therapeutic aspect through vocational considerations, as well as the role of the parents in these helping processes. Part III focuses on systems of service delivery, ranging from inpatient and day treatment models to the delivery of services in the home; at all times, the emphasis is on programs that have been successful. Part IV presents a modern perspective on the multiple challenges in training both mental health and mental retardation specialists, as well as the critical dimension of providing a well-trained cadre of paraprofessionals in both fields. And finally, Part V encompasses key current research perspectives as well as possible future directions for this rapidly growing area of professional interest and involvement.

Each of the contributors to this volume has been actively involved in—and directly focuses on—major dimensions of mental illness in mentally retarded individuals. By their direct sharing of specific information from their collective (and extensive) professional experiences, these contributors hope to aid fellow professionals to better understand and serve this complex and challenging population. We share the hope that their contributions to this volume will help extend the professional base of modern information about what *can* be done to effectively aid retarded citizens whose lives have become complicated by the inroads of mental illness.

Frank J. Menolascino
Jack A. Stark

Acknowledgments

For the last 25 years, the editors of this volume have been directly involved in clinical and research work with mentally retarded individuals who also have emotional and behavioral problems. We have been fortunate, during this period of time, to be assisted by and to learn from so many competent colleagues. We would particularly like to acknowledge the professional and paraprofessional staff members of the Nebraska Psychiatric Institute and Meyer Children's Rehabilitation Institute who have assisted in our professional development over the years. Special thanks are due to Dr. Cecil Wittson, Dr. Merrill Eaton, Dr. Robert Kugel, Dr. Louise Eaton, and Dr. Paul Pearson. In addition, we deeply appreciate the assistance, in the preparation of this volume, provided by Rose Theis, Alan Toulouse, Vicki Strampe, Barbara Tuccitto, Tammi Goldsbury, Carol Anderson, and Sue Pinkerton. Most of all, we would like to thank the thousands of families that we have worked with and tried to help over the years; they have been encouraging and have appreciated our efforts to understand and help.

FRANK J. MENOLASCINO
JACK A. STARK

Contents

Introduction

In the wake of the national deinstitutionalization movement, the personality
and behavioral dimensions of the mentally retarded have taken on a new ur-
gency and interest for mental health professionals. Increasingly, they are being
asked to assist in the understanding and the effective treatment and management of a very large group of retarded citizens who have the *combined* symptoms of mental retardation and mental illness. Yet, there are precious few
mental-health personnel who have had an extensive exposure to the didactic
or clinical dimensions of mental retardation—not to mention the appearance
of this symptom in conjunction with signs or symptoms of mental illness. Although training and ongoing clinical experiences had been an important and
integral dimension of the mental health professional's interest and involvement
in mental retardation at the turn of this century, they ceased to be so because
of three major changes in societal and professional viewpoints during the first
two decades of this century. First, the individualized psychiatric-case-study
approach became displaced by the rapid psychometric-intelligence-testing approach. Second, the retarded became erroneously viewed and labeled as rather
unsavory "deviants" in our society. And third, the fixed genetic–brain-
pathology causalities became the dominant beacons of a rather dismal view of
the field of mental retardation. This trio of professional and societal changes,
acting in concert, literally eliminated the individualized, humanistic professional postures that had produced an excellent record of help and program
achievements by mental health professionals at the turn of this century. As
mental-health training interest and ongoing professional efforts in mental retardation went into eclipse, so did the accompanying professional enthusiasm
for finding ways to help the retarded. Beyond the previous interest in maximizing the developmental potentials and personality adjustment of the retarded
(whether they were also mentally ill or not), the retreat of mental health professionals ushered in four decades of backward custodial care for the "hopeless"
in large institutional settings.

The above state of affairs, persisting as it did until the early 1960s, left the
mental health aspects of mental retardation as a narrow and "fruitless" area
for professional involvement. However, with the advent of the report of the
President's Panel on Mental Retardation and President John F. Kennedy's
benchmark federal legislation in 1963, the field of mental retardation literally
came alive once again. This renaissance of interest and involvement—actively
joined in by professionals and parent-volunteers alike—brought back (and extended) the earlier professional postures of help and hope. Improvements in

the diagnosis, treatment, and management of mental retardation flowed from the new national commitments to service, research, training, and social policy changes. Spurred onward by fresh conceptualizations of societal and professional viewpoints (e.g., the ideology of normalization and the maturational posture of the developmental model), the quality-of-life issue for the mentally retarded again became a focal point for professional approaches. For example, elucidation of a wide variety of the primary causes of mental retardation led to more rational treatment approaches, and civil rights considerations brought into question the validity of segregating retarded citizens in large, remote institutions. In addition, energetic advocacy involvement in supporting the parents of the retarded have brought an additional focus on seeking community-based services for their retarded sons and daughters. The national social policy of deinstitutionalizing the retarded, which directly flowed from the above-noted major changes in the 1960s, has successfully reduced the population of the public institutions for the retarded from 190,000 to 125,000. Yet, these major changes have ushered in a current state of affairs wherein previously institutionalized retarded citizens (or their previously unserved mirror images in the community) have had great difficulty in shifting *from* past "expected" social adjustments of passivity and dependency *to* acquiring the interpersonal skills necessary to "make it" in community-based service settings. Indeed, it is the very lack of these needed interpersonal skills (i.e., personality attributes for successfully handling interpersonal conflict, impulse control, adaptive approaches to coworkers in a sheltered work setting, and so on) that have underscored the pressing need for greatly increased professional knowledge, involvement, and research into the personality adjustments and the mental illness parameters of mentally retarded citizens.

Accordingly, the recent renaissance of professional involvement and the continuing dynamism of the field of mental retardation have illuminated the nature and types of mental illness in the mentally retarded and are providing a wide variety of appropriate answers about how best to diagnose and treat individuals with both mental illness and mental retardation. This volume, by the breadth and depth of its contributions, is an excellent example of what can be done to understand and help mentally retarded citizens whose lives have become complicated by mental illness.

Nature of the Dual Diagnosis

Introduction

The major thrust of this volume is sixfold: to provide the reader with a basic understanding of mental illness in the mentally retarded, to help the reader to acquire new knowledge about the available research and its application, to provide strategies and models for training professionals and paraprofessionals, to recommend service delivery systems and models of care and treatment, to provide new insight into therapeutic and management approaches, and to provide a framework for future directions and goals.

Thus, Part I focuses on providing the reader with a basic understanding and with the tools necessary to achieve the objectives and goals of this book. It contains three chapters that focus on the basic nature of mental illness and on mental illness in mentally retarded individuals, as well as on the planning of delivery service programs for this unique population.

Chapter 1 contains perhaps the finest chapter to date on the nature and incidence of mental illness in mentally retarded individuals, if one's major criterion is comprehensiveness of research analysis in the area. The authors of this chapter have conducted an exhaustive review of the literature and have organized information in a succinct way, so as to answer the question of why mentally retarded individuals are placed in institutions and what are the major relationships between mental illness and mental retardation.

The most serious form of mental illness, psychosis, is analyzed in its historical perspective and is presented to show those who are most affected by this type of mental illness, particularly those with schizophrenia. Other subcategories of psychoses are presented, as well as the more common neurotic conditions, particularly anxiety reactions and disorders. Suicide and alcoholism, common in the personality disorders, are also the subject of a discussion that should be helpful to the reader because these concerns are rarely reviewed.

There seems to be a great deal of confusion about the physiological factors that cause, contribute to, or exacerbate the mentally retarded individuals' emotional-behavioral problems. Seizures, metabolic dysfunctions, and chromosome and genetic disorders may all be involved but are often inappropriately diagnosed. As a result, remediation efforts are less than complete because of the many causes of the mentally retarded individual's behavior.

Chapter 1 concludes on an optimistic note with specific recommendations and implications for treatment and additional research in our ongoing efforts to understand, delineate, and remediate the psychological and physiological disorders of mentally retarded individuals.

It has been said that perhaps the greatest trait of men and women who are famous leaders is their ability to understand and comprehend the historical significance of past events and their implications for current and future events. Drs. Ruedrich and Menolascino, in Chapter 2, provide the reader with an important historical overview of the development of treatment practices for mentally retarded individuals with mental health problems. Drs. Ruedrich and Menolascino trace the social, economic, and political forces that have shaped the treatment of mentally retarded individuals from the early nineteenth century, with the initial work of Itard and Seguin, to the current emphasis on deinstitutionalization. Understanding those factors that historically resulted in misunderstanding and inappropriate care of the mentally retarded individual with mental illness is important for all who work in this area.

Special insight is provided via the exceptionally effective didactic technique of a case history analysis. An analysis of three case histories provides a fundamental understanding of the basic behaviors that constitute mental illness as well as treatment strategies for mentally retarded individuals. In short, a delineation of those behaviors that constitute mental illness and its subcomponents should prove to be extremely helpful to mental health personnel in this era of renewed commitment to citizens with this dual diagnosis.

The complex problems associated with the deinstitutionalization of mentally retarded individuals with emotional and behavioral problems are clearly evident in Chapter 3. Faced with the issue of placing large numbers of a heterogeneous group of individuals with dual diagnosis in the community, Dr. Parkhurst was forced to address the definitional issues as well as to assess the needs of this population. The following eight major objectives could serve as a model for those communities considering the integration of individuals with the dual diagnosis into the community: (1) the development of a survey instrument regarding appropriate services; (2) regional needs assessment; (3) a survey of existing services for this special population; (4) an investigation of national models with implications for local adaptation; (5) the development of a delivery-service-system model for deinstitutionalization to both rural and urban centers; (6) an estimation of the cost and an identification of personnel, equipment, and funding sources; (7) the development of legislative and policy recommendations for the delivery of services; and (8) the development of data and service information for public education and prevention packages.

The data generated in each of these steps should provide a practical approach that communities throughout the country could use almost immediately in their efforts to serve mentally ill-mentally retarded individuals and their families.

This chapter also provides a transition to Part II, which addresses the more specific service models and programs for this population.

The Nature and Incidence of Mental Illness in Mentally Retarded Individuals

Julie A. Parsons, Jack G. May, Jr., and Frank J. Menolascino

1.1. Introduction

·The presence or absence of mental illness plays a crucial role in determining the quality of a mentally retarded person's adjustment to community and family life. Mental illnesses have long been recognized as a primary factor leading to the institutionalization of mentally retarded individuals.[1,2] Study after study highlights the importance of mental illness as a factor leading to institutionalization and/or failure in community adjustment. Penrose[3] concluded that emotional instability is one of the most important contributing factors in the selection of mentally retarded individuals for institutionalization. Penrose stated,

> It may be doubted if mental illness, whether in the form of epilepsy, neurosis or psychosis, should be regarded as a true cause of intellectual defect, but it is quite certain that mental illness is a very important contributory factor in the selection of cases . . . seen in institutions "and these cases" [sic] are only a small sample of all those of comparable ability in the general population. They require care and control because they are out of harmony with their social environments, and often this is due to a mentally disordered state. (p. 198)

Foale[4] contended that the mildly retarded adolescents who are admitted to institutions are placed there not because of their low intelligence, but because of their emotional instability. Similarly, Beier[5] concluded that "Behavioral disturbance, after the degree of intellectual deficiency itself, is [sic] the single most important cause of institutionalization of the mentally retarded" (p. 479). Menolascino[6] also noted that "Currently, a frequent reason for requesting admission to these institutions is the retarded individual's ability to adjust within the primary community. Many of these 'community rejects' display an overlay of emotional disturbance which accounts for their adjustment problems" (p. 3). Similarly, Kirman[7] contended that mildly retarded individuals with an IQ greater than 50 seldom fail on the job or in social adjustment because of low intelligence; rather, many mildly retarded individuals fail because of temperamental instability, neuroses, or psychoses. Philips[8] noted that mentally re-

Julie A. Parsons • Palo Alto Center for Stress Related Disorders, 675 Forest Avenue, Palo Alto, California 94301.   *Jack G. May, Jr.* • Department of Psychology, Florida State University, Tallahassee, Florida 32306.   *Frank J. Menolascino* • Departments of Psychiatry and Pediatrics, Nebraska Psychiatric Institute, University of Nebraska Medical Center, Omaha, Nebraska 68105.

tarded individuals usually come to the attention of society because of a failure in social adaptation, not because of low intelligence. These observations have received strong support from empirical studies.

As early as 1927, Kinder and Rutherford[9] reported that, contrary to expectation, relatively little correlation was found between the degree of retardation and social adjustment. They identified the child's environment as an important factor in social adjustment for their sample of retarded children. Gardner and Giampa[10] examined the relationship between intelligence level and social-emotional behavior in institutionalized mentally retarded individuals. They concluded that inappropriate social-emotional behaviors (such as screaming and hitting) are independent of behavioral competence.

Thus, it appears that social adjustment is not directly related to global intelligence. It is, however, an important factor in leading to institutionalization. Primrose[11] analyzed 502 consecutive admissions to a mental retardation hospital and found that 64% of the admissions were for antisocial behavior and allied psychiatric reasons; severe physical disability accounted for only 17% of the admissions.

In spite of the potential, in recent years, for research on the national deinstitutionalization phenomenon and the actual community experiences of retarded persons, the recent literature on the psychiatric aspects of mental retardation is sparse. Heaton-Ward[12] pointed out that several modern psychiatric texts contain only one to two paragraphs on mental illness in mentally retarded individuals, and that scientific papers on mental retardation rarely address mental illness in this population. Clearly, there is a need to examine and draw together the scattered efforts in this neglected field, in order to provide a sound basis for current treatment–management efforts and research challenges therein.

1.1.1. A Major Problem: Definition

As Beier[5] pointed out, the first problem encountered in an examination of the literature on the association between mental illness and mental retardation is that of defining the population. Beier stated that most definitions of mental retardation and mental illness are descriptive and are often more a function of the author's biases than of the patient's etiological or behavioral characteristics.

The concept of mental retardation has changed over the years; thus, the populations studied in the early part of this century may be very different from populations studied recently. Today, mental retardation is regarded as a symptom, subsuming a heterogeneous group of etiological and functional conditions. The most commonly accepted definitions emphasize that the syndrome consists of both intellectual retardation and deficits in social adaptation, and that such deficits are apparent before adulthood. As Menolascino and Egger[13] pointed out, the term *mental retardation* implies both a symptom of an underlying developmental disorder and an assessment of an individual's potential ability to learn.

Chess[14] presented a useful system for classifying mental retardation that takes into account the varying relationships between mental retardation and mental illness. She suggested the following categories:

1. Mental retardation with no behavior disorder. In these individuals the deviance is understood only in terms of slow cognition, since their behavior is appropriate to their mental age.

2. Mental retardation with behavior disorder due to cerebral dysfunction. Although Chess admitted a hesitancy in relating these symptoms to cerebral dysfunction in all cases, she suggested that this category might subsume such symptoms as hypo- and hypermobility, shortened attention span, distractibility, imperviousness to the environment, hypo- or hyperirritability, lability or sameness of mood, dependence or independence, obsessive-compulsive behaviors, stereotyped behavior, and self-stimulatory behaviors.

3. Mental retardation with reactive behavior disorder. Overdependent, aggressive, fearful, and markedly unorganized activity is noted herein.

4. Mental retardation with neurotic behavior disorder. This pattern reflects the elaboration of a variety of personality defenses against anxiety.

5. Mental retardation with psychosis. The presence of major disorders of thinking, feeling, and very poor ability to relate to animate objects typifies these psychoses.

Only recently has there been a consensus in the definition of mental illness, as an abnormality of behavior, emotions, or relations sufficiently marked or prolonged as to both handicap the individual and distress his or her family or community. Thus, the conceptualization of mental illness and the parallel modern description of mental retardation have both evolved and changed. Accordingly, the populations subsumed by each of these diagnostic rubrics have identified—at different periods of time—populations that cannot be considered comparable. Indeed, much of the research on the relationship between mental retardation and mental illness arose in the late nineteenth and the early twentieth centuries. We hope to avoid these problems in this chapter by using the diagnostic system on mental retardation of the American Association on Mental Deficiency[15] and the recent DSM-III diagnostic system of the American Psychiatric Association.[16] The reader is referred to each of these diagnostic references, as noted in the reference section.

1.1.2. Susceptibility

The prevailing opinion in the literature is that mentally retarded individuals are more susceptible to mental illness than their nonmentally retarded peers. Numerous reasons are presented for this susceptibility. Pollock[17] identified four reasons frequently given for the perceived high rate of mental illness among the mentally retarded: (1) reduced capacity to withstand stress; (2) poor ability to resolve mental and emotional conflicts; (3) lack of social competence and, consequently, a potential for being led into difficulty by their associates; and (4) emotional instability, which may lead to loss of self-control. Pollock stated that, in most states, mentally retarded adults receive little attention unless they get into social or legal difficulties, and this factor might account for the high incidence of mental illness reported in institutionalized retarded individuals.

Cytryn and Lourie[18] noted that in the process of growing and developing, a mentally retarded person faces more hazards than does the normal person; they suggested that such hazards increase in direct proportion to the degree of retardation. They noted a number of factors that contribute to the emotional vulnerability of the retarded person: (1) the relatively lengthy process of individuation and mother recognition, which may lead to more intense feelings of dependence on the part of the child; (2) the delayed appearance and the longer duration of childhood stages, such as negativity and the development of autonomy, which may complicate the task of parenting and consequently leave the child with residual conflicts in these areas; (3) perceptual problems, which may limit social responsiveness and mental alertness, and which may significantly contribute to language delay; and (4) constitutional factors (e.g., hypersensitivity to external and internal stimuli, hyposensitivity to sensory stimulation, aggressiveness, and difficulty in coping with anxiety, frustration, and impulse), which may weaken the emotional resilience of retarded individuals, making crises more frequent and the process of recovery longer or incomplete. Cytryn and Lourie noted also that an unfavorable self-image may be brought about by frustration and failure in the mentally retarded individual, and that play may not be used in a normal developmental way by retarded children. The family may play a role in increasing the retarded child's susceptibility to mental illness because of the child's delayed early responses, which may lead to parental turmoil, grief, disappointment, or guilt. On the other hand, unawareness of their child's retardation may create overly high expectations in the parents. Denial, overprotection, infantilization, and overt or covert rejection are other family responses that may lead to the development of emotional problems in a retarded child. Cytryn and Lourie[18] also noted the role of the community in reinforcing this susceptibility. Prevailing community attitudes may influence parental reactions: the more sophisticated the community, the more emphasis it tends to place on intelligence. In addition, peers may exclude and scapegoat the retarded child, thus increasing the probability that mental illness will develop. Cytryn and Lourie emphasized that mental retardation is not a contraindication to normal personality development, but that, if the handicap is not handled properly, it may lead to a greater vulnerability to mental illness.

Philips[8] also concluded that mentally retarded individuals are more vulnerable to defects in personality development because of interpersonal experiences as well as because of constitutional endowment. Philips's emphasis on the isolation of the retarded individual was confirmed by Wortis,[19] who identified inadequate services and rejection by family, peers, and society as major factors in the development of mental illness in mentally retarded individuals.

Menolascino[20] pointed out that the high frequency of special sensory and central integrative disorders associated with moderately retarded individuals may greatly hamper their attempts at appropriate problem-solving and may thus lead to a higher probability of developing atypical or abnormal behaviors. According to Menolascino, the limited repertoire of personality defenses of the moderately retarded individual, combined with a typically concrete approach, creates fertile intrapsychic ground for excessive overreactions to minimal external stresses. He noted that proneness to hyperactivity and impulsivity, rapid mood swings, and temporary regression to primitive self-stimulation are typical of the fragile personality structures of moderately retarded individuals.

Only a handful of authors have maintained that mentally retarded individuals are less susceptible to mental illness than other individuals. Simmons[21] noted that the old misconception "to be dumb is to be happy" is being replaced by a recognition that personal-social adjustment for many mildly to moderately retarded individuals is fraught with difficulties. Nevertheless, as recently as 1966, Penrose[22] restated the optimistic view of the "happy retardate" in these terms: "Nevertheless, on the whole, a striking feature of the intellectually handicapped is their amiability, their freedom from emotional stress, and their willingness to cooperate with others" (p. 748).

Thus, it appears that theoretical arguments exist for both the increased and the decreased susceptibility of mentally retarded individuals to the development of emotional disorders. Although the debate must be settled empirically, the prevailing professional opinion is that mentally retarded individuals are more prone to mental disorder than are their nonretarded peers, for a variety of constitutional and/or psychosocial reasons.

1.2. The Nature and Relationship between Mental Retardation and Mental Illness

Menolascino[20] noted that the study of the relationship between mental retardation and mental illness is difficult because *both* mental retardation and mental illness are symptoms that may have many causes. It is not surprising, then, to find that the relationship between the two conditions may vary. Approaches to the study of the relationship between mental retardation and mental illness can generally be divided into three main categories: (1) those that examine the role of mental illness in creating the symptom of mental retardation (i.e., a pseudoretardation conceptualization); (2) those that emphasize the belief that mental retardation leads to mental illness, by virtue of an increased number of stresses encountered by retarded individuals; and (3) those that are based on the belief that underlying dysfunction may lead to both mental retardation and mental illness in the same individual. These three categories are, of course, not mutually exclusive, and a given author may subscribe to one, all, or none of these beliefs, although noting the interactions between these three processes.

1.2.1. Pseudoretardation

The study of pseudoretardation gained greatly in popularity in the period 1940–1970 and led to much research on the differential diagnosis of mental

retardation versus autism, childhood schizophrenia, and other behavior disturbances.[23,24] Chess,[14] however, cautioned that "inaccurate diagnoses of
'emotional disturbance with pseudoretardation' are often given to mentally
retarded children with behavioral disorders—especially in the absence of identified organic developmental deviance" (p. 180). She pointed out that the coexistence of mental retardation and behavioral abnormality does not necessarily
imply primary mental illness and secondary (i.e., reversible) mental retardation. Most authors have identified only a small minority of mentally retarded
children, when thoroughly studied in a clinical setting, as being functionally
retarded with a potential for normal performance.

1.2.2. Mental Retardation as a Predecessor of Mental Illness

Mental retardation does not necessarily predispose an individual to mental
illness. However, it is frequently argued that the multiple stresses that the
retarded individual commonly encounters may predispose him or her to the
development of mental illness. Cytryn and Lourie,[18] for instance, noted that
in an accepting, stimulating environment, with educational and vocational training, the majority of retarded individuals are capable of developing good social
and vocational adjustments, as well as appropriate interpersonal relations. Cytryn and Lourie pointed out that mentally retarded individuals often face hazards beyond those faced by the normal population, and that the direly needed
family and environmental supports are frequently absent.

Chess[14] noted the role of environmental stressors, such as excessive demands and constant disapproval, in leading to fixed defensive behavior systems
in mentally retarded individuals. Potter[25] noted also that mildly retarded individuals, because of their negative self-image and the competitive nature of
their environment, are especially prone to anxiety.

Philips[8] attacked what he sees as misconceptions about the association of
mental retardation and mental illness. He identified the following ideas as misconceptions: (1) that maladjusted behavior is a result of the mental retardation
rather than of disturbed interpersonal relations; (2) that mental illness in retarded children is different in kind from that in normal children; and (3) that
certain symtoms are the results of organic brain syndrome. He argued that
disturbed behavior in retarded persons is a result of delayed, disordered personality functions and disturbed interpersonal relations resulting from frustrations, separation, and trauma. He noted that behavior disturbances in mentally
retarded individuals are a function of the same processes that lead to behavior
disturbance in normal individuals. Further, Philips noted that in his experience,
the entire gamut of psychopathology seen in normally intelligent children is
also seen in retarded children. Finally, he pointed out that hyperactivity, attention span deficits, distractibility, and impulsivity—symptoms often associated with organic damage—can also appear in children without organic brain
damage. Philips concluded that, in our society, cognitive functioning is so important that intellectually retarded individuals almost always have major problems in vocational adaptation. He pointed out that these problems arise not

only from constitutional endowment, which places limits on development, but from continuing adverse interpersonal experiences with the environment. Tarjan[26] likewise noted that, although symptoms in mentally retarded individuals may differ from those in intellectually normal individuals, the basic psychopathological processes are similar and require interventions that must be modified only to accommodate the cognitive impairments that are present. He noted that stressors that may be valued as relatively trivial by persons of average intelligence may lead to overt psychiatric manifestations in mentally retarded individuals.

In summary, the prevailing professional viewpoint is that the increased number of interpersonal stressors encountered by the retarded individual, combined with his or her limited intrapsychic resources and abilities to cope, eventuates in the retarded person's increased susceptibility to the development of mental illness.

1.2.3. A Common Etiological Factor

It has long been suggested that behavior problems in mentally retarded individuals stem from the etiological factor that produced the retardation.[27] Barr,[28] for instance, considered head banging and autistic hand play a part of the underlying retardation process itself, and Bartemeier[29] noted that some mental disturbances might be the direct outcome of mental retardation (this view was later concurred with by James[27] and Jancar[30]).

Chess[14] emphasized that coexisting mental illness and mental retardation are most likely manifestations of the same underlying genetic and metabolic dysfunctions, although she also noted the major role of interpersonal and environmental stressors in producing mental illness.

1.2.4. The Extreme View

It has been suggested that the syndrome of mental retardation must include a degree of disturbed emotional development, although the nature and extent of such disturbances have not yet been adequately defined or identified. Although this represents a rather extreme view, it is not inconsistent with definitions of mental retardation that include deficits of social adaptiveness as an essential component of the syndrome. For example, Wortis[19] concluded,

> The cerebral defects and disorders that retard development also produce derangements of behavior. Hardly any retardate is the full equivalent of a normal but chronologically younger person: there are nearly always some defects and distortions of behavioral development, too. Most of these are minor; serious distortions are infrequent, and the central problem is usually the intellectual backwardness. (p. 411)

Similarly, Webster[31] noted that mental retardation is a "clinical syndrome," rather than "an intellectual defect or brain disease per se." He contended, "The mental retardation clinical syndrome regularly includes significant disturbances in emotional development which have neither been generally recognized nor as yet very clearly defined" (p. 39). He believed that the primary psychopathology of mental retardation includes emotional problems (i.e., manifested by repetitiousness, inflexibility, negativism, compulsive traits, and perservation) and contended that, in severely retarded children, thelack of flexibility and repetitiousness is so prominent and the capacity for object relations is so limited that it is very difficult to clinically distinguish true compulsive defenses from the primary psychopathology of mental retardation.

Thus, a number of clinicians have suggested that the syndrome of mental retardation must include a degree of disturbed emotional development, as well as intellectual retardation.

In brief, it seems clear that, for whatever etiological reasons, mental retardation and mental illness frequently coexist. The importance of research and treatment is clearly established in view of the significant detrimental impact of mental illness on the adjustment of mentally retarded individuals. Eisenberg,[32] in 1958, identified an important research question that remains just as salient today:

> The interdependence of emotion and intelligence is a fundamental fact of human behavior, at the psychological and biological levels of integration. We should not any longer wonder at the evidence of dysfunction of either in the presence of disorder in the other, but rather ask: By what mechanism has it occurred in this particular case and by what means may it be remedied? (quoted in Beier, 1964, p. 473)

1.2.5. Frequency of the Dual Diagnosis

A fair number of research studies have attempted to ascertain the frequency of the dual diagnosis of mental retardation and mental illness. These studies generally fall into four categories: (1) surveys of institutions for the mentally retarded; (2) surveys of institutions for the mentally ill; (3) surveys of noninstitutionalized adults; and (4) surveys of children. For reasons of space, we will note the most important studies and summarize and interpret the findings generally.

Surveys of institutionalized retarded individuals include those by Primrose,[11] Vanuxem,[33] Penrose,[34] Rohan,[35] Neuer,[36] Leck, Gordon, and McKeown,[37] Donoghue, Abbas, and Gal,[38] Williams,[39] and Reid.[40] In summarizing these surveys, estimates of the incidence of mental illness among the institutionalized mentally retarded vary considerably. The most consistent reports on the incidences of psychoses in the mentally retarded cluster around 4%–6%. Most estimates of the incidence of serious psychiatric disorder, including both the personality disorders and the psychoses, range from 8%–15%. When the minor emotional problems are included, estimates soar well above 50%.

Surveys of institutions for the mentally ill have worked from the opposite direction in order to discover the number of mentally retarded individuals whose institutionalization was apparently caused by mental illness. Most of the early studies reported high percentages of the mentally ill residents to be mentally retarded. Rosanoff, Handy, and Plesset,[41] for example, reviewed the statistics for a New York State hospital and found that 30% of the epileptic psychoses, 17% of the schizophrenias, and 10% of the manic-depressive psychoses occurred in patients who were also considered mentally retarded. Similar surveys (and findings) were reported by Pollock,[17] Duncan,[42] Hunsicker,[43] Innes, Kidd, and Ross,[44] Payne,[45] and Mercer.[46]

Few surveys of noninstitutionalized retarded adults have been conducted to ascertain the presence and frequency of mental illness. One worthy of mention is that of Weaver,[47] who reported a study of 8,000 wartime soldiers who had IQs of less than 75. Of these mentally retarded soldiers, 37% were black, and 63% were white. The mildly retarded men and women who were included were classified into three groups: (1) those who showed chronic patterns of maladjustment becoming severe enough to necessitate discharge from the military service; (2) those who demonstrated, on the whole, adequate adjustment except for minor episodes; and (3) those who adopted to military environments without any evidence of significant maladjustment. Forty-four percent of the males and 38% of the females were discharged for psychiatric, psychosomatic, or disciplinary reasons. Most of these individuals had personality deficiencies, including, in order of frequency, severe emotional immaturity and instability, severe aggressive reactions, poor motivation, lack of cooperation, severe antisocial behavior, lack of group loyalty, and schizoid and paranoid traits.

Surveys of children conducted to ascertain the prevalence of the dual diagnosis have also been rather infrequent. Chess[14] conducted an intensive study of 52 mentally retarded children living at home and found that 60% demonstrated signs and symptoms of mental illness. Menolascino[48] found that 5.2% of 616 children under age 8, who had been referred to a multidisciplinary clinic with suspected mental retardation, displayed psychotic symptoms. In 1977, Menolascino[20] reported that 37% of a group of institutionalized Down's syndrome children were also mentally ill, and that 56% of these children had demonstrated features of mental illness at the time of their admission to the institution.

Menolascino[20] noted that the findings in a series of reports covering the past 15–20 years indicate that mentally retarded children under 12, living with their families or in their communities, demonstrate a 20%–35% frequency of emotional disturbance. Menolascino pointed out that the rate of emotional disturbance in nonretarded children is 14%–18%.

1.2.6. General Findings

It is difficult to compare all of the studies on the incidence of mental illness in mentally retarded individuals. Craft,[49] for instance, pointed out that many studies have been conducted on different groups and have used different definitions; that differences have existed in environmental stressors (i.e., wartime induction versus hospitalization); that different views have prevailed regarding diagnostic labels and the point at which a diagnosis of mental disorder has been made; and finally, that some difficulties are inherent in the double diagnosis of retardation and emotional disorder, as one may be partially dependent on the other. He concluded, however, that depressive illness is rare among the mentally retarded, and that personality disturbances are common and may contribute to "psychotic outbursts."

Tizard[50] reviewed the literature and concluded that only if a descriptor trait could be objectively assessed (e.g., number of seizures) was there agreement between repeated surveys of mental illness in the retarded. He reported that, in Penrose's studies of retarded persons in institutions, about 30% demonstrated a behavior disorder. Among the mildly retarded, as many as 60% demonstrated behavior disorders, but these problems were not likely to be serious or permanent.

Pilkington[51] also reviewed the surveys and agreed that they were open to serious criticism. In spite of a lack of standardization and precision, difficulties of diagnosis, and latitude in defining psychiatric problems, Pilkington found a broad measure of agreement among studies. He concluded that approximately 10% of the hospitalized retarded suffer from some form of mental illness. The four studies that he reviewed suggested that 10%–50% of the institutionalized mentally retarded population may benefit from professional mental-health contact. Heaton-Ward[12] likewise noted that an appropriate figure cannot be quoted even on the prevalence of all forms of mental illness in all mentally retarded individuals, but that limited information is available. He noted that surveys of new admissions to hospitals for the mentally handicapped and of resident populations have yielded a psychiatric-disorder prevalence rate of up to 60%, and that, if personality disorders are excluded, the combined prevalence of psychoses and neuroses appears to be 8%–10%.

Menolascino[20] noted that most studies of the frequency and types of emotional disturbances in mentally retarded individuals contain methodological problems. He noted that the pre-1960 studies were conducted mostly in institutions or hospitals with a focus on mildly retarded residents and found mental illness frequency rates of 16%–40%. Menolascino pointed out that, as institutions were traditionally used as a social mechanism for shutting away mentally retarded individuals with major behavioral difficulties, these figures are disproportionately large unless they are compared to those for all retarded individuals. He noted that the more recent studies among community-based populations of retarded individuals, however, have reported a similar range of mental illness. Many of the current individuals, he suggested, may be "community mental retardation program rejects," and the lowered social adaptive capacities of such mentally retarded individuals (and hence their higher incidence of mental illness) may be related to low expectations by and of the individuals, cultural-social deprivation, and dissimilarity of personal expectations.

Menolascino[20] commented on a series of reports during the last 15–20 years that focused on mentally retarded individuals, especially children under 12, living with their families or in the community. Generally, 20%–35% of these individuals were found to have allied mental illness. He also pointed out that the concurrent presence of mental illness disturbance and mental retardation may partially reflect a professional bias about not treating the signs and symptoms of mental illness in the mentally retarded. Thus, biases may have facilitated the progress of mentally retarded individuals along the path to institutions as "disturbed" individuals. Menolascino noted that 10%–18% of nonretarded children are estimated to be mentally ill,[52] whereas estimates of all types of mental disturbance in the general adult population have been as high as 40%. He concluded, therefore, that the reported frequencies of emotional disturbance in mentally retarded individuals suggest a "moderately increased susceptibility" to mental illness for them as a group.

1.2.7. Conclusions

Research appears to rather consistently indicate that approximately 10% of the institutionalized mentally retarded adult population demonstrate severe mental illness, such as the psychoses. When minor mental illnesses are included, estimates rise to as high as 60%. Although it is usually thought that these estimates of mental illness among institutionalized mentally retarded individuals grossly exaggerate the actual incidence of mental illness among the retarded as a whole, community studies tend to suggest otherwise. Many of the community studies conducted on mentally retarded children suggest a 20%–35% frequency of mental illness. Few studies focus on adults in community settings, however, and child studies should not be taken as being representative of adult populations. It is possible that many of the childhood mental-health problems are greatly ameliorated by adulthood.

These findings suggest that mentally retarded individuals are slightly more susceptible to mental illnesses than are nonretarded individuals, although the reasons for this finding are not clear. Mentally retarded individuals may face more frustrations and conflicts than do other individuals, because of their handicaps or cognitive abilities. However, as Menolascino[20] pointed out, the higher rate of mental illness noted in mentally retarded individuals may also reflect the backlog of cases that have stemmed from professional unwillingness, in the past, to treat mental illness in mentally retarded individuals.

One conclusion can be stated with confidence. It is clear that the myth of "dumb, but happy" and the allied belief that mentally retarded individuals are immune to emotional problems may be laid to rest, once and for all. Hopefully, this burial of old myths will lead to increased responsiveness on the part of professionals to the recognition and the treatment of mental illness in mentally retarded individuals.

1.3. Psychoses

1.3.1. Historical Perspectives

MacGillivray[53] credited Seguin[54] with first suggesting that a psychotic disorder might complicate the clinical picture of mental retardation. Seguin[54] divided such psychoses into two main types (hyperkinetic and hypokinetic), depending on the degree of motor activity. Griesinger[55] presented a similar classification, dividing the psychoses of the mentally retarded into apathetic and excitable types. He described the symptoms of the excitable psychoses as including biting, destructiveness, aggression, and extreme fretfulness, and he regarded these as clinical signs of "pure mania."

Contrary to the early recognition of the coexistence of psychosis and mental retardation, as well as the allied ongoing attempts at classification, some authors steadfastly maintained that psychoses did not occur in the mentally retarded; that the described psychotic episodes in the lowest levels of retardation could not be regarded as mental illness; that psychoses only in "high-grade" retarded persons are similar in nature to those occurring in persons of normal intelligence; and that psychoses in the mentally retarded appear with greatly modified symptoms.[34,56-58]

In spite of previous controversy, by the early twentieth century the majority of American and English authors recognized the presence of psychoses in mentally retarded individuals. Opinions differed, however, regarding the susceptibility of this population to psychoses, as well as regarding the incidence, the course, the prognosis, and the nature of the symptomatology.

In summary, by the early twentieth century, it was an established fact that mentally retarded individuals can and do suffer from psychotic disturbances. These disturbances appear to fall into two categories: (1) psychotic disturbances similar in kind to those observed in persons of normal intelligence, which are most often described in persons of mild to moderate levels of mental retardation; and (2) psychotic disturbances unique to mentally retarded persons, colored by their low intelligence and associated deficiencies. There is little agreement about what behaviors should be included in this last category, as well as about their meanings. Most attempts to delineate these psychotic reactions have emphasized the atypical form that such disorders manifest themselves in severely and profoundly retarded individuals.

1.3.2. Susceptibility to Psychoses

Although a few early authors, such as Bartemeier,[29] contended that mentally retarded individuals were less susceptible to psychoses than individuals of normal intelligence, the prevailing arguments emphasized an increased susceptibility. Common arguments included a focus on physiological inadequacies, especially in the lower IQ individual, and on psychogenic factors in higher IQ individuals. Information regarding the precipitating factors in such psychoses is limited and contradictory. Some authors, however, contend that most psychoses in mentally retarded persons have clear precipitating factors, often not of sufficient magnitude to have precipitated a psychosis in a person of normal intelligence. Others believe that the precipitating factors are of relatively little importance, and they emphasize inherent constitutional inferiority.

1.3.3. Incidence of Psychoses in the Mentally Retarded

The first three decades of this century saw very little effort to ascertain the frequency with which psychoses occurred in mentally retarded persons, although it was slowly being recognized that these two conditions coexisted. This paucity of studies, prior to 1930, did include an excellent study by Gordon.[59] He reported on 37 cases of psychosis in mentally retarded persons, and he categorized them descriptively. He found that 15 of the patients suffered psychotic disorders that reflected an intensified distorted mode of thinking, feeling, and acting (i.e., schizophrenia disorders). The remaining 22 patients had signs and symptoms characteristic of the classical psychoses: manic and depressive disorders (12 patients), paranoid disorders (3 patients), and delirious or confusional states (7 patients).

The 1930s and the early 1940s saw several large-scale efforts to identify the frequency of psychoses in mentally retarded individuals. Scattered efforts in this field have continued until the present time. Jackson and Pike[60] estimated that the incidence of psychoses occurring with mental deficiency was 6.3% in a state hospital in Pennsylvania. Greene[61,62] found evidence of a similar incidence rate in a much more elaborate analysis of admissions to Walter E. Fernald State School in Massachusetts. Of 1,900 admissions from 1920 to 1930, Greene regarded 233 (12.4%) as showing evidence of psychosis. Of these cases, 36% demonstrated symptoms that were so bizarre as to merit commitment to a hospital for the mentally ill.[61]

Pollock[17] found 39.6% of the 444 mentally retarded patients admitted to civil state hospitals in New York in 1942 to be diagnosed as "psychoses with mental deficiency." An additional 18.4% were diagnosed as schizophrenia, and 9.9% as psychoses with convulsive disorders. Leck, Gordon, and McKeown[37] identified 618 mentally retarded institutionalized individuals with psychiatric disorders and found 28.6% of the disorders to be psychotic. Of a total of 1,652 hospitalized subnormal patients, 618 were considered psychiatric. Williams[39] reported that a medical assessment of 752 hospitalized subnormal patients indicated 153 adults as being psychotic.

In a more recent study, Heaton-Ward[12] investigated the incidence of psychotic mental illness among 1,251 mentally retarded patients in four hospitals. He noted that the diagnosis of psychosis in retarded individuals presents special problems and that some definitions of psychosis would allow all profoundly and some severely retarded individuals—who have no speech, are emotionally labile, and demonstrate purposeless actions and meaningless patterns of destruction—to be considered psychotic. He asserted that the criteria of an impaired sense of reality and lack of insight must require the capacity for intelligible communication with the patient if one is to ascertain their presence.

Beier[5] reviewed studies on the incidence of psychoses in mentally retarded persons and concluded that there is a paucity of literature on the association of nonschizophrenic psychoses and mental retardation and that most articles are case studies, presenting few general inferences. For the most part, these conclusions remain valid today, with the exception of the emergence of a recent body of literature on manic-depressive psychoses in mentally retarded individuals.

1.3.4. Conclusions Regarding the Incidence of Psychoses

The methodological problems inherent in epidemiological studies are compounded when dealing with two symptom clusters such as mental retardation and psychosis. A prevalent problem in many of the early studies stems from the use of a diagnostic manual that contained the heterogeneous "wastebasket" category of "Mental Deficiency with Psychosis" and did not allow the specification of the presence of coexisting mental retardation when "classical" psychotic reactions were present. In spite of the obvious limitations in the existing studies, a few conclusions appear to be warranted. Studies based on admissions to institutions for mentally retarded individuals find 5.6%–12.4% of the patients displaying psychotic symptomatology. Of admissions to hospitals for the mentally ill, the incidence of "Psychosis with Mental Deficiency" appears to approximate 3% for the first admissions, a percentage that is consonant with the estimated frequency of mental retardation in the population as a whole.

1.3.5. Schizophrenia

The literature on the relationship between schizophrenia and mental retardation is extensive. Undoubtedly, Penrose[3] was correct in concluding that the type of psychosis most intimately associated with mental defect in actual clinical practice is some form of schizophrenia. Beier[5] overviewed the literature on the incidence of psychoses in mentally retarded individuals and found that schizophrenia (and psychotic episodes of excitement) is the psychosis most frequently associated with mental retardation. Like Penrose, he concluded that, from almost any point of view, schizophrenia is the psychosis most intimately associated with retardation. Beier's conclusions appear to be accurate assessments of both the past and the current situation with regard to the literature on the relationship between schizophrenia and mental retardation.

Several authors have emphasized the similarity of the clinical pictures of schizophrenia occurring in mentally retarded and in nonretarded individuals. Heaton-Ward,[12] for instance, stated that he was able to make a confident diagnosis of schizophrenic illness on the basis of the usually accepted clinical criteria. Herskovitz and Plesset[58] also contended that schizophrenic reactions in the mentally retarded are "much the same as in persons of normal intelligence." They noted some differences in that "the pre-psychotic personality may be typically schizoid . . . but it is often strongly colored by the lack of normal intelligence and a general lack of personality integration" (p. 582). A number of authors argued against the term *pfropfschizophrenia*, maintaining there is nothing distinctive about schizophrenic psychoses in mentally retarded individuals.[63-65]

However, some authors have flatly argued that schizophrenia does not occur in severely and profoundly mentally retarded individuals. Reid[66] stated, "In the author's opinion, the inability of most idiots to communicate verbally precludes the possibility of diagnosing schizophrenic and paranoid psychoses in these patients'' (p. 214). Herskovitz and Plesset[58] believed that schizophrenic psychoses could not occur in persons with IQs less than 50; Hayman[57] reached similar conclusions. Penrose[3] noted that isolated schizophrenic symptoms (i.e., catatonic waxy flexibility, stuporous states, outbursts of violence, stereotypy, negativism, and mannerisms) are often found in the severely retarded, and he emphasized that their psychiatric significance is difficult to determine. He noted that Earl[67] considered these symptoms indicative of psychosis, but Penrose argued, ''Alternatively, they can be regarded as modes of reaction of an infantile nature, which imply that instinctual and emotional development has been retarded along with intellectual development'' (p. 214).

Kirman[7] argued for the possibility of schizophrenia in profoundly retarded individuals; Reid was of the opinion that, because the profoundly retarded cannot speak, it is not possible to diagnose schizophrenia in them reliably. The present writers are of the opinion that an assessment based on changes in behavior is valuable. The more severely mentally handicapped, like the mildly retarded, may develop a definite personality and an elaborate system of social relationships. These may then deteriorate relatively suddenly in some cases, and the patient may regress to a simple level, withdraw actively from social contacts, lose interest, and become apathetic and unproductive. In some cases, such a picture may reasonably be interpreted as the onset of a schizophreniform illness superimposed on the original intellectual deficit, despite the absence of expressed hallucinations, delusions, or thought disorder.

Given that the two conditions coexist, a number of authors have noted differences between schizophrenic symptoms occurring in mentally retarded and nonretarded individuals, whereas others believe that the clinical signs are essentially the same. Reid[66] described in detail schizophrenic symptomatology based on observations of a small number of mentally retarded patients. The prevailing opinion appears to be that the same clinical signs are present in schizophrenia that co-occur with mental retardation (with slight modifications) as in other schizophrenia. This generalization applies only to verbal, moderately to mildly retarded persons. The picture is somewhat different with respect to profoundly and severely retarded individuals. Some authors have flatly denied that schizophrenic processes occur in such individuals. Others have described schizophrenia-like syndromes occurring in profoundly and severely retarded persons. Kirman[7] outlined guidelines for diagnosing schizophrenia in profoundly retarded individuals that appear to be useful. A practical and conceptual approach to the identification and the treatment of emotional disturbance in this population was noted in the work of Menolascino,[6] who described and explained the development of ''primitive behaviors'' in severely and profoundly retarded individuals.

In summary, schizophrenia clearly occurs in mentally retarded individuals. The prevailing opinion is that verbal, moderately to mildly retarded individuals demonstrate only slight modification in the traditional clinical signs of schizophrenia. There is greater disagreement over the nature of schizophrenic symptoms in more severely retarded individuals. Guidelines for diagnosing schizophrenia in mentally retarded individuals tend to focus on the significance of rapid deteriorative changes in behavior. This appears to be a useful approach to the identification of serious emotional disturbances in severely and profoundly retarded individuals. Similarly, Menolascino's[6] concept of "primitive behavior" also provides a practical, treatment-oriented conceptualization of serious mental illness in profoundly and severely retarded individuals.

1.3.6. Affective Disorders

Wolpert[68] pointed out that the modern view of affective disorders departs sharply from Kraepelinian concepts. He noted that affective disorders are currently divided into two groups—(1) bipolar and (2) unipolar (solitary and recurrent depressive illnesses)—which exhibit two different types of heritability. This division should be kept in mind when examining the previous literature in the field. In spite of advances in recognizing two distinct types of affective disorders, he pointed out that there are still many disparate formulations of the underlying processes, based on intrapsychic, interpersonal, genetic, and/or biochemical points of view. These various approaches to affective illnesses are reflected in the writings of those concerned with mentally retarded individuals.

1.3.7. Manic-Depressive Equivalents

Descriptions of "affective storms" and maniclike excitements in mentally retarded individuals appear frequently in the literature. As early as 1937, Milici[69] concluded that one of the most common psychoses in mentally retarded individuals was transitory excitement alternating with depression. Beier[5] noted that episodes of excitement are one of the most frequent psychoses associated with mental retardation in the literature. Reid[40] speculated that these reported transient effective storms may be fast, brief attacks of manic-depressive psychosis, possibly with florid mixed affective symptoms. Revill[70] also discussed the possible relationship of these affective storms to manic-depressive illness. He noted that such symptoms are more common than manic-depressive psychosis in mentally retarded patients and described these "storms" as states of excitement, lasting from hours to weeks. They sometimes reach a psychotic level, with associated thought disorder, delusions, and hallucinations. Revill made the following comment regarding the relationships of these affective storms to manic-depressive illnesses:

> It is thought that they represent two entities. Because of the greater vulnerability of the retarded patient, due to his relatively poor integration of personality, reactions to stress may take a severe form. Also because of the lesser degree of integration of the personality, internal stress (i.e., endogenous illness) will not often produce a typical clinical picture, but an atypical undifferentiated one. Such outbursts can therefore be regarded in this light as manic-depressive equivalents.

1.3.8. Manic-Depressive Psychosis

Early reports of manic-depressive psychoses in mentally retarded individuals were most frequently descriptions of recurrent depressions, although

Wildman[71] reported that the course and activities of manic-depressive episodes were the same in the mentally retarded as among the "constitutionally normal." Hurd,[56] as early as 1888, described cases of mania, melancholia, and *folie circulaire* in the mentally retarded; and Clouston[72] wrote, "Congenital imbeciles may have attacks of maniacal excitement or of melancholic depression—in fact are subject to them."[40] p. 205. Kraepelin[73,74] believed that "Imbecility may form the basis for the development of other psychoses such as manic-depressive insanity."[40] p. 205. Several recent studies have recognized and described the occurrence of manic-depressive psychotic symptoms in mentally retarded individuals. Reid,[40] for example, noted,

> It is important to recognize the presence of manic-depressive psychosis in mental defectives. There is an association between mental illness and disturbed behavior in mental defectives, and the first step towards effective treatment is, of course, correct diagnosis. In imbeciles, feebleminded, and borderline mental defectives it is relatively straightforward. The symptomatology may at times be unusual, but knowledge of the patient and close study of the symptoms and natural history of the illness should suggest the correct diagnosis. (p. 211)

Similarly, Hucker[75] concluded that "more recent studies suggest that while bipolar illnesses do occur in the subnormal, the diagnosis may be difficult to reach in patients who have a serious degree of mental handicap" (p. 36). According to several recent authors, then, manic-depressive disorders can be diagnosed in mildly and moderately retarded individuals.

There appears to have been a surge of interest in the association between mental retardation and manic-depressive illness within the past several years. Emphasis has been placed on investigating the etiologies of such affective disorders, as well as their possible relationships to mental retardation. Many authors accept heritability of manic-depressive illness as a fact. There is, however, no evidence of a specific genetic link between mental retardation and manic-depressive disorders. Efforts have been made to link specific chromosomal abnormalities with both mental retardation and manic-depressive illnesses; this relationship has not been established. Enough information is available, however, to suggest that further research be conducted. Biochemical factors have also been identified as a possible etiological component in the development of manic-depressive disorders in mentally retarded individuals.[76] Psychogenic factors are infrequently mentioned, partially because of the Freudian belief that mentally retarded individuals lack the prerequisite intelligence for developing manic-depressive illness. It seems, however, that psychogenic factors may play a role in initiating manic-depressive episodes.

Unipolar depression undoubtedly occurs in mentally retarded individuals, although there is a common belief that such depression is rare. It seems probable that most cases of depression in mentally retarded individuals go unnoticed or undiagnosed, for a variety of reasons. Symptoms of depression are too often regarded as intrinsic elements of retardation or as typical of institutional behavior. Depressive symptoms may also appear to be secondary to more obvious problems. Finally, the nondisruptive nature of depressive symptoms lessens the likelihood that institutional staff will view the behavior as a problem.

1.3.9. Paranoid Psychoses

As with most other mental illnesses, the coexistence of paranoia with mental retardation was at one time doubted. Both Berkley[77] and Gordon[59] questioned whether paranoia could appear in mentally retarded individuals in view of "their defect in ideational processes."[66] Although paranoid psychoses are infrequently associated with mental retardation, it seems that mildly and moderately retarded individuals can display all the classical signs of paranoid psychoses. The most prominent symptoms, however, are features other than delusional systems. Intellectual limitations appear to preclude the development of systematic delusions in profoundly and severely retarded individuals. There is little agreement over what etiological factors produce paranoia in mentally retarded individuals. Tredgold and Soddy[78] emphasized the functional nature of paranoid reactions as methods of coping with environmental stress. Reid,[66] on the other hand, speculated on the relationship of paranoid psychoses to chromosomal abnormalities and sensory deficits. Heaton-Ward[12] noted that the typical onset is during or after the fourth decade, and he speculated on the etiological role of menopause.

1.3.10. Conclusions

Psychotic behavior clearly occurs in mentally retarded persons. At the lower levels of intelligence, there is professional disagreement over the nature and meaning of psychotic symptoms. There seems to be an agreement, however, that mildly and moderately retarded individuals demonstrate classical psychoses, which are identifiable via standard diagnostic criteria. Descriptions of psychotic behavior in severely and profoundly retarded individuals generally emphasize abnormal levels of motor activity and sudden changes in personal habits or lifestyles.

Most authors agree that mentally retarded individuals are more susceptible to psychoses than are individuals of normal intelligence. Incidence studies, however, suggest that mentally retarded individuals account for approximately 3% of all psychotic cases, a number consistent with the incidence of mental retardation itself in the general population. Studies regarding the precipitating factors of psychoses in mentally retarded individuals have yielded contradictory findings. Incidence studies are, in general, fraught with numerous methodological problems, not the least of which is institutionalization. Approximately 5%–12% of institutionalized mentally retarded adults demonstrate psychotic symptomatology. Schizophrenic symptoms are the most frequently reported psychotic symptoms in mentally retarded individuals, and manic-depressive symptoms are also frequently noted. Little information is available on noninstitutionalized mentally retarded adults.

Little is known about the course and prognosis of psychosis in mentally retarded individuals. The picture is by no means as bleak as it is usually painted, however, as there is some evidence that the course of psychosis in such individuals is more benign and that the prognosis for recovery is more favorable than in individuals of normal intelligence.

Lastly, there is little experimental research on the differences between psychotic and nonpsychotic mentally retarded individuals. Such research could provide valuable, empirically based direction in an area that is currently fraught with excessive subjective observations and methodologically inadequate studies.

1.4. Neuroses

Psychoneuroses in mentally retarded individuals have been less frequently reported than the psychoses. Nevertheless, early in this century, neuroses were recognized and described in mentally retarded individuals. Several early studies also discussed "instability" in mentally retarded individuals, a concept that was related to, but not identical with, neuroses.

Periodic reviews of this topic have appeared in the literature. Feldman[79] found the literature on psychoneuroses in the mentally retarded to be sparse and indicated that efforts in this area were limited to itemizing surface neurotic symptoms in large groups of institutionalized residents, or to emphasizing the concomitance of hysteria and low intelligence.

Menolascino[20] found little literature on the relationship between mental retardation and neuroses prior to 1950. He noted that previous reviews on the subject suggest that the frequency of neurotic disorders in mentally retarded individuals is low, and that there are apparently few varieties of neurotic manifestations noted in retarded individuals.

1.4.1. Relationship of IQ to Neuroses

The literature[40,80–82] seems to indicate that neuroses are associated more frequently with below- or above-average intelligence than would be expected on the basis of change. The type of neurosis most frequently associated with low intelligence is the dissociative reaction.

1.4.2. Neurotic Manifestations in General

Menolascino[20] defined neurosis as a condition wherein "Internalized symbolic responses to anxiety are chronically utilized to handle recurring patterns of interpersonal friction" (p. 134). He noted that the neuroses are classified as minor mental illnesses in mentally retarded individuals for several reasons: (1) the neuroses are separate from the mental retardation itself (in contrast to the etiological relations that are implied with some of the major mental illnesses); (2) the extent of these disorders does not appreciably interfere with social and vocational adjustment for prolonged periods; and (3) traditionally, such disorders have been viewed as more treatable. Menolascino noted that many early reports suggest a higher frequency of neuroses in moderately and mildly retarded individuals than in severely retarded individuals. Such reports led to speculation that the development of neuroses is beyond the limits of severely retarded individuals. He noted that the low incidence of neuroses identified in the severely retarded may be partially due to the fixed professional belief that mentally retarded individuals are unable to view their interpersonal world in a sufficiently complex manner so as to develop the typical defense mechanisms that comprise a psychoneurosis. He noted a second viewpoint, which holds that neurotic-like adjustment or constructs, such as displaced aggression, are manifested as a general behavioral turmoil in mentally retarded individuals living in the community. This viewpoints tends to suggest that psychoneurotic reactions in mentally retarded individuals are similar in type and frequency to those in the nonretarded population.

1.4.3. Hysterical Reactions

Hysteria (variously referred to as *conversion, histrionic*, or *dissociative disorders*) is frequently cited as one of the most common neuroses occurring in moderately and mildly retarded individuals.[5,83] Several writers have suggested that hysterical reactions, especially blatant and primitive manifestations, are more common among individuals of mildly retarded or borderline intelligence.[80,83,84] Indeed, this was the general conclusion emerging from the neuropsychiatric work during the two world wars. Only a handful of writers have maintained that hysteria is not common in the moderately retarded[74] or the mildly retarded.[85]

1.4.4. Anxiety Reactions

Anxiety reactions are frequently noted in mentally retarded individuals.[3,5,59,83,86,87] Hutt and Gibby[88] noted that acute anxiety states in mentally retarded children are usually accompanied by depression or phsycial complaints, and that such anxiety centers on the fear of rejection. Much has been written on the susceptibility of mentally retarded individuals to the anxiety reactions. Many authors have commented on the increased number of problems faced by mentally retarded individuals and/or their lessened ability to tolerate such stressors.[45,80,81,88,89] This view is typified by Hutt and Gibby[88]: "Due to his more severe problems and lesser capacities to tolerate stress, his anxieties are more readily aroused, and he has more need to engage in defensive reactions" (p. 151).

1.4.5. Depressive Reactions

Depressive symptoms (e.g., sadness, difficulty in initiating sleep, and anxious perplexity about the future) are usually reported as secondary to traumatic or crisis situations in the mentally retarded; they are only infrequently reported in the literature. More recent studies[90] are beginning to more closely view the interrelationship between depression and the symptom of mental retardation.

1.4.6. Incidence of Neuroses

Many authors note that psychoneuroses in mentally retarded individuals are common,[78,86,91] and at least as frequent as among nonretarded individuals.[3] Tizard and O'Connor[92] reviewed the studies that compared the distribution of neuroses in the mentally retarded with that of neuroses in the nonretarded and concluded that a general consensus emerges: in highly stressful situations, such as army induction, the percentage of neuroses among the retarded in just under 50%,[47] and in more normal circumstances, the incidence is just over 20%. They noted that the percentage of neuroses in the nonretarded population is seldom above 20%.

In summary, early studies commonly reported incidences of neuroses in mentally retarded individuals in the area of 20%. Wartime data suggest that as many as 50% of mildly retarded/borderline individuals may become neurotic when faced with severe stress. Recent studies, however, report much lower estimates in the range of 4%–6%.

It seems clear that psychoneuroses occur among retarded individuals at a rate frequently equal to or greater than that found in the general population. Such neuroses are most likely a response to the greater pressures encountered by mentally retarded individuals, as precipitating factors can frequently be identified. In times of great stress, such as wartime induction, mentally retarded individuals may more easily succumb to neurotic conditions than nonretarded individuals. The precipitating factors, although sometimes dramatic, may also include smaller events such as laboratory blood tests or intelligence testing.

Manifestations of neuroses in mildly and moderately retarded individuals appear to be similar to those in nonretarded individuals. Hysterical reactions have been most frequently associated with mental retardation in the literature, and this association may be partially due to the bizarreness and obviousness of such reactions when they do occur. Anxiety reactions, obsessive-compulsive states, and phobic conditions have also been reported in retarded individuals. Psychosomatic and physical complaints appear to play a very large role in the symptom picture of these conditions.

There is a strong belief that neurotic anxiety in mentally retarded individuals may be directly expressed as behavior disorders (e.g., aggressive behaviors). In addition, the concept of "institutional neurosis" does have great utility and should be kept in mind in interpreting all research conducted in institutions: what is adaptive in an institution all too often is maladaptive in the community, and vice versa.

1.5. Personality Disorders

Personality disorders have been rarely identified in psychiatric incidence studies of mentally retarded populations. As early as 1928, Harris[83] identified a probable reason for this finding. While noting that anomalies of temperament and character are much more important than psychoses and psychoneuroses, he noted also the difficulties in measuring such disorders. Menolascino[20] noted

also that personality disorders other than antisocial personality are rarely reported in mentally retarded individuals. Menolascino defined such disorders
as chronic maladjustments of behavior patterns that are qualitatively different
from psychotic or neurotic disorders. He emphasized the magnitude of this
category, which includes passive-dependent and acting-out individuals, as well
as antisocial personalities. Reid[93] maintained that a diagnosis of personality
disorder requires a close evaluation of past history of maladaptive behaviors,
in conjunction with the current clinical findings.

Studies that attempt to identify personality disorders among retarded individuals generally report a relatively high rate of such disorders, compared
to neuroses and psychoses. Craft,[49] for instance, found that schizoid personalities and emotionally unstable personalities were the most frequently observed psychiatric disorders among 324 inpatient mentally retarded individuals;
he identified 30 schizoid personalities, 31 emotionally unstable personalities,
3 dependence reactions (resulting from physical ailments), 4 aggressive personalities, 2 compulsive personalities, and 10 antisocial personalities.

Menolascino[20] offered the following contrasting conclusion regarding personality disorders in retarded individuals: "In summary, personality disorders
do occur in the mentally retarded, are primarily based on extrinsic factors,
have no distinct etiological relationship to mental retardation, and despite persistent folklore, are not increased in their frequency in the retarded population"
(p. 210).

For a variety of reasons, personality disorders are rarely diagnosed in
mentally retarded individuals. A major reason is the difficulties involved in
identifying the relatively subtle symptoms of personality disorders. However,
when the incidence of personality disorders among mentally retarded individuals have been closely assessed, relatively high rates have often been noted.
The diagnosis of personality disorders in retarded individuals would appear to
be useful in identifying characteristic maladaptive modes or responses. A retarded individual may demonstrate, for instance, schizoid personality traits that
are not of psychotic proportions, yet require attention and treatment. Care
must be taken, of course, not to over-diagnose personality disorders, and mere
developmental lags must not be viewed as evidence of such disorders.

1.5.1. Suicide

There is not a systematic body of knowledge regarding the incidence of
suicide or suicidal behaviors in mentally retarded individuals. Sternlicht, Pustel, and Deutsch's 1970 study stands as a key intensive investigation into this
phenomenon. Nevertheless, scattered references have been made to this subject beginning as early as 1845, when Wells described a suicidal form of mania
in a retarded individual wherein the patient attempted self-destruction by
fire.[132]

Sternlicht, Pustel, and Deutsch[94] undertook an extensive investigation at
the Willowbrook State School in New York State in an effort to shed light on
this neglected topic. They indicated, first of all, that in spite of the "plethora"

of material written on suicide, an exhaustive survey of this literature failed to locate a single research investigation or theoretical treatise on suicide in mentally retarded individuals. They noted that this lack of research may be partially due to the fact that suicide has always been considered a marginal problem among retarded individuals. Sternlicht and his associates defined *suicidal behavior* as acts of attempted or suggested suicide, as no successful suicide attempts were identified in their population studies. They noted, "There is every reason to believe, however, that were staff supervision and surveillance less vigilant and effective than they are, many of the attempted suicides would have eventuated in committed suicides" (p. 95). They found an incidence of attempted suicide of 0.9% of the total Willowbrook population, or 9 per 1,000 patients. They noted that this incidence closely approximates the rate of 1% (10/1,000) that exists among the general population of the United States. In contrast to the general finding that females attempt suicide more frequently than males, Sternlicht, Pustel, and Deutsch found twice as many attempts by mentally retarded males. Their findings with respect to age also reflect a reversal of the general population trend, with retarded adults attempting suicide five times more frequently than retarded adolescents. They noted, however, that these attempts might indeed have been actual suicides in the absence of close and constant supervision.

In summary, although suicide and suicide attempts are not generally regarded as problems among populations of mentally retarded individuals, scattered reports indicate that suicide attempts do occur, and suicide threats should be taken seriously. Truly, this dimension of mental illness in the retarded *does* need further and extensive clinical attention and research focus.

1.5.2. Alcoholism

Almost nothing has been written regarding the relationship between alcoholism and mental retardation, and most of what has been written has been based on speculation and ignorance. Historically, alcoholism was considered a cause of mental retardation. Barrett[95] suggested that alcoholism commonly was found as an antecedent in the parents of retarded persons and thus served as an underlying cause of the retardation. Howe[96] reported that the "most prominent and prolific" theory of degeneracy is that of "intemperance" as a cause of family deterioration.[97] Of 359 retarded individuals, Howe reported that 99, by conservative estimates, were "children of drunkards." Tredgold[98] likewise noted that alcoholism was a contributory factor in mental retardation, contending that its effects showed up after the first successive generation.

Surveys of psychiatric problems among mentally retarded populations seldom comment on the frequency of alcoholism. The only factual information available suggests that an outstanding feature of mental retardation is an "apparent antagonism to alcoholism."[99] Bailey, Williams, and Komora[99] found that, among groups of soldiers during World War I, a high rate of mental retardation was associated with a low alcoholism rate. Although the percentage of moderate drinkers among the mentally retarded was slightly higher than that found in neuropsychiatric patients as a whole, the mentally retarded group was sixth in order of frequency with respect to intemperance. Similar low correlations were found between drug addiction and mental retardation.

In summary, it appears that, during the first half of this century, it was rather commonly believed that descendants of alcoholics were likely to be mentally retarded, as a direct consequence of their ancestors' alcoholism. "Insanity attacks" in mentally retarded individuals were also attributed to alcoholism, and mentally retarded persons were commonly considered more prone to the effects of alcohol than nonretarded persons. Objective evidence, however, suggests that clinical alcoholism has only rarely been reported in mentally retarded individuals. Pollock,[17] for instance, identified only 17 cases of alcoholism among 444 mentally retarded patients admitted to a New York civil state hospital in 1942. Very little objective evidence is available on this subject, but what little evidence there is suggests that alcoholism is only rarely associated with mental retardation. It is not clear whether this finding relates to characteristics of retarded individuals, or whether it is a function of the fact that alcohol has not traditionally been available to many retarded individuals in this society.

It should be noted that the fetal alcohol syndrome, which is often associated with subsequent mental retardation, is a direct consequence of excessive drinking by the mother-to-be. There is, however, no evidence that mental retardation and alcoholism are associated in any other manner.

1.6. Seizure Disorders, Mental Retardation and Mental Illness

Epilepsy can be defined as "a sudden and excessive disorderly discharge from the nerve cells within the brain . . . accompanied by a marked disturbance of consciousness, an excess or lack of muscle tone, convulsive movements, disorders of sensation, or major irregularities in the automatic functions of the body" (p. 367),[13] and it occurs more frequently among mentally retarded individuals than in the general population. Menolascino[20] reported that the incidence of epilepsy in the general population is approximately 5 in 1,000, and Cytryn and Lourie[18] estimated that as many as 20%–25% of all institutionalized mentally retarded individuals have epilepsy.

Bakwin and Bakwin[100] pointed out that some epileptic persons have normal to superior IQs, although a higher proportion (compared to nonepileptic persons) have IQs less than 100. Studies consistently indicate that at least 15% of the epileptic population is seriously retarded. Menolascino and Egger[13] seemed justified in concluding that "The occurrence of convulsive disorders in combination with mental retardation is not coincidental, but that both result from the same underlying central nervous system disorder" (p. 375).

1.6.1. Symptoms of Epilepsy

Ervin[101] noted that there are few psychopathological phenomena that have not been observed during epileptic seizures, including disorders of affect (depression, anxiety, terror, and rage); disturbances of thought (forced thinking, obsessive rumination, fragmentation, and neologisms); perceptual changes (hallucinations); and disturbances of behavior.

1.6.2. Mental Disturbances Associated with Temporal Lobe Epilepsy

Approximately 20% of all epileptic patients demonstrate psychomotor seizures[101] of temporal lobe origin. Dongier[102] noted that confusion is not always present, but that mood swings and disturbances in affect may occur. Anxiety and depression in association with normal consciousness, as well as marked paranoid ideation, may be observed.

Bakwin and Bakwin[100] noted that temporal lobe seizures are characterized by episodes of bizarre, automatic, stereotyped movements; clouding of consciousness; and partial or complete amnesia for events. Such episodes may last for moments or for hours and may be manifested in a variety of ways, including perceptual changes; self-awareness changes; forced or disorganized thought, mood, and affect changes; complex hallucinations; and complex stereotyped automatisms. It is to be noted that these behaviors are similar to those associated with schizophrenia. However, the exact mechanisms or role of temporal lobe epilepsy in producing psychiatric disorders remains unclear.

According to Dongier,[102] centrencephalic epileptic patients frequently show psychotic episodes of relatively brief duration (several hours). Such episodes are not chronic, do not lead to permanent mental disturbance or dementia, are usually of a confusional nature, and are not to be regarded as psychotic episodes. Dongier did conclude that these lobe cases demonstrate a propensity for severe psychiatric disturbances. O'Gorman[103] identified psychotic features in epileptic patients that he considered indistinguishable from those of schizophrenia.

In a study of 83 epileptic patients, Ervin[101] noted that 30% of the generalized cases and 65% of the psychomotor seizure cases demonstrated psychotic episodes. Ervin suggested that such individuals might be misdiagnosed as schizophrenic, and that some children with episodic behavior disorder, poor impulse control, and affective lability might also demonstrate temporal-lobe EEG abnormalities.

1.6.3. "Epileptic Personality" and Behavior Disorders

Tizard[104] conducted a comprehensive review of the literature and concluded that there is no evidence that epileptic individuals have a characteristic personality. Ervin[101] noted that individuals with epilepsy exhibit a wide range of personality types and abnormalities. Bakwin and Bakwin[100] also noted that the concept of an "epileptic personality" has generally been discarded.

Nevertheless, behavioral disorders are often identified in association with epilepsy. Bakwin and Bakwin[100] pointed out that opinions differ with respect to whether such behaviors are caused entirely or in part by the cerebral disorder underlying the epilepsy, or whether they are a result of the reaction to the illness and subsequent treatment interventions. They pointed out that some individuals use their seizures to get attention or to avoid uncomfortable situations; they may do this through conscious inducement of a seizure (via hyperventilation) or through a conditioned reflex to stress. Bakwin and Bakwin noted that 60% of all epileptics experience their first seizure before age 10 and thus grow up with this handicap. As the majroity of seizures can be controlled by medication,[13,101] it seems likely that behavior problems can also be reduced upon the effective control of the seizure activity.

In summary, epilepsy and mental retardation are clearly related, although the nature of this relationship is still unspecified. Epilepsy occurs more frequently among more severely retarded individuals, in comparison to mildly retarded individuals. When epilepsy coexists with mental retardation, the two probably stem from the same underlying CNS pathology (e.g., at the more severe levels of retardation), and as an associated handicap in others. When mental retardation and epilepsy occur together, behavior problems appear to be compounded. Mentally retarded children with seizures demonstrate more behavior disorders than nonretarded children with seizures. They also demonstrate more behavior disorders than do retarded children without seizures.

1.7. Special Relationships Between Mental Retardation and Mental Illness

Occasionally, reports appear in the literature linking specific mental retardation syndromes to mental illness.

1.7.1. Metabolic Disorders

Jancar[30] noted that a number of the inborn errors of metabolism have been identified and described in mentally retarded individuals and are closely allied (i.e., may be a part of the symptom complex) to mental illness.

1.7.1.1. Phenylketonuria

Phenylketonuria (PKU) is the metabolic disorder most frequently discussed in relationship to mental illness. The classical clinical picture of untreated PKU is severe mental retardation, seizures, and psychotic behavior.[13,105]

Penrose[106] described PKU patients as generally pleasant and "good-tempered," whereas Benda[107] noted frequent aggression and "wild" behavior. Most often, schizoid and withdrawn behavioral traits are described.

Cytryn and Lourie[18] noted that the clinical picture varies, but they reported that patients do display hyperactive, erratic, unpredictable behaviors and that they exhibit frequent temper tantrums and bizarre movements of the body and the upper extremities. Himwich and Himwich[108] reported that many institutions' records reveal that PKU children are often admitted with a diagnosis of "childhood schizophrenia."

Penrose[3] cautioned that the psychiatric significance of isolated schizophrenic symptoms in PKU patients is difficult to determine. Menolascino[87] warned that, although a number of symptoms may be found, they might be more characteristic of severe mental retardation and institutionalization than of PKU specifically. The salient question appears to be identification of behavior disturbance, if such exists, in metabolically untreated and treated (i.e., appropriately regulated on the PKU diet) PKU patients. It has been noted that effectively treated PKU patients do not show psychotic behavior; it tends to be absent, as are the retardation and seizure phenomenon also. Accordingly, it appears that the psychotic feature of the nontreated PKU patient reflects a metabolic toxic psychosis.

1.7.1.2. Hartnup's Disease

Himwich and Himwich[108] note that Hartnup's disease is a metabolic disorder associated with intermittent and variable malfunctions. One manifestation of the disorder is psychosis, and occasionally, progressive mental retardation occurs. Accordingly, Hartnup's disease appears to be one of the rare instances in which a common etiological factor is strongly suggested for both mental retardation and mental illness, even though one or the other disorder, rather than both, appears to be manifested in a given individual.

1.7.1.3. Wilson's Disease

Wilson's disease is a condition of genetic origin characterized by degeneration of the brain stem and breakdown of the liver, resulting from abnormal copper metabolism. Menolascino and Egger[13] noted that it is frequently characterized by associated emotional and mental abnormalities.

1.7.1.4. Lesch-Nyhan Syndrome

Menolascino and Egger[13] described this X-linked recessive syndrome as including elevated levels of uric acid in the blood, developmental retardation, spastic cerebral palsy, distinctive body movements, and self-mutilative behavior (such as biting fingers, toes, and lips). The level of mental retardation noted is variable and is not always severe. These patients do feel pain, according to Menolascino and Egger, and often plead with observers to keep them from biting themselves. They are often quite aggressive to others, use foul language, strike, bite, and spit.[109] A recent report by Nyhan[110] notes the continuing untreatable states of the behavioral aspects of this syndrome to date.

In summary, the Lesch-Nyhan syndrome appears to be an instance wherein mental retardation and behavioral disorder are so closely allied as to form essential parts of the same syndrome.

1.7.2. Chromosomal Disorders

It should be noted that there are two types of chromosomal abnormalities, which are frequently—though not always—associated with different classes of manifestations. As Penrose[22] pointed out, "Autosomal aberrations seem to produce defect rather than insanity, but the situation is somewhat different with respect to the sex chromosomes. The effects of sex chromosomal aberrations are more noticeable in relation to alterations in character and stability than they are in relation to intellectual loss" (p. 753).

1.7.2.1. Abnormal Sex-Chromosome Arrangements

Abnormal sex-chromosome arrangements may be manifested only by mental retardation, rather than by personality disorders or mental illness. In general, the greater the number of extra X chromosomes, the more severe is the level of concurrent mental retardation.

1.7.2.2. Extra X Chromosome in Males

Jancar[30] concluded that males with supernumerary X chromosomes are more liable than others to mental retardation, mental disorder, epilepsy, and antisocial conduct. Klinefelter's syndrome (XXY instead of XY karyotype) occurs in about 1 in 4,000 males, according to Shapiro and Ridler[111] and Menolascino and Egger.[13] In institutions for the mentally retarded, however, the rate is 1 in 2,000.[111] Shapiro and Ridler noted that the retardation associated with Klinefelter's syndrome is usually mild. Rainer[105] noted that 1% of the male mentally retarded institutionalized patients have Klinefelter's syndrome. The syndrome is typically not recognized until puberty.[13,112]

Among the seriously disturbed, the criminally insane, or the institutionalized mentally retarded, between 1% and 2% of males have Klinefelter's syndrome. According to Forssman and Hambert,[113] the Klinefelter's personality spectrum evidences passive aggressiveness, episodic confusion, schizophreniform disorders, paranoia, manic-depressive psychoses, epilepsy, and obsessional disorders. Cytryn and Lourie[18] emphasized psychogenic factors, social withdrawal, and body-image distortion in the etiology of mental illness in these individuals. However, further research is direly needed to clarify the puzzling behavioral pictures seen in Klinefelter individuals.

1.7.2.3. Extra X Chromosome in Females

Forssman and Hambert[113] reported that it can be considered an established fact that females with extra X chromosomes are more liable to both mental retardation and mental illness. Polani[114] reported that the frequency of XXX females is five times greater among schizophrenic women than among females in hospitals for the mentally retarded.[114]

1.7.2.4. Extra Y Chromosomes in Males

Jacobs, Brunton, and Melville[115] surveyed 197 mentally retarded male patients who were residing in a maximum security hospital as a result of "violent, dangerous, and criminal propensities." Twelve chromosomal abnormalities were identified, including eight cases of extra Ys, yielding an incidence of 3.5%. Jacobs *et al.* assumed that this was a higher incidence than in the general population. Parker, Mavalwala, Weise *et al.*[116] reviewed the literature on clinical manifestations on XYY males and found that tallness, aggressive behavior, and mental retardation were frequently mentioned.

The extra Y chromosomes in males appear to distinctly increase the probability of antisocial behavior or mental illness. This condition is also associated with mental retardation, although less so than Klinefelter's.

1.7.2.5. XO Females (Turner's Syndrome)

Forssman and Hambert[113] reported that Turner's syndrome occurs in 0.03% of newborn girls, and in 0.06% of mentally retarded girls. Turner's syndrome is associated with mental retardation, but mental illness appears to occur less frequently with this XO karyotype than when extra Xs occur. There is strong evidence that XO/XX mosaic karyotypes are associated with schizophrenia.

1.7.3. Autosomal Abnormalities

Autosomal abnormalities are typically associated with mental retardation. Reid[66] presented interesting findings regarding autosomal and sexual aberrations found in mentally retarded paranoid psychotic individuals and concluded that "The association of paranoid psychoses with chromosomal abnormalities (and with disorders of vision as well as of hearing) is of interest and should be followed up" (p. 217).

1.7.3.1. Down's Syndrome

Menolascino[117] found that institutionalized Down's syndrome (DS) individuals fit the oft-repeated behavioral stereotype of "Prince Charming" behavior, being given to mimicry and appearing to be overtly happy and friendly. He considered this behavior, however, secondary to affect hunger, secondary in turn to lack of early mothering and to early labeling as a "deviant."Menolascino[118] reported that 11 of 86 DS outpatient children examined by a clinical team were deemed to be mentally ill. About half as many cases of emotional disturbance were identified in the Down's syndrome children as in most studies using varied populations of mentally retarded individuals, however. Moore, Thuline, and Capes[119] compared the maladjusted behavior of DS individuals from all the institutions in Arizona and Washington with a matched control group of residents. They found the DS group to be significantly less maladjusted on 14 to 21 measures. Moore, Thuline, and Capes[119] concluded that DS individuals, as a group, tend to exhibit less maladjustment than their mentally retarded peers. Similarly, Webster[120] reported that DS was the only diagnostic category in his study of 159 preschool mentally retarded children in which no cases of severe disturbance in emotional development were identified. Johnson and Abelson[121] found that DS individuals demonstrated a higher proportion of socially adaptive and socially competent behaviors in 7 of 11 comparisons, even though, as a group, they were slightly younger and duller than the comparison group. This type of study is also consistent with the outstanding work of Domino concerning the social-adaptive and behavioral dimensions of DS. Heaton-Ward[12] commented that of all the autosomal chromosomal aberrations, trisomy-21 is the one in which psychoses are most frequently reported. It should be remembered, of course, that trisomy-21 individuals outnumber all of the other mental-health-associated chromosomal aberrations combined, and that trisomy-21 is an easily recognized syndrome.

Psychoses have been consistently reported in DS individuals, commencing with the extensive work of Earl[67] on the "larval catatonic form of schizophrenia." Rollin[122] described a catatonic psychosis in 23.3% of his cases in which autism and emotional disorder were evidenced. He described previously docile and affectionate individuals' becoming excited, near-manic, wild, and noisy. The onset of the illness was followed by a rapid deterioration in toilet and speech habits and in social relations. Rollin described the final clinical picture as being that of a fully developed catatonic psychosis, characterized by huddling in corners, vacant, fixed stare, loss of volition, automatic obedience, and flexibilitas cerea. Beier[5] concluded that DS individuals, as a group, are probably no more homogeneous in terms of adjustment factors or problems than other unselected groups of normal or mentally retarded individuals. In one area, however, DS individuals appear to be at a disadvantage: Jancar[30] reported that DS individuals appear to show an increased frequency of premature senile dementia.

In conclusion, although there is strong evidence to suggest that, although Down's syndrome individuals, as a group, are better adjusted and more socially competent than other mentally retarded groups, they also are not immune to serious psychological disturbance. They appear to suffer the same emotional disturbances as other mentally retarded individuals, although the prevalence of such disturbances may be somewhat less than in non–Down's syndrome retarded individuals.

1.8. Other Genetic Disorders

1.8.1. Tuberous Sclerosis

Tuberous sclerosis (epiloia) is a congenital disorder manifested by tumor-like masses in numerous organs, which are most frequently noted in the brain and the skin.[13] The term *epiloia* was coined by Sherlock[13] in 1911 to refer to the mental retardation accompanying this condition.[133]

Broffenbrenner[123] noted that the behavior of epiloiac patients is different from that of the majority of retarded individuals. Characteristic behaviors, according to Broffenbrenner, include moroseness, sullenness, unwillingness to associate with others, negativistic behavior, rhythmic movement of the limbs and the fingers, humming, and unresponsiveness. Cytryn and Lourie[18] noted that the degree of mental retardation in epiloiac patients ranges from mild to very severe, and that psychotic symptoms are sometimes associated with the condition. Although the idea persists that tuberous sclerotic patients frequently manifest psychotic behaviors, new studies appear to be needed to reveal the degree to which this finding holds true today.

1.9. Infectious Diseases

1.9.1. Encephalitis Lethargica

Bakwin and Bakwin[100] noted that idiopathic encephalitis is not frequently followed by cerebral impairments, mental retardation, sleep disturbances, and/or emotional outbursts. Mautner[85] likewise observed, "Behavior disorders following encephalitis may resemble schizophrenic reactions and it remains a hair-splitting discussion whether they have to be called schizophrenia or not, as long as we have no objective diagnosis" (p. 188–189). Penrose[3] argued that the frequently noted organic psychoses associated with mental retardation are an aftermath of encephalitis lethargica. The very nature of the encephalitis disorder tends to disrupt major areas of the central nervous system. Thus, it should not be surprising to note a multiplication of signs and symptoms in postencephalitic disorders. Beyond the encephalitis disorders, it should be noted that the meningitis disorders can also produce major behavioral pictures of a similar type. The common feature results from major brain impairment (with resultant behavioral disorganization) secondary to an infectious viral or bacterial process. In other words, an organic brain syndrome is produced by the infection process, and a superimposed psychotic behavioral picture is frequently noted in association with it.

1.9.2. Congenital Syphilis

Penrose[3] argued that congenital syphilis (or juvenile general paresis) leads to progressive mental deficiency in children, in which the child becomes "increasingly stupid, neurotic, indifferent to its surroundings, dirty in its habits and eventually bedridden, with contracted limbs, marked emaciation . . ." (p. 215). Sometimes, euphoria and mildly grandiose ideas are observed in the early stages, according to Penrose. Although the exact causal relationship between congenital syphilis and mental retardation has not been established, many clinical studies provide a useful reminder that undiagnosed and/or untreated congenital (or postnatal onset) syphilis is associated with a high incidence of psychotic behavior. The types of psychosis that syphilis most typically present are ones that feature signs of organic brain syndrome and rather grandiose delusions of omnipotence.

1.10. Severe Disorders of Childhood

Several severe behavioral-developmental disorders of childhood have been identified that seem to occur in mentally retarded, as well as in nonretarded, children. These disorders include early infantile autism, as well as childhood schizophrenia. These terms are sometimes used interchangeably, although they have been rather carefully differentiated by many professionals. These disorders all serve to severely limit a child's adaptive capacity. In addition, there is strong evidence that such severe disorders of childhood are caused by CNS dysfunction, rather than by psychogenic factors.

1.10.1. Infantile Autism

The primary pathology of infantile autism is an inability—from the very start of life—to relate to people in an ordinary or appropriate manner; other key symptoms include obsessiveness, motor stereotypy, and echolalia.

Rutter[124] identified the current use of the term *infantile autism* as denoting

> disorders beginning before the age of 30 months, in which there may or may not be associated intellectual retardation or neurological dysfunction, but in which the key clinical features are a particular form of impaired social and language development (which must have a number of specific characteristics and which must be out of keeping with the child's general intellectual level), together with an "insistence of sameness" as shown by stereotyped play patterns, abnormal preoccupations, and resistance to change. (p. 12)

The prevailing professional opinion[125] is that a wide variety of CNS impairments are the causes of infantile autism and not "emotionally cold" parents, as was previously contended.

1.10.2. Mental Retardation and Autism

In the original description of early infantile autism, Kanner[23] felt that the retarded intellectual functioning of autistic children was secondary to their failure to establish basic human relationships. This belief was based partly on their rote memory skills, occasional verbal skills, lack of physical stigmata, and serious facial expression. However, there is evidence that autism is found at all levels of intelligence, and that the syndrome varies with different IQ levels. For instance, autistic children who are also mentally retarded are not likely to gain speech and academic skills, nor are they likely to proceed to higher education or paid employment.[126] They are also more likely to develop seizures than are nonretarded autistic children.[124] Further, the austic child with mental retardation demonstrates a wider range of deficits than the nonretarded autistic child, whose deficits are primarily verbal. Mentally retarded autistic children demonstrate the more severe disorders of social development, as well as a greater amount of deviant social behavior. Thus, the prognosis for the mentally retarded autistic child is considerably more limited than that of an autistic child with normal nonverbal intelligence.

1.10.3. Differential Diagnosis of Autism

Research indicates that most severely retarded children are able to relate to adults, to communicate, to vocalize, and to use expressive speech better than autistic children, for the most part.[127] There is also evidence suggesting that severely and profoundly retarded children demonstrate uniform deficits, whereas the symptom picture of autism is fragmented.[128] The differential diagnosis between autism and childhood schizophrenia is usually made on the basis of onset and course, although, in practice, the differential diagnosis is quite difficult.

In summary, the current professional assessment (1983) of autism is that it emanates from a very wide variety of underlying neuropathological and neuropsychological causes—rather than functional interpersonal causes—and that it manifests some atypical behaviors that tend to have many similarities to the behaviors noted in moderate to mildly retarded individuals (usually in conjunction with a major controlled language disorder).

1.10.4. Childhood Schizophrenia

Current views of childhood psychoses tend to focus on the description of behaviors,[20] such as bizarre manners or gestures, uncommunicative speech, lack of differentiation between objects and people, a persistent lack of interest in animate objects, lack of eye contact, minimal response to interpersonal or structured play interactions, unusual speech patterns (i.e., echolalia, with otherwise normal language development), and stereotyped motor habits. Though it may appear difficult to differentiate early infantile autism from childhood psychosis on the basis of symptoms, a key consideration is the typical percentage of personality regression that is noted in childhood schizophrenia. Herein, the DSM-III nomenclature[131] of the American Psychiatric Association has greatly aided in clarifying the recent diagnostic confusion between autism and the syndrome of schizophrenia when it appears in childhood.

1.10.5. Idiot Savants

Idiot savantism[129] is a condition in which an otherwise retarded individual demonstrates a phenomenal or marked special aptitude in comparison to normal as well as to retarded persons. It has been argued that idiot savantism is a condition characterized by deficiencies in abstraction, along with abnormal concretization and channeling of abilities.[130] Similarly, it has been viewed as an atypical form of schizophrenia wherein the ego has overfocused on portions of the external environment that still prove to be enjoyable to these terribly ill individuals. Lastly, it is not unlikely that idiot savantism is based on a CNS dysfunction that has unequal effects on various cognitive abilities. This is a very rare syndrome, and the available information suggests that a wide variety of causal entities produce the final pathway of the rather dramatic symptoms typically noted.

1.11. Conclusions and Implications for Treatment and Research

It can no longer be maintained that mentally retarded individuals escape the debilitating effects of mental illness by virtue of their "simple approach" to life. Mental illness and behavioral disturbances clearly occur in many mentally retarded individuals and interfere, to varying degrees, with their ability to adjust.

The prevailing professional opinion is that—for a wide variety of reasons—mentally retarded individuals are more susceptible to mental illness than are nonretarded individuals. Research rather consistently indicates that approximately 10% of mentally retarded institutionalized individuals demonstrate symptoms of severe emotional disturbance (psychosis and neurosis). When minor behavior disturbances are included, estimates rise as high as 60%. Studies conducted on mentally retarded children and adults in the community confirm that 20%–35% demonstrate evidence of mental illness (compared to 14%–18% of nonretarded children). The evidence as a whole suggests that mentally retarded individuals display an incidence of mental illness that is moderately increased over that of nonretarded individuals. Psychogenic factors, as well as an increased exposure to psychological stressors, appear to play a primary etiological role in mildly and moderately retarded individuals, whereas CNS disorders and sensory deficits are frequently nominated as etiological factors in the more severely retarded population.

Professsionals who are well acquainted with both conditions—mental illness and mental retardation—experience little difficulty in making a differential diagnosis. Much confusion arises, however, when a professional with experience only in the field of mental health (or mental retardation) attempts to untangle the factors contributing to a presenting clinical picture of both mental retardation and mental illness. Only professionals trained and clinically experienced in both fields are able to sort out what types of behavior are due to limited intelligence and what signs and symptoms are the result of inadequate adjustment or instances of mental illness.

Flexible behavioral approaches are seen as extremely effective treatment interventions with emotionally disturbed mentally retarded individuals. The value of such approaches, however, is contingent on the manner in which they are applied. Openminded and flexible clinicians develop behavioral treatment programs based on current behaviors and specific goals, reassess the efficacy of such programs, and continually modify them to best assist the patient in developing new (i.e., more adaptive) behaviors while simultaneously eliminating maladaptive behaviors. True, a particular patient may indeed lack the capacity to reach a given goal, but a flexible behavioral treatment program allows this conclusion to be based on ongoing behavioral observations and analyses rather than on preconceived ideas regarding the abilities of the mentally retarded as a group.

The important elements of any treatment plan are an openminded approach, a periodic reassessment of treatment efficacy, and the willingness to continually modify treatments until a useful and effective one is found. Although behavior modification approaches lend themselves easily to this model, it is clear that a more balanced treatment–management program is most often necessary to provide maximal treatment benefits. A professional who can bring extensive knowledge of both mental retardation and emotional disturbance to bear on the formulation of treatment plans can help to ensure that professional judgment will work for the good, rather than to the detriment, of retarded individuals.

Thus, two general conclusions can be drawn with respect to the diagnosis and treatment of mental illness in mentally retarded individuals. First, there is a pressing need for professionals who are trained in both mental retardation and mental health. Second, the focus should move from an emphasis on diagnoses based on etiological factors, to diagnoses that rely on descriptions of symptoms and allied specific formulations of treatment plans that can maximize treatment response and future prognosis.

Implications for research are also clear. Incidence studies that investigate the frequency of mental illness among mentally retarded individuals have served their purpose. It seems unlikely that a definitive statement can ever be made regarding the exact incidence of mental illness among mentally retarded individuals in general. Any incidence study must clearly specify diagnostic criteria for the nature of the mental illness noted in mentally retarded individuals. Studies that investigate the incidence of specified behaviors or mental illnesses provide significantly more information than do studies that focus on identifying incidence rates by utilizing vaguely defined terms.

Descriptive studies of mental illness in mentally retarded individuals can provide useful and practical information to the clinician. Such studies can serve to dispel myths, can help lay foundations for data-based classification systems, and can contribute to a wider appreciation of the fact that mental retardation and mental illness can and do often coexist to complicate (and at times obfuscate!) the symptom pictures of each other. Further research could, for example, more clearly establish the manner in which the various levels of mental retardation modify expressions of mental illness. Research is also needed to provide an empirical basis for the differentiation of mental illness in mentally retarded individuals, in a way that is tied to treatment and prognosis. Currently, we do not have available the treatment technology to warrant the pouring of large amounts of time and effort into differential diagnoses in the clinical setting, especially if such diagnoses are based only on etiological factors.

The contribution of institutionalization to the development of mental illness is unknown, although it is presumed to play a role. There is, therefore, a need for studies that assess maladjusted behaviors at the time of institutionalization and at later dates. There is increasing and strong evidence of metabolic substrates of psychotic disorders, and there is no reason to believe that individuals with mental retardation should be excepted from this finding. It appears fruitless to continue debating whether mental illness in retarded individuals is a result of psychogenic factors or of CNS dysfunction. In addition, the argument over what causes mental illness in mentally retarded individuals is nonproductive, because of the inability to determine to what degree CNS dysfunction accounts for an individual's behavior. In some cases, however, CNS dysfunction can be identified; and in these cases, the etiological role of these dysfunctions should actually be investigated.

1.12. Conclusion

Mental retardation is a syndrome and need not carry with it immutable assumptions about etiology or prognosis. Professional attitudes of the past may have contributed as much as any other factor to the unfavorable outcomes and the pessimistic prognoses in cases where mental retardation and mental illness coexist. A sensitivity on the part of clinicians to the presence of mental illness in mentally retarded individuals, a willingness to treat such disorders, and a preference for flexible and balanced treatment approaches can go far toward decreasing the incidence of mental disorders currently found in mentally retarded individuals. Professionals must recognize that mentally retarded individuals who suffer from mental illnesses, regardless of their ultimate intellectual potential, have the same rights of treatment as any other group of human beings. Only then can the mental health field begin to fully meet the complex needs of retarded individuals.

References

1. Maney AC, Pace R, Morrison DF: A factor analytic study of the need for institutionalization: Problems and populations for program development. *Am J Ment Defic* 69;374–384, 1964.
2. Shellhaas MD, Nihira K: Factor analysis of reasons retardates are referred to an institution. *Am J Ment Defic* 74;171–179, 1969
3. Penrose LS: Biology and Mental Defect, rev. ed. New York, Grune and Stratton, 1962.
4. Foale M: The special difficulties of the high grade mentally defective adolescent. *Am J Ment Defic* 60;867–877, 1956.
5. Beier DC: Behavioral disturbances in the mentally retarded, in Stevens HA, Huber R (eds): *Mental Retardation*. Chicago, University of Chicago Press, 1964.
6. Menolascino FJ: Emotional disturbances in institutionalized retardates: Primitive, atypical and abnormal behaviors. *Ment Retard* 10;3–8, 1972.
7. Kirman BH: Clinical aspects, in Wortis J (ed): *Mental Retardation and Developmental Disabilities: An Annual Review*. New York, Brunner/Mazel, 1973.
8. Philips I: Psychopathology and mental retardation, in Menolascino F (ed): *Psychiatric Aspects of the Diagnosis and Treatment of Mental Retardation*. Seattle, Special Child Publications, 1971.
9. Kinder DJ, Rutherford EJ: Social adjustment of retarded children. *Mental Hygiene* 11;811–833, 1927.
10. Gardner JM, Giampa FL: Behavioral competence and social and emotional behavior in mental retardation. *Am J Ment Defic* 75;168–169, 1970.
11. Primrose DA: A survey of 500 consecutive admissions to a subnormality hospital from 1st January 1968 to 31st December 1970. *Br J Ment Subnormality* 17;25–28, 1971.
12. Heaton-Ward A: Psychosis in mental handicap. *Br J Psychiat* 130;525–533, 1977.
13. Menolascino F, Egger ML: *Medical Dimensions of Mental Retardation*. Lincoln, University of Nebraska Press, 1978.

14. Chess S: Treatment of emotional problems of the retarded child and of the family, in Menolascino FJ (ed): *Psychiatric Aspects of the Diagnosis and Treatment of Mental Retardation.* Seattle, Special Child Publications, 1971.
15. Grossman HJ: *Manual of Terminology and Classification in Mental Retardation.* Washington, American Association on Mental Deficiency, 1973.
16. American Psychiatric Association: DSM-III (*Diagnostic and Statistical Manual of Mental Disorders*), ed 3. Washington, D.C., Author, 1980.
17. Pollock HM: Mental disease among mental defectives. *Am J Psychiat* 101;361–363, 1944.
18. Cytryn L, Lourie RS: Mental retardation, in Freedman A, Kaplan H (eds): *Comprehensive Textbook of Psychiatry.* Baltimore, Williams and Wilkins, 1967.
19. Wortis J: The role of psychiatry in mental retardation services, in Mittler P (ed): *Research to Practice in Mental Retardation,* Vol 1: *Care and Intervention* (Proceedings of the Fourth Congress of International Association for the Scientific Study of Mental Deficiency). Baltimore, University Park Press, 1977.
20. Menolascino F: *Challenges in Mental Retardation: Progressive Ideology and Services.* New York, Human Sciences Press, 1977.
21. Simmons J: Emotional problems in mental retardation. *Pediatr Clin North Am* 15;957–967, 1968.
22. Penrose LS: The contribution of mental deficiency research to psychiatry. *Behav J Psychiatr* 112;747–755, 1966.
23. Kanner L: Autistic disturbances of affective contact. *Nervous Child* 2;217–250, 1943.
24. Bialer I: Emotional disturbance and mental retardation: Etiological and conceptual relationships, in Menolascino FJ (ed): *Psychiatric Approaches to Mental Retardation.* New York, Basic Books, 1970.
25. Potter HW: Mental retardation: The Cinderella of psychiatry, in Menolascino F (ed): *Psychiatric Aspects of the Diagnosis and Treatment of Mental Retardation.* Seattle, Special Child Publications, 1971.
26. Tarjan G: Mental retardation and clinical psychiatry, in Mittler P (ed): *Research to Practice in Mental Retardation,* Vol 1: *Care and Intervention.* Baltimore, University Park Press, 1977.
27. James SG: The relationship of dementia praecox to mental deficiency. *J Ment Sci* 85;1194–1211, 1939.
28. Barr M: *Mental Defectives.* Philadelphia, P. Blakiston's Son (cited in MacGillivray, 1956).
29. Bartemeier L: Psychoses in the feebleminded. J Psychoasthenics 30;314–324, 1925.
30. Jancar J: Psychiatric aspects of mental retardation, in Mittler P (ed): *Research to Practice in Mental Retardation,* Vol 1: *Care and Intervention* (Proceedings of the Fourth Congress of International Association for the Scientific Study of Mental Deficiency). Baltimore, University Park Press, 1977.
31. Webster TG: Problems of emotional development in young retarded children. *Am J Psychiatr* 120;34–41, 1963 (cited in Menolascino, 1972).
32. Eisenberg L: Emotional determinants of mental deficiency. *Arch Neurol Psychiatr* 80;114–121, 1958.
33. Vanuxem M: Prevalence of mental disease among mental defectives. *Proceedings of the American Association on Mental Deficiency* 4;242–249, 1935 (cited in Herskovitz et al.).
34. Penrose LS: A clinical and genetic study of 1280 cases of mental defect. Special report series of Medical Research Council, Number 229, 1938. Reprinted as *The Colchester Survey.* London, Institute for Research into Mental and Multiple Handicap, 1975.
35. Rohan JC: Mental disorder in the adult defective. *J Ment Sci* 92;551–563, 1946.
36. Neuer H: The relationship between behavior disorders in children and the syndrome of mental deficiency. *Am J Ment Defic* 52;143–147, 1947.
37. Leck I, Gordon WL, McKeown T: Medical and social needs of patients in hospitals for the mentally subnormal. *Br J Prevent Soc Med* 21;115–121, 1967.
38. Donoghue EC, Abbas KA, Gal E: The medical assessment of mentally retarded children in hospitals. *Br J Psychiat* 117;531–532, 1970.
39. Williams CE: A study of the patients in a group of mental subnormality hospitals. *Br J Ment Subnorm* 17;29–41, 1972.

40. Reid AH: Psychoses in adult mental defectives: I: Manic-depressive psychoses. *Br J Psychiatr* 120;205–212, 1972.
41. Rosanoff AJ, Handy LM, Plesset IR: The etiology of manic-depressive syndromes with special references to their occurrences in twins. *Am J Psychiatr* 91;725–762, 1935.
42. Duncan AG: Mental deficiency and manic depressive insanity. *J Ment Sci* 82;635–641, 1936.
43. Hunsicker HH: Symptomatology of psychosis with mental deficiency. *Proceedings of the 62nd Annual American Association on Mental Deficiency*, 43;51–56, 1938.
44. Innes G, Kidd C, Ross HS: Mental subnormality in northeast Scotland. *Br J Psychiatr* 114;35–41, 1968.
45. Payne R: The psychiatric subnormal. *J Ment Subnorm* 14;25–34, 1968.
46. Mercer M: Why mentally retarded persons come to a mental hospital. *Ment Retard* 6;8–10, 1968.
47. Weaver TR: The incidence of maladjustment among mental defectives in a military environment. *Am J Ment Defic* 51;238–246, 1946.
48. Menolascino F: Emotional disturbance and mental retardation. *Am J Ment Defic* 70;248–256, 1965.
49. Craft M: Mental disorder in the defective: A psychiatric survey among in-patients. *Am J Ment Defic* 63;829–834, 1959.
50. Tizard J: Individual differences in the mentally deficient, in Clarke AM, Clarke ADB (eds): *Mental Deficiency*. Glencoe, IL, Free Press, 1958.
51. Pilkington TL: Symposium on the treatment of behavior problems: 1. Psychiatric needs of the subnormal. *Br J Ment Subnorm* 18;66–70, 1972.
52. Joint Commission on Mental Health in Children (JCMHC): *Crisis in Child Mental Health: Challenge for the 70's*. New York, Harper and Row, 1969.
53. MacGillivray RC: The larval psychosis of idiocy. *Am J Ment Defic* 60;570–574, 1956.
54. Seguin E: Idiocy and Its Treatment by the Physiological Methods. New York, 1866, reprinted by the Teachers College of Columbia University, New York, 1907.
55. Griesinger W: Mental Pathology and Therapeutics. Transl Robertson CL, Rutherford J. London, 1867 (cited in Hayman, 1939).
56. Hurd HM: Imbecility with insanity. *Am J Insanity* 45;261–269, 1888.
57. Hayman M: The interrelations of mental defect and mental disorder. *J Ment Sci* 85;1183–1193, 1939.
58. Herskovitz HH, Plesset MR: Psychoses in adult mental defectives. *Psychiatr Q* 15;574–588, 1941.
59. Gordon A: Psychoses in mental defects. *Am J Insanity* 75;489–499, 1918.
60. Jackson JA, Pike HV: The classification and percentage of psychoses represented in the population of a state hospital for mental diseases. *Med J Rec*, 1930 (cited in Greene, 1930).
61. Greene RA: Psychoses and mental deficiencies, comparisons and relationships. *J Psychoasthenics* 35;128–147, 1930.
62. Greene RA: Conflicts in diagnosis between mental deficiency and certain psychoses. *Proceedings of the American Association for the Study of the Feebleminded* 35;127–148, 1933 (cited in Schilder, 1935).
63. Brugger K: Die erbbiologische Stellung der Propfschizophrenie. *Z Neurol Psychiatr* 113;348–378, 1928.
64. Irle G: Zur Problematik der sogenant Propfschizophrenie. *Schweiz Arch Neurol Psychiatr* 35;209–217, 1950 (cited in Reid, 1972).
65. Katzenfuss H: Beitrag zum problem de propfschizophrenie. *Schweiz Arch Neurol Psychiatr* 35;295–316, 1935 (cited in Reid, 1972).
66. Reid AH: Psychoses in adult mental defectives: II: Schizophrenia and paranoid psychoses. *Br J Psychiatr* 120;213–218, 1972.
67. Earl CJC: The primitive catatonic psychosis of idiocy. *Br J Med Psychol* 14;230–253, 1934.
68. Wolpert EA: *Manic-Depressive Illness: History of a Syndrome*. New York, International Universities Press, 1977.
69. Milici P: Propfschizophrenia: Schizophrenia engrafted upon mental deficiency. *Psychiatr Q* 11;190–212, 1937.

70. Revill MG: IV. Manic-depressive illness in retarded children. *Br J Ment Subnorm* 18;89–93, 1972.
71. Wildman HV: Psychoses of the feebleminded. *J Nerv Ment Dis* 42;529–539, 1915.
72. Clouston TS: *Clinical Lectures on Mental Diseases*. London, 1883 (cited in Reid, 1972).
73. Kraepelin E: Psychiatrie. Leipzig, 1896. Published as *Clinical Psychiatry*, transl Diefendorf AF. New York (cited in Reid 1972, Heaton-Ward, 1977).
74. Kraepelin E: Lehrbuch der Psychiatrie, 1902, trans and rev as *Clinical Psychiatry*, Diefendorf AR. New York, Macmillan, 1921.
75. Hucker SJ: Pubertal manic-depressive psychosis and mental subnormality—A case report. *Br J Ment Subnorm* 21(40);34–37, 1975.
76. Keegan DL, Pettigrew A, Parker F: Amiqriptyline in the psychotic states of Down's syndrome: The comparison of two cases. *Dis Nerv Syst* 35;381–383, 1974.
77. Berkley HJ: The psychoses of the high imbecile. *Am J Insanity* 72;305–314, 1915.
78. Tredgold RF, Soddy K: *Textbook of Mental Deficiency*, ed 10. Baltimore, Williams and Wilkins, 1963.
79. Feldman F: Psychoneuroses in the mentally retarded. *Am J Ment Defic* 51;247–254, 1946.
80. Ebaugh FG: Major psychiatric considerations in a service command. *Am J Psychiatr* 100;28–33, 1943.
81. Dewan JG: Intelligence and emotional stability. *Am J Psychiatr* 104;548–554, 1948.
82. Mayer-Gross W, Slater E, Roth M: *Clinical Psychiatry*. London, 1969.
83. Harris G: Mental deficiency and maladjustment. *Br J Med Psychol* 8;385, 1928 (cited in Beier, 1964).
84. Thorne FC: Hysterical manifestations in mental defectives. *Am J Ment Defic* 48;278–282, 1943.
85. Mautner H: *Mental Retardation: Its Care, Treatment and Physiological Base*. New York, Pergamon Press, 1959.
86. Skottowe JA: *Clinical Psychiatry for Students and Practitioners*. London, Practitioner Series, 1953. Ed 2, Boston: Little, Brown, 1964.
87. Menolascino F: Emotional disturbance in mentally retarded, in Enzer NB, Goin KW (eds): *Social and Emotional Development: The Preschooler*. New York, Walker and Company, 1978.
88. Hutt ML, Gibby RG: *The Mentally Retarded Child*. Boston, Allyn and Bacon, 1958.
89. Earl CJC: *Subnormal Personalities*. London, Balliere, Tindal and Cox, 1961.
90. Menolascino FJ, Eaton LF: Future trends in mental retardation. *Child Psychiatr Human Devel* 10;156–168, 1980.
91. Prideaux E: The relation of psychoneuroses to mental deficiency. *J Neurol Psychopathol* 2;209–220, 1921.
92. Tizard J, O'Connor N: The employability of the high-grade mental defectives. *Am J Ment Defic* 55;144–157, 1950.
93. Reid W: *The Psychopath: A Comprehensive Study of Antisocial Disorders and Behaviors*. New York, Brunner/Mazel, 1978.
94. Sternlicht M, Pustel G, Deutsch M: Suicidal tendencies among institutionalized retardates. *J Ment Subnorm* 16(32);93–102, 1970.
95. Barrett AM: *Heredity in Nervous and Mental Disease*. Association for Research in Nervous and Mental Disease, 1923, published in 1925.
96. Howe SG: *Report Made to the Legislature of Massachusetts upon Idiocy*. Boston, Presented from the State Edition by Collidge and Wiley, 1848 (Senate No. 51. Feb., 1848) (cited in Sarason and Doris, 1969).
97. Sarason SB, Doris J: Psychological Problems in Mental Deficiency, ed 4. New York, Harper and Row, 1969.
98. Tredgold AF: *Mental Deficiency*. London, Ballier, Tindall and Cox, 1908.
99. Bailey P, Williams F, Komora P: *The Medical Department of the U.S. Army in the World War, Volume 10: Neuropsychology*. Washington, Government Printing Office, 1929.
100. Bakwin H, Bakwin RN: *Clinical Management of Behavior Disorders in Children*, ed 4. Philadelphia, W.B. Saunders, 1972.

101. Ervin FR: Brain disorders, IV: Associated with convulsions (epilepsy), in Freedman AM, Kaplan HI (eds): *Comprehensive Textbook of Psychiatry*. Baltimore, Williams and Wilkins, 1967.

102. Dongier S: Statistical study of clinical and electroencephalographic manifestations of 536 psychotic episodes occurring in 515 epileptics between clinical seizures. *Epilepsia* 1;117–142, 1959 (cited in Ervin, 1967).

103. O'Gorman G: Psychosis as a cause of mental defect. *J Ment Sci* 100;934–943, 1954.

104. Tizard B: The personality of epileptics: A discussion of the evidence. *Psychol Bull* 59;196–210, 1962.

105. Rainer JD: Basic biological sciences, in Freedman AM, Kaplan HI (eds): *Comprehensive Textbook of Psychiatry*. Baltimore, Williams and Wilkins, 1967.

106. Penrose LS: *Biology and Mental Defect*, rev ed. London, Sidwick and Jackson, 1954.

107. Benda CE: *Developmental Disorders of Mentation and CPs*. New York, Grune and Stratton, 1952.

108. Himwich WA, Himwich HR: Neurochemistry, in Freedman AM, Kaplan HI (eds): *Comprehensive Textbook of Psychiatry*. Baltimore, Williams and Wilkins, 1967.

109. Fujimoto W: Mental retardation and self-destructive behavior: Clinical and biochemical features of the Lesch-Nyhan Syndrome, in Murray RF, Rosser PL (eds): *The Genetic Metabolic and Developmental Aspects of Mental Retardation*. Springfield, Il, C.C. Thomas, 1972 (cited in Menolascino and Egger, 1978).

110. Nyhan WL: Behavior in the Lesch-Nyhan syndrome. *Annual Progress in Child Psychiatry and Child Development* 175–194, 1977.

111. Shapiro A, Ridler MAC: The incidence of Klinefelter's syndrome in a mental deficiency hospital. *J Ment Defic Res* 4;48–50, 1960 (cited in Penrose, 1966).

112. Forssman H: The mental implication of sex chromosome aberrations. *Br J Psychiatr* 117;353–363, 1970.

113. Forssman H, Hambert G: Incidence of Klinefelter's syndrome among mental patients. *Lancet* 1;1327, 1963.

114. Polani PE: Abnormal sex chromosomes and mental disorders. *Nature* 223;680–686, 1969 (cited in Adams et al, 1970).

115. Jacobs PA, Brunton M, Melville MM: Aggressive behavior, mental subnormality and the XYY male. *Nature* 208;1351–1352, 1965 (cited in Clark et al., 1970).

116. Parker CE, Mavalwala J, Weise P, et al: The 47 XXY syndrome in a boy with behavior problems and mental retardation. *Am J Ment Defic* 74;660–665, 1970.

117. Menolascino F: Changing developmental perspective in Down's syndrome. *Child Psychiatr Hum Dev* 4;205–215, 1974.

118. Menolascino F: Psychiatric aspects of mental retardation in children under 8. *Am J Orthopsychiatr* 35;852–861, 1965.

119. Moore BC, Thuline HC, Capes LU: Mongoloid and nonmongoloid retardates: A behavioral comparison. *Am J Ment Defic* 73;433–436, 1968.

120. Webster TG: Problems of emotional development in young retarded children, in Menolascino F (ed): *Psychiatric Aspects of the Diagnosis and Treatment of Mental Retardation*. Seattle, Special Child Publications, 1971.

121. Johnson RC, Abelson RB: The behavioral competence of mongoloid and non-mongoloid retardates. *Am J Ment Defic* 73;856–857, 1969.

122. Rollin HR: Personality in mongolism with special reference to catatonic psychoses. *Am J Ment Defic* 51;219–237, 1946.

123. Broffenbrenner AN: Correlating morbid anatomy and clinical manifestations in the feebleminded. *Proceedings of the American Association on Mental Deficiency* 38;180–196, 1933.

124. Rutter M: Diagnosis and definition, in Rutter M, Schopler E (eds): *Autism: A Reappraisal of Concepts and Treatments*. New York, Plenum Press, 1978.

125. Rutter M, Schopler E: *Autism: A Reappraisal of Concepts and Treatments*. London, Plenum Press, 1978.

126. Rimland B: *Infantile Autism*. New York, Appleton-Century-Crofts, 1964.

127. Wolf E, Wenar C: A comparison of personality variables in autistic and mentally retarded children. *J Autism Child Schizophr* 2;92–108, 1972.
128. Menolascino FJ: Infantile autism: Descriptive and diagnostic relations to mental retardation, in Menolascino F (ed): *Psychiatric Approaches to Mental Retardation*. New York, Basic Books, 1970.
129. Tredgold AF, Soddy K: *Textbook of Mental Deficiency*, ed 9. Baltimore, Williams and Wilkins, 1956.
130. Scheerer M, Rothman E, Goldstein K: A case of an "Idiot Savant": An experimental study of personality organization. *Psychol Monogr* 58;1–63, 1945.
131. American Psychiatric Association. *Diagnostic and Statistical Manual of Mental Disorders*, ed 3. Washington, D.C., 1980.
132. Wells RA: *Cretinism and Goitre*. Oxford Press, London, 1845 (cited in Reid[40]).
133. Sherlock EB: *The Feebleminded*. MacMillan & Co., London 1911 (cited in Broffenbrenner[123]).

Dual Diagnosis of Mental Retardation and Mental Illness

An Overview

Stephen Ruedrich and Frank J. Menolascino

2.1. Introduction

The recent national movement removing the mentally retarded from institutional settings into the community has literally changed the definitions of normal and abnormal behavior in these individuals. Specifically, the impact of deinstitutionalization not only has changed the physical site of service delivery but has also dramatically altered the need for mental health services for the mentally retarded. Behaviors that were traditionally viewed as "expected" in institutionalized retarded citizens are often viewed as abnormal within the mainstream of society.[1] For example, the clinical phenomena of rocking, rumination, and head banging are frequent in the institutionalized retarded; within the institutional setting, they are traditionally viewed as "expected" behaviors, and their abnormalities are tolerated. Such behaviors are rarely seen in retarded citizens raised at home. That certain behaviors occur more frequently in certain settings can be explained either by a difference in the individuals in the two settings or by an environment that promotes, allows, or expects such behavior.

When one combines the uncertainty of the primary causes of mental retardation with the problems of the clinical description of mental illness, one has large areas of possible clinical confusion: symptoms or behavior for which it is difficult, if not impossible, to assign an identifiable etiology or pathophysiological process. For example, the origins of a retarded child's hyperactivity may range from motor expression of anxiety to manifestations of cerebral dysfunction, or both. Similarly, a shortened attention span may be the end product of determinants ranging from inadequate parental relationships in infancy (suggesting that the parents were unable to operate as a selective stimulation barrier for this child) to impaired (i.e., neurological) midbrain screening of stimuli. The moderately retarded adult can surely have both a seizure disorder and schizophrenia. If we expand on this concept, it can be argued that mental

Stephen Ruedrich • Department of Psychiatry, Nebraska Psychiatric Institute, University of Nebraska Medical Center, Omaha, Nebraska 68106.   *Frank J. Menolascino* • Departments of Psychiatry and Pediatrics, Nebraska Psychiatric Institute, University of Nebraska Medical Center, Omaha, Nebraska 68105.

retardation is itself a *symptom*, or that mental retardation *per se* is asymptomatic. Most current diagnostic thinking regarding mental retardation describes both (1) retardation of intellectual development and (2) deficits in social adaptation skills. If we pursue this line of reasoning, it would appear that abnormal behavior occurring in these individuals that is not attributable to (1) or (2) above can and should be ascribed to the presence of a concurrent psychiatric disorder. Further evidence of this line of thought may be found in a recent definition of mental retardation: "He gets along reasonably well with his parents (or mate), siblings, and friends, has few overt manifestations of behavioral disturbance, using his apparent intellectual potential close to its estimate, and contented for a reasonable portion of time" (p. 32).[2] Thus, combined diagnoses become more clearly indicated in frequent instances of mixed disorders. Failure to describe and/or delineate these multiple disorders in the same individual sharply limits both professional understanding and effective treatment. However, mental retardation itself, coupled with possible multifactorial causes of associated behavior and/or psychiatric disorders, not only increases the possible number of causes but also presents possibilities for professionals to initiate a wide array of specific treatment interventions in these complex dual diagnostic challenges.

These issues underscore the need for bridging the gap between the roles of mental-retardation and mental-health programs in meeting the individual needs of all retarded citizens. Increasingly, one notes joint rehabilitation efforts between mental-retardation and mental-health colleagues. These efforts include crisis mental-health intervention services, the provision of back-up inpatient mental-health facilities for regional mental-retardation programs, the provision of mental-health outreach consultative services (e.g., patient-centered and program-centered consultations) to community-based mental retardation programs, specialized mental-health programs solely for mentally retarded–mentally ill persons, and the use of parents of the retarded as paraprofessionals for other parents and their retarded–mentally ill sons or daughters.

Thus, mental retardation by itself does not necessarily imply abnormal or deviant behavior, although many symptoms may be attributable to the observed intellectual or social deficits. The diagnostic system of the American Psychiatric Association[3] embraces the symptomatic and developmental parameters that are such important considerations here. Clinically, vigorous efforts must therefore be made to diagnose psychiatric disorders that if unrecognized and untreated can result in ongoing suffering and regression in a retarded individual. Descriptions of mental illness in the mentally retarded should include the behavioral patterns that produce serious conflicts within retarded individuals, in their families, and in the greater circle of their community transactions. Only by considering the dual diagnosis can the clinician effectively treat these patients and, in doing so, maximize their intellectual and social-adaptive capabilities.

2.2. Historical Overview

Prior to the present century, it is difficult to speak of the scientific study of mental retardation because, like that of mental illness, its early history was dominated by primitive thinking that tended to attribute the problems to various supernatural causes. Except for the work of Hippocrates and a few of his contemporaries, mental retardation or any identifiable description of it does not appear in the medical writings of antiquity. The caregivers of the first 18 centuries of the Christian era had little interest in mental retardation (or mental illness) and its manifestations. Readers who are particularly interested in the early historical aspects will find relevant materials in Kanner[4] and Menolascino.[5]

At dawn of the Nineteenth century, a French psychiatrist, Jean-Marc-Gaspard Itard,[6] published a report on his five-year project of "educating the mind" of Victor, known as the "Wild Boy of Aveyron." Itard's report sparked the beginnings of widespread scientific and professional concern with "idiocy" (mental retardation). His interest and professional involvement arose from his earlier successful efforts to educate the deaf; he was convinced that Victor's mind could be educated by a segment in a training system of special sensory inputs and allied habit training. Itard's work clearly illustrates what a creative, humanistic, and highly structured approach could help a developmentally delayed individual to accomplish. He recognized the significance of motivation, transference, and what we would today call ego development and the strengthening of ego controls through the use of identification. Accordingly, Itard's *De l'Education d'un homme sauvage*[6] can be viewed as the first detailed report on dynamic psychotherapy.*

Édouard Seguin's book *The Moral Treatment, Hygiene, and Education of Idiots and Other Backward Children*[7] is another landmark professional contribution to the behavioral-developmental aspects of mental retardation. Seguin, also a psychiatrist who had specialized in the education of the deaf, was inspired by Itard's reported work with Victor. Under the leadership of Samuel G. Howe, a Boston psychiatrist specializing in the education of deafmutes, Seguin's system was introduced to America in the mid-1800s, when Dr. Howe became the director of the first state-supported school for the retarded in Boston. At the same time, for political reasons, Seguin fled France and, with Howe's encouragement, came to the United States. From then on (circa 1850), he was active in assisting nineteenth-century Americans in establishing schools for "idiots and other feebleminded persons" and residential centers for their humane care.

During this second half of the nineteenth century, mental health professionals further involved themselves with some of the key issues of retardation. The American Association on Mental Deficiency was founded in 1876; all of its charter members were psychiatrists. They and many other psychiatrists who followed in their footsteps were dedicated to the proposition that, through the application of psychotherapeutic principles and dynamically oriented education, "idiotic" and "imbecile" children could be substantially improved.

---

* An excellent review of Itard's benchmark work is provided by Harlan Lane in his book *The Wild Boy of Aveyron*, 1976.

However, in the last decade of the nineteenth century, another fateful trend developed. The Parisian School of Psychiatry and Neurology turned its attention to the possible causative factors in the symptom of mental retardation. Although describing mental retardation in psychological and behavioristic terminology, this group firmly adhered to the thesis that the ultimate nature of these conditions lay in some form of brain impairment. This one-dimensional view was expressed in a variety of "defect" theories that implied a distinct limitation in the retarded person's learning and/or adaptive ability. Because of "damaged internal mechanisms," the symptom of retardation was seen as being beyond the scope of extrinsic (i.e., educational or treatment) manipulations. There is no doubt that this particular defect concept played a dominant part in shifting the professional posture and role of mental health workers from positive therapeutic intervention to custodial gatekeeping.

The defect concept was also utilized to "explain" some occasional manifestations associated with mild mental retardation, which were being recognized more frequently. One particular area drew a great deal of attention: maladaptive social behavior. Most retarded individuals with such problems were identified in adolescence and came to the "idiot asylums" as social misfits, neglected children, or both. Evident limitations in the "learning of letters" and the frequent association with social failure prompted the English psychiatrists to term these individuals "moral imbeciles." For all practical purposes, Goddard[8,9] later equated "moral imbecility" with his definition of the "moron," attributed the condition to heredity, and speciously pronounced that these "defective deviants" were untreatable.

In summary, borne along on the crest of a dawning social conscience, the nineteenth century initially witnessed the recognition of mental retardation as a condition in which the intellectual faculties had never developed sufficiently. It witnessed "educating the minds of idiots," and for almost 90 years, mental health workers had a well-established and well-documented role of leadership in promoting the humane care, treatment, and management of the mentally retarded. It should be noted that many of today's "new developments" in the care, training, and education of the mentally retarded were anticipated (and practiced!) with sophisticated skill by nineteenth-century mental-health professionals. As the twentieth century approached, two trends were noted: the rise of the "brain impairment" concept in professional thinking, and a move away from the concept of sheltering the retarded from society. This latter approach was then drastically altered to one of protecting society from the retarded. Concomitantly, the attitude of benevolence toward the retarded faded away.

At the beginning of the twentieth century, important trends coalesced into a tragic interlude that left a lasting imprint on the professional mental-health worker's involvement in the field of mental retardation. In a time span of only 20 years (1900–1920), the interest and involvement of mental health professionals shifted away from mental retardation. The following three crucial developments, operating in a symbiotic relationship, administered the *coup de grâce* to the earlier enthusiasm about and challenge of mental retardation for the mental health profession in the United States: (1) the introduction of the

Binet Test to America in 1908; (2) the publication of Goddard's[8] monograph on *The Kallikak Family* in 1912; and (3) the interest and involvement of mental health personnel in the burgeoning field of psychoanalysis. Let us explore how these three developments served to alienate the mental health professionals' interest from mental retardation.

Almost overnight, the Binet Test and its subsequent modifications gained acceptance as a crucial diagnostic technique for mental retardation. Indeed, it soon came to be utilized as the one and only guide for educational purposes and even for the prognosis of social effectiveness. The mental status interview and the assessment approach were replaced by the mental-test approach, and professional mental-health services became viewed as expendable. The discovery of vast numbers of "morons in our midst" through the use of mental tests soon became a matter of widespread concern, especially because so many of the mildly retarded appeared to be "social misfits." The fact that is was mostly the "social misfits" who came under scrutiny was overlooked, and the conclusion was drawn that all retarded individuals were social problems, or potentially so.

Goddard was not alone in sounding this "eugenic alarm." Others contributed to the growing consensus, which in time reached four distinct conclusions: (1) there were more retarded persons in our society than people realized; (2) the mentally retarded accounted for virtually all of the current social ills; (3) heredity was the major cause of mental retardation; and (4) because the "decadent" retarded appeared to reproduce faster than nonretarded citizens, society would soon be destroyed unless drastic measures were taken.

While these societal and "genetic" concepts about mental retardation were taking hold, American mental-health professionals were rapidly assimilating the dynamic concepts of psychoanalysis into mental health evaluation and treatment. Psychotherapeutic efforts with the psychoneuroses served to entice mental health professionals away from the more prosaic activities in mental retardation, and Itard's psychotherapeutic and educational efforts with Victor were forgotten.

It is interesting to note that the child psychiatry in America had its early beginnings in this same time period at the Judge Baker Clinic in Boston. Here, some of the same "morons" were being evaluated as juvenile delinquents! Yet, the evaluation setting (community-based) of this clinic and the professionals involved (the prototype of the multidisciplinary professional diagnostic-treatment team of today) were not greatly different from current models of diagnosis and treatment. The resultant psychodynamic formulations and treatment recommendations were both welcome and helpful. Indeed, it appears that the previously noted mental-health ferment in the mental retardation institutions was transposed directly to the community-based work in juvenile delinquency, though the retarded were often not viewed as "good treatment candidates" in this new family-based and community treatment model and locale of service delivery.

The tragic interlude stimulated major financial commitments on a national scale to the construction of even larger institutions in which to incarcerate "dangerous" retarded citizens. In rapid succession, restrictive marriage and sterilization laws and lifelong segregation ("warehousing") of retarded individuals in inexpensive institutions produced what Vail[10] aptly described as the professional mental-health worker's posture of "dehumanization." The role of mental health professionals in mental retardation rapidly became that of a jailer, and the prevailing professional-societal expectations left little room for the humane and therepeutic models that had typified the earlier role of mental health professionals in mental retardation. This change alone was enough to repel many professionals who earlier had been motivated by a humane ambition to rehabilitate retarded persons.

As noted by Wolfensberger,[11] the period from 1925 to the very recent past was characterized by the prevailing institutions' practices and a continuation of the practices that had evolved from these outdated professionals rationales. The pictorial overview, entitled *Christmas in Purgatory*, by Blatt and Kaplan,[12] and recent reports of the President's Committee on Mental Retardation[13-17] document this aimless continuity in pictures and words. During this same period, major organizational changes occurred in the structure of professional mental-health organizations, which also reflected these changes. The bulk of our nation's rapidly evolving child psychiatry services became noninstitutionally oriented—a trend that has continued and strengthened during the last 25 years. The previously noted rapid drift of mental health professionals away from mental retardation in the 1920s and 1930s culminated in a significant organizational restructuring in the American Psychiatric Association; its section on Mental Deficiency was formally replaced by a new section on Child Psychiatry in 1959. This change gave organizational support to psychiatry's disenchantment with mental retardation, and a formal separation resulted. The work of many dedicated mental-health professionals in the area of mental retardation continued, but they became lost voices in a wilderness in which national professional mental-health organizations simply tolerated mental retardation as their Cinderella[18-20] and gave little else to it.

In summary, it is clear that mental retardation attracted the interest and participation of outstanding mental-health professionals throughout the nineteenth century and for the first decade of the twentieth century. By the 1920s, the interest of mental health professionals in the mentally retarded had begun to deteriorate. From then until 1960, the topic of mental retardation and the clinical challenges of the mentally retarded occupied only a peripheral position in the training and practice of mental health professionals.

2.3. Current Period of Mental Health Reinvolvement

The last three decades have witnessed increased efforts on the part of professionals of all disciplines to identify and label the various etiological agents (or processes) that can produce the symptom of mental retardation. Research toward this end has been uncovering biological (including hereditary, genetic, metabolic, traumatic, and neuroanatomical), educational, and psychosocial (intrapsychic, familial, economic, and cultural) determinants of mental retardation. Instrumental in this area has been the dedication of citizen advocacy groups (for example, the National Association for Retarded Citizens), which have actively joined forces with professionals to demand that more effort, interest, and financial support be devoted to research in this previously relatively neglected arena.

Recent contributions, noting the interrelationships between mental retardation and mental illness, have reflected this renaissance of professional interest. Indeed, the bulk of the literature on this topic has appeared since 1960.[5,21–26] Particular professional focus has been placed on (1) the frequency and types of psychiatric disorders in the retarded and (2) the treatment–management approaches that have been employed to ameliorate these coexisting entities.

2.3.1. The Nature of Mental Illness in the Retarded

The examination of the coexistence of mental retardation and mental illness in an individual has necessitated the creation of definitions of these two entities. That for mental retardation has been described above; for mental illness, more controversy exists, but various definitions are currently gaining widespread consensus regarding their accuracy. In the DSM-III,[3] a mental disorder is conceptualized as a "clinically significant behavioral or psychological syndrome or pattern associated with either a painful symptom (distress) or impairment in functioning (disability)" (p. 6).[3] One other definition of mental illness is that of Chess, who noted it to be "an abnormality of behavior, emotion, or relationships—in which abnormalities are sufficiently marked and/or prolonged as to handicap the individual himself and/or distress his family or the community—and which continue up to the time of assessment" (p. 34)[27] Using such definitions, one can clearly see that mental illness can be expected to coexist with and complicate mental retardation and that most mentally retarded individuals are already hanidcapped with limitations in the areas of intellectual functioning and/or social adaptation and therefore can be expected to react or respond less than optimally to the demands of everyday life. That is, such individuals begin "at risk" for the development of psychiatric disorders, and it is clear that any condition that renders one *less* capable of handling reality-based demands makes one *more* susceptible to the development of mental illness. Table 1 enumerates the "at-risk" factors that make retarded individuals vulnerable to mental illness.

It should be further noted that efforts directed at decreasing the level of risk can be expected to lower the frequency and severity of mental illness in these persons. That is, optimum treatment of coexisting medical disorders (e.g., control of seizure disorders and increased locomotion with physical medicine rehabilitation) and attempts to reverse or modify adaptive deficits (e.g., individual instruction and use of sign language in mutism) will lessen the likelihood of concurrent psychiatric disorders.

Table 1. At-Risk Status of Mentally Retarded for Mental Illness

1. Medical fragility --- sees many professionals
2. Reflections of parental concerns --- what is wrong
3. Peer group expectations to perform
4. Frustration from repeated failures
5. Humiliation of being ridiculed
6. Fears generated in trying to survive in a highly complex and impersonal world
7. Overprotectiveness → dependency
8. Push toward superachievement → beyond intellectual/emotional capacity

2.3.2. Influences of the Level of Retardation

Expanding on the above, it can be seen that the degree of impairment of social and intellectual functioning profoundly affects both the frequency and the types of psychiatric disorders appearing in retarded individuals. For example, those persons with severe or profound retardation are more likely to have gross CNS dysfunction and severe language impairment. These deficits often lead to an inability to participate normally in interpersonal and social transactions or to develop complex personality, respectively. As a result, severely retarded persons, when stressed beyond their adaptive capabilities, are often noted to respond with stereotyped and out-of-contact behavior, which may mimic "autism." A study by Chess, Horn, and Fernandez[28] clearly noted that if severely retarded infants (who were also blind and deaf secondary to rubella) were provided with early and ongoing interpersonal developmental stimuli, they tended to show delayed and primitive behavior that was consistent with their level of retardation. However, these authors also noted that, in those instances where these early sets of experiences were *not* provided, the infants displayed "blindisms," rocking, obstinancy, and "organic autism." If intervening treatment experiences are absent, then these personality impacts are often displayed as persistent disturbed and out-of-contact behavior. Similarly, the moderately retarded are affected by varying levels of intellectual and social impairment, but to a somewhat lesser degree. Retardation at this level can often produce its own set of personality characteristics, including such traits as relative inflexibility and passivity. In fact, Webster[29] noted a consistent set of personality characteristics in moderately retarded children that he considered the basic psychopathology of this group of individuals (see Table 2).

One must be careful, however, in working with this group to separate these basic traits (which are based on the level of impairment) from the signs and symptoms of specific psychiatric disorders (which may result from or may be superimposed on a person with these characteristics). The few available autobiographies of moderately retarded individuals may be helpful in this regard (for example, Nigel Hunt[30]). Here, these basic personality features are noted *without* the presence of symptoms or signs of allied mental illness.

Table 2. Primary Psychopathology in the Mentally Retarded

1. Benign autism
2. Repetitiousness (nonobsessive)
3. Relative inflexibility (rapid change → personality disorganization)
4. Passivity: A protective posture secondary to perceived failure
5. Simplicity of the emotional life
6. Language delay
7. Level of retardation
8. Nature of family support system
9. Nature and extent of helpful service alternatives
10. Attention to subjective responses

Mildly retarded individuals have a unique set of stresses. Their often nearly normal appearance tends to preclude their easy identification by others as being handicapped individuals and can lead to unrealistic expectations on the part of the individual and/or his or her loved ones, as well as to a series of major interpersonal failures. At the same time, these individuals are capable of developing some insight into their limitations. Emotional disturbances in the mildly retarded often result when the individual is labeled as deviant and is enmeshed in the dynamic interplay of disturbed family transactions. The frequent delay in establishing that these youngsters have a distinct handicap (usually not confirmed until age 6–9) is a common source of anxiety for the mildly retarded individual. Low self-esteem is very frequent in the mildly retarded; the stigma of attending special classes, as well as adverse encounters with the social interpersonal environment, tends to make them feel ineffective and "different." This reaction may be compounded by the individual's inability to integrate the normal developmental sequences at the appropriate time in his or her life. For example, during the late childhood period of personality integration, the mildly retarded person has considerable difficulty understanding the symbolic abstractions of schoolwork and the ongoing complexities of social adaptive expectations from both the family and the peer group. It is at this stage that the mildly retarded often gain some understanding of their limitations. Unfortunately, by early adolescence, they have all too often established an identity that incorporates both retardation and deviance. The mildly retarded are not as likely to be buffered by loved ones or to be redirected by them into new interpersonal coping styles that can help correct earlier misconceptions about the self. Without a source of ongoing family or community support and direction, the mildly retarded are at high risk to develop mental illness or marginal identities in our society.

2.4. Frequency and Types of Mental Illnesses in the Retarded

Before discussing the prevalence of mental illness in the mentally retarded or the form that such illness takes, one must address the problems special to this difficult diagnostic area. Only by doing so can the mental health (or other medical) professional hope to maximize her or his diagnostic accuracy in dealing with this group and, what is more important, not to overlook the presence of a psychiatric disorder and, in doing so, add to the psychic suffering (or increase the intellectual or adaptive deficits) that can occur when these diagnoses occur together. As mentioned above, in the past this has been an area of much confusion and little reward for many professionals working with the mentally retarded. It is often difficult to utilize the usual diagnostic knowledge, skills, or techniques in the clinical assessment of such people, and the professional can become lost, dismayed, or both when confronted with the myriad potential determinants of abnormal behavior in retarded persons, especially in those with severe or profound deficits in social–intellectual functioning, and even more in those with limited or no language (production or comprehension). The mental health professional often finds that her or his most valuable tool, the standard diagnostic interview and mental status examination, becomes unwieldy, unworkable, or useless in attempts to assess these individuals. For this reason, it should be stressed that the mental status examination of a mentally retarded individual—whether to confirm the primary diagnosis of mental retardation, to assess whether it is an instance of "pseudoretardation," or to confirm the coexistence of emotional disturbance and mental retardation—cannot be used successfully in isolation from general diagnostic procedures.

It should be noted here that when attempting to accurately diagnose the presence of mental illness in the mentally retarded, the clinician must obviously rely more on the *signs* (disturbed behavior) and less on the *symptoms* (verbally reported distress or dysfunction) that characterize the various psychiatric disorders, especially in those individuals at the severe to profound end of the intellectual–social spectrum. This is a distinct difference in approach from many clinicians' usual diagnostic framework, which often focuses on symptoms as determinants of diagnosis. Another difference (less marked) is the degree to which the clinician must obtain diagnostic information (current and past history, social and family history, and even mental status) from third parties and must make an effort to elicit this information from those persons (family, friends, or caregivers) who have lived and worked most closely with the mentally retarded individual. This is to say not that mental status examinations of retarded persons are useless or unnecessary, but that they may form a somewhat smaller (but still important) part of the overall diagnostic assessment of this group. Thus, the mental health professional should (ideally) carry out his or her own physical and neurological examinations and should be able to interpret pediatric–internal medicine and neurological consultations, as well as such studies as psychological evaluations and electroencephalograms. Following this process, the mental health professional is in a much better position to see the whole person and thereby to piece together the diagnostic puzzle that emotional disturbance can present in the mentally retarded person. To cast the mental health professional in the role of a "complete professional" may be viewed as "asking too much," but failure to assess clearly all parameters of a child's or an adult's behavior can result in many of the major diagnostic errors made with the retarded.* It seems that exclusive focus on the mental status examination has perpetuated the classic split between the "psyche" and the "soma" in evaluating and treating the retarded.

Early studies of the prevalence and the specific form of psychiatric disorders in the mentally retarded reported an incidence ranging from 16%[31] to 28%[21] to 40%.[32] However, these pre-1960 investigations suffer from some major methodological problems, the most notable of which is that most, if not all, of them were carried out in institutional and/or hospital settings. Because institutional settings have *traditionally* been used as societal mechanisms for managing (in addition to giving care to and isolating) retarded persons with social-adaptive difficulties or more *recently* have been used for "community program rejects,"[33] such studies may not accurately reflect the incidence of psychiatric disorders in this group. More recent studies,[33-37] which are also institutionally based, although more methodologically sound, can be similarly criticized.

That such investigations may reveal an over-representation of mental illness in the mentally retarded is illustrated by Menolascino,[38] who studied the incidence of mental illness in a sample of institutionalized individuals with Down's syndrome. Of the total sample, 35% were mentally ill at the time of the study, but there were clear indications that 56% of the total sample had had emotional disturbances at the time of admission to the institution, which had figured in their admission. Hence, 21% of the total sample no longer evidenced the psychiatric disorder but remained institutionalized. The question arises, "Why were they sent to an institution for the mentally retarded rather than to a mental health institute?" The same individual with Down's syndrome and concurrent pneumonia or malignancy would probably not be similarly institutionalized, nor should the prevalence of these disorders in Down's patients be assessed solely on their presence in an institutionalized sample. The same should be true for mental illness and mental retardation, which will otherwise appear overrepresented if the psychiatric disorder has led to an inappropriate admission, less-than-adequate treatment, or a delayed return to the community.

Directly addressing this issue are a number of recent reports on mentally retarded individuals who lived with their primary families and/or their primary community at the time of the study.[2,38-49] These studies report that the mentally retarded fall prey to the same types of mental illness that befall people with normal intellectual abilities. Recent professional literature repeats the theme that, in the retarded, the full range of psychoses, neuroses, personality disorders, behavioral disorders, and adjustment reactions exist as are noted in the general population. However, some studies dealing with the noninstitutionalized retarded have revealed a higher incidence, a different spectrum, or unique qualitative differences in the psychiatric disorders that appear concurrently with mental retardation.[21,22,50-53] Indeed, it can be postulated that even if mentally retarded persons are emotionally well adjusted, they will experience

---

* If a university-affiliated program diagnostic team or a similar team in a community mental-health center is available, then an in-depth professional background in the individual diagnostician is not an essential element.

Table 3. Most Frequently Reported Mental Illnesses in the
Mentally Retarded

Psychoses
    Schizophrenia (paranoid, catatonic, undifferentiated, propfschizo-
        phrenia)[a]
    Manic-depressive psychosis
    Psychotic depression (unipolar)
Anxiety disorders
    Conversion reaction
    Anxiety reaction
    Depressive reaction
Personality disorders
    Schizoid personality
    Passive aggressive
    Antisocial personality
Transitional-situational
    Adjustment reaction to stress
    Adjustment disorders
    Symptomic alcoholism
    Suicide gestures
Syndrome-associated
    Stereotyped behaviors (e.g., Lesch-Nyhan: self-destructive acts)
    Confusional-aggressive episodes (e.g., seizures disorders)

[a] See reference 83.

some difficulty functioning independently or semi-independently in their community. If their lives are complicated by a psychiatric disorder, their adjustment
difficulties are obviously complicated. Recent studies have reported rather consistently a 20%–35% frequency rate of mental illness in the noninstitutionalized
mentally retarded and have strongly suggested that clinical focus must be placed
on the diagnosis and the subsequent treatment of the combined finding of mental
illness and mental retardation—a point that is comprehensively reviewed, along
with the specific types of disorders noted in Chapter 1. This extensive review
notes that nearly all psychiatric disorders known to occur in the general population have been described in the mentally retarded; these are synopsized in
Table 3.

The following case histories illustrate each of the major areas of psychiatric
disturbance noted in Table 3.

Miss A. was a 23-year-old female with severe mental retardation who
had been living in group homes since the age of 19. The staff had noted a
distinct behavioral change over the preceding seven months, with decreased
socialization and poor job performance at her sheltered workshop placement. They reported occasional episodes of giggling and stated that she had
been observed talking and gesturing to herself for the first time. On several
occasions, she awakened in the middle of the night, appearing very fright-
ened, and twice she had been found asleep under her bed in the morning.
On examination, she appeared disheveled and distracted. She often giggled

for no apparent reason, often tilted her head for prolonged periods of time on several occasions as if straining to hear something. Her answers to questions were often inappropriate and revealed a decrease from a previously documented higher level of functioning. Physical, radiologic, and metabolic examinations were unremarkable. Evaluation by the psychiatric consultant eventuated in a diagnosis of schizophreniform psychosis; hospitalization at a local psychiatric institute was recommended and accomplished. Treatment was initiated, utilizing a combination of milieu therapy, group psychotherapy, and antipsychotic medication. Over the next three weeks, there was a gradual reduction in inappropriate laughter and hallucinations and an improvement in spontaneous vocalization, sleep, and emotional contact with others. Her freehand drawings had initially been marked by pictures of knives, bloody scenes, and religious themes; it was noted that she slowly began to produce the animal and flower themes that she had excelled in in the past. As she improved, she was slowly reintroduced back into her sheltered work setting and did very well in that setting. She was discharged six weeks following admission and continued on a low dose of thiothixene for outpatient follow-up.

Mr. B. was a 52-year-old white male with mild mental retardation. He was committed to a psychiatric hospital by the police after an altercation surrounding his refusal to leave the house in which he had been living. The house belonged to his uncle, who had allowed him to live there following the death of his mother two years previously. At that time, Mr. B. had suffered a depressive episode that had been successfully treated with ECT. His uncle had reported that he had told Mr. B. that he wanted to sell the house six months before admission, but that Mr. B. had refused to leave or cooperate with the uncle in making other living arrangements. During that time, he had been having daily crying spells and difficulty falling asleep, had increased his food intake and gained 30 pounds, had broken furniture, had cursed at visitors, and believed that his uncle was conspiring to put him in prison. On examination, he was moderately obese, and his speech was characterized by a significant dysarthria. His responses to most questions were monosyllabic, and he repeatedly angrily talked about "taking me to jail." Otherwise, his affect was flat and his mood appeared depressed. When asked about his feelings and his family, he quickly became tearful and would talk less. The physical examination and allied laboratory evaluation were within normal limits. The diagnosis of major depressive disorder, recurrent, with psychotic features, was made, and treatment was initiated with individual psychotherapy, group psychotherapy, and tricyclic antidepressant medication. He slowly responded and began to be able to talk about his fears about being on his own and the possibility of ending up in prison because he had no home or family. By the third hospital week, his sleep had improved, his crying spells had disappeared, and he had no further delusions of persecution. A guardian was obtained who was able to help the patient participate in ongoing decision-making challenges. He was discharged to a group home–sheltered workshop in his community and received outpatient psychiatric follow-up.

Mr. C. was a 19-year-old moderately retarded white male who had been residing in group homes most of his life. He had been in his current place-

ment for the preceding three years and had done quite well there in a sheltered work setting until two months prior to his admission. At that time,
two simultaneous events took place that were disruptive to him: two of the
caretakers at the group home setting left and were replaced within one week
by two strangers; additionally, because of an intercurrent medical problem,
Mr. C.'s roommate was hospitalized, and Mr. C. received a new roommate
who was significantly older and displayed persistent behavioral problems.
The new roommate would often remain awake throughout the night, pacing
or playing his radio loudly in spite of staff admonitions. Over the subsequent
two months, there was a gradual change in Mr. C.'s behavior in that he,
too, became sleepless at night and began roaming around within the group
home or leaving it at night, necessitating staff's following him to return him
to the home. At the same time, his performance in the sheltered work setting
deteriorated, and he became increasingly involved in minor verbal altercations with several of his co-workers and staff members there. He became
more generally active and spent more time in seemingly purposeless motor
activity; he was also noted to be somewhat irritable and would often engage
in verbal bating of some of his acquaintances in the community residence.

At the time of admission, he stubbornly discussed the above conditions
and noted that he was upset; he wondered what had happened to his roommate and to former friends (the staff members). Initially, in the hospital,
he had difficulty falling asleep, less than optimum appetite, and much purposeless motor behavior. He also seemed to be quite anxious and would
spend extended periods of time muttering to himself. There were no apparent psychotic symptoms and no other symptoms of depression. Physical
and laboratory examinations were unremarkable. He was treated with a
combination of individual and group psychotherapy as well as a continued
highly structured work program. Within 10 days of his admission, most of
his presenting symptoms had fallen away, and he began to be reintroduced
into his community group-home placement and seemed to do much better
than prior to admission. During this time, his original roommate had returned, and on discharge, he was able to resume his old relationships with
his former roommate. Final diagnoses were Axis I—mental retardation,
mild; Axis II–adjustment disorder with mixed disturbance of emotions and
conduct.

Mr. D. was a 35-year-old mildly retarded male who was admitted to
the psychiatric hospital for the second time. His history revealed a chaotic
childhood involving termination of his parents' rights when he was 2 years
old and multiple transfers between a series of foster homes and orphanage
placements between the ages of 2 and 16. During this time, there had been
numerous incidents of running away from various foster homes, arrests
during runaways for drug taking and shoplifting, some minor vandalism,
poor school performance, and several physical altercations with peers—
and on one occasion, with a police officer. His chaotic lifestyle had persisted, and he had been arrested on two occasions for theft and had spent
a brief time in a county jail following the theft of an automobile. He had
continued to abuse drugs and alcohol and had gathered a reputation as a
barroom brawler, especially when intoxicated. He had been married and
divorced once and then had lived with and left a second partner after im-

pregnating her. He had managed to maintain limited employment, usually working as a laborer, but on one occasion, he had managed to be involved as a helper in a local truck-driving operation for a period of seven months. He had spent a great deal of his adult life, between his marriage and involvement with his second partner, living in missions, panhandling, and generally traveling around the country.

The current hospitalization had been precipitated by some similar out-of-contact behavior that had occurred during a period of intoxication, and he had been transferred by police officers from a local jail to the psychiatric hospital. The above history had been obtained from the patient, who seemed to take a certain delight in recounting some of his past illegal or shady activities, and from a family member who was willing to give a history but unwilling to have any other contact with the patient, "Because he has burned me too many times before." The diagnostic impression was anti-social personality and mild mental retardation. He was singularly uninterested in treatment opportunities and, following his court appearance for the problems that had prompted his admission, he was discharged to an uncle in a distant state who felt that farm work would "straighten him out real quick." The prognosis for this gentleman was considered poor.

Finally, it must be emphasized that the presence of mental retardation in a person with a psychiatric disorder does not proscribe and should not prevent successful treatment of the concurrent mental illness. All too often in the past, this paradoxical professional bias has been used as a justification *not to treat* the retarded person's accompanying emotional disturbance. This bias was clearly identified by Woodward, Jaffee, and Brown[54] in 1970 when they noted,

> There are two prevalent attitudes on the part of many practicing child psychiatrists in the New York area with which we differ strongly: 1) there is the attitude that a psychiatric diagnosis must be made in terms of either "organicity" or "non organicity." Those holding this view seem unable to conceive of a mixed picture. Our experience would suggest that a mixed picture is common. To us it is irrational to say that a child with brain damage can have only one form of pathology, and this explains everything. Why can't a child have mild brain damage and a psychoneurosis? 2) There is the attitude that a child who has any evidence of mixed brain damage at all, even an isolated abnormal electroencephalogram without other evidence of central nervous system involvement, should not be denied psychotherapy. This attitude exists in spite of the known fact that many disturbed children respond poorly to psychotherapeutic programs, and have no evidence of organic lesions. We believe that the decision whether a child should have psychotherapy depends on the estimate of his ability to profit by it, regardless of the presence of organic pathology. (p. 290)

This pair of attitudinal biases may have added unduly both to the past and to the current reports of high-frequency mental illness in the retarded, with little evidence of effective efforts to treat the mental illness in these individuals. Indeed, these professional blind spots may have incorrectly pushed some retarded citizens into institutional patienthood as "chronically disturbed retarded persons."

2.5. The Mentally Retarded Offender

The mentally retarded individual who displays delinquent or criminal behavior has, like the antisocial personality, raised questions about the etiology
and the nature of these behaviors in clusters as signs or symptoms of mental
illness in the retarded. However, there is little reported information available
to support this hypothesis. During the first three decades of this century, it
was believed that virtually every mentally retarded individual was a potential
juvenile delinquent, and that most criminals had overt manifestations of mental
retardation.[9] Since the time of Goddard's "scientific" investigations, approximately 450 separate studies on the intelligence of juvenile delinquents have
been published; in fact, it is probable that no other single characteristic of the
juvenile delinquent has been so thoroughly studied. Still, these investigations
have not provided conclusive evidence regarding the relationship between general intelligence and delinquent or criminal behavior. There has been considerable divergence of conclusions in the various studies: (1) the retarded are a
type of "born criminal" (i.e., "moral idiots"); (2) retardation is a hereditary
characteristic, and this factor accounts for the preponderance of male retarded
offenders; (3) the retarded characteristically commit antisocial crimes of assault
and sexual assault; (4) retarded individuals commit crimes in the absence of
inhibiting social factors because they lack the capacity to grasp the social values
of their culture, including its social and legal definitions of right and wrong;
(5) because of their lowered general cognition, the retarded cannot be deterred
by the threat of punishment; (6) the retarded are suggestible, and so they respond to the criminal leadership of intellectually brighter persons; and (7) retarded individuals are more frequently reared in families and neighborhoods
where their day-to-day identification with delinquent models is common.[34]

The rationale for these opinions ranges from the biological to the biosocial.
The biological concept of the retarded person as a "moral idiot" or a genetic
"criminal type" historically preceded the biosocial view of the mentally retarded offender as the product of negative social interactions. During the early
decades of this century, there was a predisposition to view the triad of mental
retardation, delinquency, and dependency as inevitably associated with the
biosocial phenomena. Even Sumner,[55] in his brilliant sourcebook *Folkways*,
cited these three characteristics as representative of the "submerged" (i.e.,
maladjusted) tenth of the general population who are at the bottom of the social
class ladder.

As Beier[21] noted in a review of this topic, the early estimates of the frequency of mental retardation in the offender ranged from 0.5% to 55%, with
the majority of the earlier studies reporting estimates in the higher percentage
range. These widely divergent points of view have persisted to the present
time.[56,57] The literature on this topic is interesting to review because the conclusions range from one extreme to the other: (1) delinquency and criminality
are frequent phenomena in the mentally retarded population and the treatment
potentials are low; (2) delinquency and criminality are infrequent phenomena

in the retarded and are dependent on environmental-familial factors, and proper treatment will effectively quell these acting-out behaviors.

Studies have indicated that the types of crimes most often committed by the retarded are qualitatively different from those most frequently committed by nonretarded offenders, with the former showing a significantly higher incidence of crimes against the person.[58] These studies point to the relatively higher incidence of mental retardation among the socially, economically, and culturally deprived segment of our population (which also produces a greater proportion of prison inmates than does the general population), and they suggest that mental retardation and crime are more significantly related to these environmental factors than they are to each other. This literature also generally concludes that there is a relatively higher percentage of arrests and convictions of mentally retarded persons charged with crime than of the total criminal population. Both points are well taken, and additional research is necessary before any judgments can be made about cause-and-effect relationships on this topic.

Brown and his co-workers have brought a new perspective to this old problem of retarded offenders.[59] Their methodology and resultant findings are most commendable, especially in contrast to the armchair viewpoints that have seemed to dominate discussions of this topic in the past. Allen[58] recommended an "Exceptional Offenders Court" for the early identification of those mentally retarded offenders in need of treatment, rather than criminal prosecution, in order to expedite their appropriate diversion to other community resources. He also provided the following summary of a modern view of the mentally retarded offender:

> Historically, society has pursued three alternative courses with the mentally retarded offender: we have ignored his limitations and special needs; or we have sought to tailor traditional criminal law processes to fit them; or we have grouped him with psychopaths, sociopaths, and sex deviates in a kind of conventicle of the outcast and hopeless. What is suggested here is a "fourth way" (e.g., the "Exceptional Offenders Court")—a way not of rejection and despair, but of acceptance and hope. (p. 607)

Another critical problem in the provision of services stems from the rejection of responsibility for retarded offenders on the part of many health and correctional professionals. For different reasons, each group rejects the mentally retarded as unsuitable for its respective treatment programs. As noted by Brown and Courtless,[59]

> Mental hospitals claim such an offender is not mentally ill; the traditional institutions for the retarded complain that they do not have appropriate facilities for the offender . . . correctional institutions would like to move such persons from their population on the grounds that programs available in the correctional setting are totally inadequate and in many cases inappropriate for application to retarded persons. (p. 373)

Three current viewpoints regarding retarded offenders that appear to be most consistent with the findings of the reported studies are worthy of note:

1. The mentally retarded are as capable of delinquent criminal acts as are the intellectually normal; however, factors other than intellectual ones appear

to be more important in the etiology of such behavior, and these factors are those commonly cited as important in the development of delinquent and criminal behavior in the general population.

2. The lowered social adaptive abilities of the retarded (e.g., lack of concrete thinking and social insight), coupled with a relative lack of supervision, may make him or her more prone to such acts.

3. Societal views of specific behavioral maladjustments (especially sexual acting-out in girls who come from broken homes or lower socioeconomic levels)[60] may result in legal charges against, or institutionalization of, a retarded person. However, the same behavior in a retarded individual of a different socioeconomic class or family background may not result in legal action. For example, delinquent behavior in a retarded girl from an intact home and the upper socioeconomic class typically eventuates in referral to a child guidance clinic, whereas her counterpart from a broken home and a lower socioeconomic class is admitted to a juvenile detention facility.[61]

There is an evolving treatment–management focus that stresses clarification of the community-based treatment and management of the retarded offender. One of the new models of community-based approaches to this challenge is the "Structured Correctional Service" of the Eastern Nebraska Community Office of Retardation.[25] This service is specially staffed with personnel experienced both in corrections and in mental retardation; its treatment and management approaches are reviewed by Strider and Menolascino.[84]

In summary, the relationship of intelligence and delinquency is still the subject of some dispute, but the areas of controversy today differ from those prevailing prior to and shortly after the first investigations into the subject. The developments that have led to the gradual acceptance of a more humanistic attitude toward the retarded offender are inextricably bound to an improved understanding of mental retardation and juvenile delinquency, as well as to advances in the methodology of social science research.

2.6. A Suggested Framework for Viewing Mental Illness in the Mentally Retarded

An alternative approach to current professional thinking concerning types of mental illness in the mentally retarded will now be discussed. Though the conceptual framework proposed here is nontraditional in terms of current diagnostic systems in mental health, it has been helpful as an approach to everyday clinical challenges in both the diagnosis and especially in the treatment and management of individuals with *both* mental illness and mental retardation. This approach is based on the authors' extended clinical experiences with three general types of mentally retarded individuals with associated mental illness: those with *primitive* behavior; those with *atypical* behavior; and those with *abnormal* behavior. These three types, with the typical diagnostic-treatment challenges that each presents, will now be reviewed.

2.6.1. Primitive Behavior

Primitive behavior is usually manifested by severely or profoundly retarded individuals who also display gross delays in their behavior repertoires. Primitive behaviors include very rudimentary utilization of special sensory modalities, particularly touch; position sense; oral explorative activity; and minimal externally directed verbalizations. In the diagnostic interview, primitive behaviors such as mouthing and licking of toys, excessive tactile stimulation, "autistic hand movement," and skin picking and body rocking are noted. From a diagnostic viewpoint, the very primitiveness of the child's overall behavior, in conjunction with much stereotyping initially, may suggest a psychotic disorder of childhood. However, these children do make eye contact and interact with the examiner quite readily, despite their very minimal behavioral repertoire.

Similarly, one might form the initial impression that both the level of observed primitive behavior and its persistence are secondary to intrinsic and/or extrinsic deprivation factors; however, at the same time, these children display multiple indices of developmental biological arrest that is of primary or congenital origin. It should be noted that these children do not possess a functional ego at the appropriate chronological age, and there is an amorphic (or minimal) personality structure. The following case history illustrates this primitive behavior type:

A 6½-year-old boy was seen at the request of the ward team (i.e., a developmental specialist, a social worker, a physician, and a psychologist); the purpose of the psychiatric consultation was to provide diagnostic clarification and treatment recommendations. The youngster had been admitted for observation at the request of both his parents and the staff of the previous treatment setting, with the following transfer impression: "Functions at the severely retarded level, but physically he looks so normal. He is not a very warm child. We wonder if he isn't an autistic child."

The personal history revealed that he was the last of three children, born after an uneventful pregnancy to a 26-year-old mother who had had no prior history of obstetrical complications; the family history was negative for hereditary disease. His birth weight and clinical status in the early neonatal period were all within normal limits. By the age of 6 months, the child was described as passive; early developmental milestones were markedly delayed, and he displayed generalized muscle hypotonicity. By the end of the first year, his developmental attainments were those of a 4-month-old child, and he had undergone a variety of medical evaluations. No definite diagnostic impressions were obtained, and the parents were counseled to provide general stimulation for their youngster. Because this family placed a high premium on child care, they were not satisfied with such nonspecific diagnostic and management recommendations. Accordingly, between the ages of 12 months and 48 months, the boy underwent six more evaluations in different parts of the country. By the age of 5 years, formal psychometric assessment indicated that the child was functioning at the 12- to 16-month developmental level; his family was perplexed and still shopping for diagnostic-treatment recommendations that would "really help him to grow like he should'' (mother's statement). Medical reevaluation at age 6 was followed by parental rejection of the diagnosis of severe mental retardation. The boy had been admitted to the present institution for the retarded for further diagnosis, observation, and possible treatment. As previously noted, the admitting impression was "possible autism."

Psychiatric examination of this youngster revealed no physical signs or symptoms of delayed development except for primitive finer hand movements, dull and vacant eyes, and the absence of any structured language. He occupied himself continuously with quick hand movements approximately 12 inches from his eyes, and he periodically picked at a spot on his left wrist. Initially, he was only passively compliant with the examiner. However, with a little inducement, he interacted with the examiner through eye contact and gingerly participated in attempts at playing "patty cake" and rolling a ball back and forth. The previously noted hand movements promptly disappeared as his attention was occupied.

Treatment recommendations focused on stopping the diagnostic "merry-go-round," while stressing the need for closer interpersonal relationships (e.g., foster grandparent contacts on a regular basis), continuity of similar passive-dependent relationships, and involvement in a highly structured, developmentally oriented program to stimulate and develop self-help skills. During a follow-up observation period, the child-care workers had begun to work actively with this youngster on self-help skills and small-group interactions, and they showed rather remarkable success. Simultaneously, ongoing family interviews helped to relieve the parents' anxiety and gave them more realistic expectations for their child.

· This type of primitive behavior is frequently seen in severely and profoundly retarded children who are from rather perplexed families, and who have received "the works" in diagnostic procedures. This type of emotionally disturbed–mentally retarded child essentially is an "untutored child" whose primitive behavior has been allowed to persist while parents and professionals have focused their concern on differential diagnostic issues. The family slowly loses its tolerance and empathy for the child as their initial high expectations and ongoing investments of energy result only in a slow dissolution of their hopes.

There is a lingering myth that retarded children, especially the more severely retarded, must "look retarded." It would seem that normal physical appearance in the presence of markedly delayed developmental milestones (e.g., in motor and language) and primitive behavior are viewed as incongruous (and/or incompatible) by both lay and some professional observers alike. Yet, a number of severely and profoundly retarded children have won "beautiful baby" contests. Frequently, the initial physical impression of these children and the complexity of their family interpersonal transactions, against the backdrop of severe mental retardation, result in an erroneous diagnosis of a psychotic disorder of childhood. This error is compounded by the treatment–management approaches that accompany such a diagnosis, and by their effects on the attitudes of the child, the parents, and professionals. In contrast, realignment of parental and professional expectations, clarifications of diagnoses, and focus on specific treatment are the keys to providing effective help for retarded individuals who display primitive behaviors.

2.6.2. Atypical Behavior

Another frequently referred to behavioral challenge is that of the adolescent retarded person who is committed to an institution because of ongoing adjustment difficulties within his or her home community, but not necessarily within his or her primary family structure. Atypical behaviors displayed by such retarded persons including poor control (as evidenced by emotional outbursts), impulsivity, sullenness, stubbornness, mild legal transgressions, and generally poor adaptation to prevocational or vocational training programs.

After such an individual arrives at the institution, psychiatric consultation most commonly is requested because (1) the youngster refuses to cooperate with the training or group social-living expectations of the institutional setting; or (2) continual abrasive comments and/or contact from the family belittle the institution's ability to help their family member. A result of such family conduct is the retarded person's questioning, "Why was I put here?" and, "Why are you keeping me?" The family denies the reality of the youngster's social-adaptive problems, and at the same time, they harass the institutional staff for focusing on and attempting positive modification of their son's or daughter's major problem behaviors.

These instances of "atypical behavior" are *atypical only for the institutional settings in which such youngsters find themselves* (i.e., they are really quite typical within the primary family subculture). Etiological diagnosis usually is in the area of "cultural-familial mental retardation" or "idiopathic mental retardation." The following case history (a response to complex intrafamilial communication patterns) is illustrative of this clinical challenge.:

> The patient was a mildly retarded 14-year-old boy whose parents had a common-law marriage. His delayed development became more obvious when he entered school; then increasing behavioral difficulties were noted. Later, a series of minor altercations with the police occurred, culminating in a car theft that necessitated his removal from the community. His parents tended to blame the school for his poor performance and subsequent maladjustment; his institutionalization was very much against their wishes, and they felt that they were being persecuted (e.g., "The law is against us. He is a good boy if other people will just leave him alone."). His adjustment to institutional placement was characterized by frequent temper outbursts when demands were made on him. He manifested continual sullenness and refused to involve himself in any of the institution's programs, except to demand that his parents be allowed to visit him weekly. Psychiatric consultation was requested to identify methods that the staff might use to motivate the boy toward a more positive role in his ongoing treatment and training program.
> Psychiatric examination revealed a tall young man of awkward physical appearance who was rather dressed up for the interview. he opened the interview by asking, "Who put you up to talking to me? Why? I'm not

retarded and don't belong here despite what *they* say, or what *you* try to get me to say!'' Following this initial salvo, he tended to limit his remarks to monosyllabic answers, nods, and grunts. He did state, ''I was sent for training, but they can't teach me nothing here. I know as much as they do!'' He would anticipate and/or avoid questions about his personal history by sullenly staring at the examiner, looking toward the door, or appearing to be greatly bored by the entire transaction. Sullen defiance, personality immaturity, and interpersonal manipulations were very much in evidence. At the end of this rather exasperating interview, he stated, ''You talk to my folks; they know me and they don't like the crap I've been getting from these jerks around here.''

Discussions of the case with staff revealed that they had minimized the importance of the family's anger toward the institution and the negative effect of this attitude on their son's adjustment. Collectively, members of the treatment team provided information gleaned from letters, telephone calls, and family visits, all of which repeated the common theme that the family was not responsible for his placement and continued to convey the message to him, ''You can come home whenever they will let you.''

It would have been extremely difficult for any individual staff member to be aware of the total clinical picture and the associated treatment challenges. However, with clarification and direction, staff members were able to devise some imaginative intervention techniques. In a planned conference with both the parents and the boy present, the parents were told that they could take their son home if they so desired. The family responded by listing numerous factors that they would have to consider; they then became quite uncomfortable and announced that they would telephone their decision to the boy. When the staff insisted that the boy be told of their decision in person and in the presence of staff members, the mother asked the boy to leave the room; she then stated that she couldn't tell him that she didn't want him to live at home because ''He will be mad at me.'' When the boy was told of the family's decision by the mother, he responded (as predicted) with an angry outburst directed toward his family. In the follow-up plan, the family's visits were restricted in number; a specific member of the treatment team was present during these visits. The staff was instructed to meet his angry outbursts with the disclaimer that they were there only to help him and were not holding him against the wishes of his parents.

Cultural-familial mental retardation is far more frequent than all other causes of retardation combined; yet, 90% of these cultural-familial retarded persons are not institutionalized. Many of the youngsters who are institutionalized are admitted to protect them from severe emotional and material deprivation.[62-64] Unfortunately, they usually are the last to be identified as mentally retarded and may already have spent their formative years in deprived settings. Not only have they been identified with dissocial and antisocial pathological living conditions, but their attitudes, defenses, and personality patterns usually are well entrenched by the time of institutionalization.

It would appear that formerly institutionalized mentally retarded individuals with atypical behavior are increasingly ''flunking out'' of community-based service programs and continue their persistently atypical behavior within a social system other than their primary family. Management is difficult unless very close coordination exists between the administrative segments of institutional or community-based systems of service.[65] Yet, it is in these very cases that the total psychosocial environment can modify motivational potential, effect changes in the patient's value systems, and achieve more positive and social-adaptive approaches to interpersonal transactions and the world of work.[66]

2.6.3. Abnormal Behavior

Most of the clearly abnormal behavior challenges encountered in institutionalized or community-based samples of retarded individuals encompass instances of psychotic behavior. It is truly remarkable that, in the eighth decade of the twentieth century, one still sees psychotic children and adolescents who have literally been dumped into institutions for the mentally retarded because of the lack of specific treatment programs in their home communities, or because of treatment nihilism toward the psychoses of early life. Treatment nihilism is a major problem because one typically notes a clinical history of great enthusiasm when treatment is initiated; then the slowness of the child's response "wears out" the treatment team, and the child is referred to another setting with the prognostic label that she or he is "untreatable." The frequently accompanying major personality regression is extrapolated to imply mental retardation, and the prognosis is viewed as "hopeless." A broad view of these individuals' developmental potentials and psychotic characteristics must be wedded to specific treatment goals if this type of treatment failure is to be avoided.

In the clinical interview, children with psychotic disorders present the following behavioral dimensions: (1) bizarreness of manner, gesture, and posture; (2) uncommunicative speech; (3) little or no discrimination between animate and inanimate objects (one of the primary signs of psychosis in childhood, an entity sharply delineated from the primitive behavior previously noted); (4) identification with mostly inanimate objects; (5) display of deviant affective expressions; (6) little, if any, relationship with peers; (7) passive compliance to external demands or stimuli; and (8) marked negativism (e.g., if pushed in an interpersonal setting, the child initially exhibits negativism, followed in rapid succession by withdrawal and out-of-contact behaviors, i.e., psychosis).

A case history is presented here to illustrate the features of a psychotic reaction in late childhood:

> The patient was a 12-year-old boy who had been admitted to an institution for the retarded at age 7 because of frequent temper tantrums, noisy screeching, carrying a large screwdriver at all times, and cruelty to animals. The personal history review noted that at age 3 he was considered somewhat precocious by his parents, but was noted to display periodic elective mutism; a hearing loss was suspected. Shortly thereafter, he became mute and regressed in his intellectual and motor achievement. At the time of admission, he was considered "different and slow" and had been unable to func-

tion in the available community-based special-education options. The staff was concerned about his withdrawal as well as his bizarre behavior, reporting that he watched the linoleum tile patterns quite carefully and would repeatedly turn to the right at every twenty-second tile interval.

On direct examination, he grimaced frequently, making no effective contact despite the lengthy interview period; he made bizarre hand movements and alternately chewed on a small ball or his left wrist, while mumbling incoherently to himself. When pushed to interact, he physically withdrew to a corner of the room and excitedly addressed the walls in a high-pitched voice; "Elephant dogs, elephant dogs . . ." The diagnosis was mental retardation secondary to a major psychiatric disorder, schizophrenia of childhood.

A treatment plan was devised for this patient that included the use of psychotropic drugs and the provision of a milieu that focused on activities and closer interpersonal contacts. The chronicity of the boy's psychosis and his interpersonal unavailability were approached via a behavior modification paradigm with a focus on reestablishing both self-help skills and interpersonal contacts. Specific management foci included developing a repertoire of skills that would permit him to function in a less restrictive environment (e.g., a community-based sheltered workshop and/or a residential hostel facility).

The treatment results noted in this case example provide much greater personal fulfillment than the passive participation in an endless merry-go-round of residences in an institution for the mentally retarded, followed by referral to a mental hospital, and then discharge (after having obtained "maximal hospital benefits") back to the institution for the mentally retarded. Many institutions for the retarded have built up large backlogs of such psychotic patients, whose definitive treatment needs have gone unmet. These patients are referred elsewhere during their acute episodes and are typically returned to a subacute remission state. Because institutional staff personnel frequently view these psychotic patients as "odd or dangerous," often the individual patient's psychotic process is refueled by apprehensive staff members, until she or he is pushed once again into an acute state.

A major current trend in institutions for the mentally retarded is to provide regional resource programs and facilities to back up the emerging community-based programs. Because mentally ill–mentally retarded individuals are often rejects from community-based programs, they present a major challenge to members of the institutional staff. This challenge demands that the focus of professional staff members be sharply attuned to the behavioral dimensions of mental retardation and to the allied needs of families who have been literally worn out by the primitive-atypical-abnormal behaviors of their mentally retarded sons and daughters.

The previously reviewed descriptive diagnostic considerations and the general/specific treatment–management plans strongly suggest that a variety of treatment approaches must be utilized to help these individuals. For example, a mentally retarded individual with a psychotic disorder may need a specific type of milieu setting, psychoactive drugs to reduce motor overactivity and mood fluctuation, behavior shaping to simulate the positive reinforcement of specific adaptive behaviors, ongoing citizen-advocate contacts, and active involvement of the family support system. Because of the complexity of these treatment ingredients, the team approach is a prime pathway for providing a wide spectrum of individualized services for these mentally ill–mentally retarded individuals.

In summary, three patterns of behavior noted in individuals with both mental retardation and mental illness have been presented. The increasing admission rate of such individuals to institutions for the mentally retarded demands a reevaluation of the individuals so referred, the way in which they are evaluated, and the spectrum of global and specific treatment–management modalities that are available for them. Finally, some administrative implications and suggested guidelines for implementing necessary diagnostic and treatment approaches are presented within the context of redirected goals for institutions for the mentally retarded—as regional resource centers—for the rapidly developing community-based programs for the mentally retarded.

2.7. Treatment and Management Modalities

It is not surprising that the professional literature regarding the treatment of psychiatric disorders in the mentally retarded has closely reflected the attitudes that characterized society's approach to the retarded in general. This can be seen in early humanistic educational approaches, followed in the late nineteenth century by a change to an overall negative posture, as professional thinking embraced the "defect position" and the sound of the "eugenic alarm." This "tragic interlude" led to a falling away of all treatment, including psychiatric treatment, of the mentally retarded, and to an emphasis solely on custodial care and isolation, in order to shield society from the retarded person perceived as a deviant or an offender. It has taken until the midway point of the twentieth century for the pendulum of public and professional opinion to swing in the direction of renewed interest in the welfare of retarded persons; fortunately, this renewed interest has also sparked increased activity, both clinical and research, in the treatment of psychiatric disorders in this group.

A review of professional reports concerning the treatment of mental illness and the mentally retarded over the last 150 years reflects a gradual evolution in treatment approaches, beginning with the early focus on viewing mental retardation as "amentia" (leading to some early educational attempts at treatment) and progressing to a "dementia" prototype (resulting in custodialism). Closely tied to institutionalization and custodial care was the widespread use of isolation, as well as physical and chemical restraints (the suppressive approach), which has persisted in some areas into the present. However, at the same time, there has been renewed interest in the treatment of specific subsets of retarded persons with behavioral problems (for example, the psychotic, the delinquent, and the brain-damaged), and since 1960, there has been increasing specificity of diagnosis and subsequent treatment of persons with both diagnoses. It is interesting to note the paradox of treatment approaches that took place between 1915 and 1960 as regards mental retardation and child psychiatry: the former was increasingly relegated to institutional settings with low expectations of improvement, the latter blossoming in the form of countless child guidance clinics focusing optimistically on individual and family psychotherapeutic approach toward children and adolescents with mental illness (but not mental retardation).

Since 1950, there has been an increasing stream of reports on the treatment and management of psychiatric disorders in the mentally retarded. Therapeutic approaches have encompassed the entire range of psychiatric treatment utilized for nonretarded persons and have included (but are not limited to) psychoanalytically oriented individual psychotherapy, therapeutic nursery schools, family therapy, group therapy, play therapy, various behavioral approaches, somatic therapy, and psychotropic medications, as well as combinations of these modalities (see especially Chapters 4, 6, 8, and 16 in this volume; also Menolascino[5]).

An in-depth review of each of the above modalities constitutes several later chapters; only an overview is given here. All of these approaches are based on a treatment plan that begins with a comprehensive study of the child and his or her family in order to determine the nature and extent of their adjustment difficulties, and then to refine intervention techniques to resolve them. Psychoanalytically based psychotherapeutic approaches have persisted but have remained sharply focused in the area of severe and complex disorders of early childhood. The relative lack of professional concentration of counseling or psychotherapy activities in the mentally retarded reflects the work of Rogers and Dyamond,[67] and others who felt that psychotherapy was not indicated or useful for mentally retarded persons with psychiatric disorders because it (psychotherapy) requires insight, high levels of verbal communication, capacity for self-reliance, and other factors inherent in normal intelligence. Such a position has been refuted by other authors,[68-71] who have described the successful use of individual psychotherapy, and still others[66,72,73] (and Monfils, Chapter 16 in this volume), who have successfully utilized group psychotherapeutic approaches in both institutional and community-based programs. Indeed, current clinical thinking embraces a wide range of psychotherapeutic treatments for mentally retarded persons with concurrent mental illnesses; the old view that the mentally retarded are not psychotherapy candidates must be discarded. Psychotherapeutic approaches that stress warmth and acceptance and that are keyed to differing developmental levels of personality functioning are not only successful but serve to illustrate that therapeutic relationships, and not level of intellectual or cognitive functioning, may be the key to successful psychotherapy.

Behavioral modification is a treatment–management approach that has been applied in a wide range of diagnoses. This approach has been used for over three decades in individual and group approaches to the retarded. Because another chapter (see Chapter 4) in this book address this treatment approach, only a brief description of its potential impact is presented here. The use of behavioral modification to treat the mentally retarded–mentally ill individual can serve both to unite past viewpoints and to illuminate new horizons of potential treatment. In contrast to past therapies, the behavioral modification approach (1) strongly focuses on the precise descriptions of simple or complex behaviors; (2) describes predictable phenomena; and (3) does not regard formal diagnostic dimensions as sacrosanct and hence does not permit them to limit full descriptive analyses of observed behavior. However, as with any treatment approach, its overutilization, in a vacuum, can be predicted to be less beneficial than a combined approach addressing all of the pertinent determinants of behavior in an individual case. As a result, isolated behavioral-modification approaches have been criticized as simplistic and symptom-bound, occasionally not recognizing the presence of specific symptoms as components of *syndromes* that may also be responsive to alternate treatment methods. Interestingly, most retarded persons and their families have, in our experience, shown a singular lack of interest in such professional debates and are more impressed by the results of treatment—regardless of professional beliefs and the resultant choices of treatment techniques.

Somatic methods, primarily the use of psychopharmacological agents, have been used through many eras for the treatment and management of retarded persons. In the past, they have often taken the form of nonspecific sedation or, more recently, the limited use of the antipsychotic medications in the psychotic retarded individual. Only in the last 20 years has there been a move toward the more directed use of psychotropic agents, including antipsychotics, antidepressants, anxiolytics, and lithium carbonate, in treating specific psychiatric disorders occurring in retarded individuals.[74] These psychopharmacological agents currently utilized in the treatment of mentally ill persons all affect neurotransmitter activity, either blocking or decreasing specific neurotransmitters, or enhancing the activity of others. As a result of experience with these medications over the past three decades, in recent studies of the metabolism of neurotransmitters in various psychiatric disorders, there has developed an improved understanding of probable neurotransmitter abnormalities in certain psychiatric conditions.[75,76] For example, it appears that children without physiological signs of anxiety who exhibit impulsive motor hyperactivity tend to be catecholamine-deficient; they are likely to respond positively to stimulant or antidepressant medication. Similarly, physiologically anxious, hyperalert children tend to have high norepinephrine levels; they generally respond selectively to the more sedative phenothiazine antipsychotics, whereas children with stereotyped or ritualistic behavior appear to have high dopamine levels and tend to respond best to the more potent, less sedating antipsychotics. Thus, as the clinician is more able to correlate probable neurotransmitter abnormalities in given psychiatric disorders with the pharmacological activities of various psychotropic medications, the probability of selecting an appropriate medication is increased.

Many clinicians might argue (correctly) that medication is not the "ultimate answer" to the presence of emotional or personality problems in the retarded[77–79]; such medications may adversely affect individuals via potential toxicity, or because of their extensive use, to the exclusion of developmental or other treatment approaches. Thus, at times, the disadvantages of medication may outweigh their advantages.[80] Although these cautions are undeniably valid, the proper use of medication by the physician can often provide an excellent entry into treatment via the rapid diminution of the offending symptoms when unacceptable behavior has caused the family or the school to demand an immediate movement toward more restrictive placement. This entry into treatment via psychoactive drug prescription must always be only the first step toward a total program of treatment, and not the final step (toward a narrow chemical restraint approach), as has taken place in the past.[81,83,84]

A more extensive view of this complicated and challenging treatment modality is provided by Dr. Donaldson in Chapter 6.

2.8. A Systematic Approach to Management

Systematically organized models of problem solving in medicine are generally superior to those that are not so structured, and this is especially true in approaching the diagnosis and treatment of the mentally retarded.[85] Areas of potential diagnostic pitfalls are compounded by difficulty with language, generally less-than-optimal opportunity for examination, and confusion regarding the nature and the natural course of the symptom of mental retardation itself. This diagnostic challenge becomes more difficult when a psychiatric disorder is superimposed, and makes a systematic approach to diagnosis and treatment mandatory if the multiple determinants of a mentally retarded individual's behavior are intelligently addressed.[53] Key elements of the proposed systematic model appear below:

1. *Careful diagnosis and treatment.* The medical adage that the "history is 90% of the diagnosis" is nowhere more true than in the treatment of the emotionally disturbed mentally retarded. As previously noted, the usual diagnostic parameters may be clouded, or inappropriate, and patient-reported symptomatology may be inaccurate or absent. It is thus imperative that the clinician remain openminded throughout the diagnostic process and focus strongly on the sequential history of the highest level of intellectual and adaptive functioning, changes in either of the above parameters, and specific primitive, atypical, or abnormal behavioral patterns. Of utmost importance in this process is the necessity of close contact with the family (or other caregivers) as those are most likely to furnish an accurate history and assessment in the individual's level of functioning (see below). Attention to the social, psychological, and biological factors contributing to the dysfunction must be clearly identified and addressed in the diagnostic assessment. Additionally, periodic reevaluation and reexamination often reveal diagnostic surprises not originally present and necessitate flexibility in approach. Finally, but perhaps most difficultly, comes the need to allow sufficient *time* for any diagnostic impression—and its subsequent treatment approach—to effect a change in the individual in the area of less subjective distress, improved intellectual or psychological functioning,

Table 4. Suggested Individualized Treatment Approach[a]

1. Clearly identify the problem(s).
2. Define it objectively in writing.
3. Identify and list three possible *alternative* treatment interventions.
4. Select *one* and implement; observe outcome.
5. Take your time! Has the proposed treatment(s) been fully implemented: have data been collected and analyzed; attitudinal problems addressed (e.g., burned-out staff with countertransference problems); or have intercurrent (i.e., new) factors recently occurred?
6. If not satisfied with outcome of number 5:
   a. Either generate another treatment focus that has resulted from the information obtained during the initial intervention attempt, and implement; or
   b. Select an alternative from the original list (number 3) and implement.
7. Take your time!
8. Repeat Step 6 if necessary.

[a] As with any human development variable, behavior slowly changes in a directional manner over time, and thus, #5 and #7 should be adhered to closely.

or normalization of behavior. These points are summarized in Table 4 and provide a systematic diagram to management, without which adequate treatment may be avoided, delayed, or missed entirely.

2. *Active family involvement.* The second principle in treatment and management is to engage the family or the family surrogate in an active participation from the outset. These persons are crucial not only for accurate diagnosis, but often also for large segments of the treatment itself, and certainly for periodic reassessment of the individual and his or her response to the treatment interventions. The clinician's attitude and level of interest frequently determine the success of this endeavor; thus, the future cooperation (or lack of it) on the part of the family may reflect his or her unspoken, as well as spoken, attitudes at the time of initial contact. The therapist needs to convey to the family his or her willingness to share the facts (and insights) that he or she obtains as the first step in such cooperation, as well as his or her expectation that the family will reciprocate (with reports, responses, and attitudes), if treatment interventions are to be optimally successful. It is valuable to indicate in an early contact that treatment planning rarely results in a single recommendation; it is something that may shift in focus and alter its course as the retarded individual continues to develop. This attitude[86] ensures the flexibility of approach that allows for the total view of the individual and promotes timely consultation and referral as the diagnostic picture changes.[87] Only in this way is it possible to avoid the "doctor shopping" that often occurs as caregivers become frustrated with new developments, problems, or crises over time. Much has been written concerning grief reactions in families with handicapped members, and these occur frequently in the parents and siblings of mentally retarded individuals. Clinicians evaluating these children (or adults) must remain vigilant for such reactions, not only at obvious junctures (e.g., the initial interpretation to parents regarding a family member's status or limitations) but also in future interactions (as reality supersedes denial and magical thinking) or surrounding

special events (specific ages in the parent or the child, certain developmental milestones, holidays, changes within the family itself, or onset of a superimposed medical or psychiatric disorder). Not surprisingly, the same grief reactions can and do occur in similar situations within the surrogate family of the retarded individual, whether in a community-based or an institutional setting, and the clinician must be sensitive to the effect that these reactions can have on ongoing treatment programs and strategies. An assessment of family interaction and strengths is a necessary part of the total evaluation because these assets are essential to planning a comprehensive treatment program.

3. *Principles of primary and secondary prevention.* Primary prevention of mental retardation has been widely discussed elsewhere and will not be addressed here. Primary prevention of psychiatric disorders in the retarded has been less well addressed, but general principles promoting mental health in the individual and her or his family, and modifying the environment so as to provide maximum opportunity for growth and development, also apply to the mentally retarded. This may take the form of mental health professionals' taking the lead in providing public education on modern dimensions on the causes of mental retardation, pushing for the establishment of newborn screening programs, and the general improvement of educational opportunities for children of all socioeconomic groups.

Secondary prevention is of perhaps more importance in this discussion, as early diagnosis and treatment can result in appropriate programs, realistic expectations, reduced frustration and alienation, and hence fewer secondary psychiatric disorders in the mentally retarded. In the severely to profoundly retarded, this process is likely to occur in conjunction with medical evaluation during infancy or in the preschool years. In the borderline, mildly, or moderately retarded, screening programs prior to or in the initial stages of formal education become relatively more important and can often prevent the frustration, the alienation, and the subsequent behavioral problems that occur in these children. Such an approach helps at all levels of involvement, preventing suffering in the mentally retarded individual, promoting realistic expectations on the part of the family and the teachers,[88] and identifying for the school those children who will need and benefit from appropriate special programs. In this sense, secondary prevention becomes a cohesive part of the ongoing work with the child and his or her family. This total approach requires continual follow-up, and periodic reevaluation must be done so that appropriate shifts in treatment and overall levels of expectation may be carried out.

4. *Principles of tertiary prevention.* As much disability can often result from the treatment of a condition as from the condition itself; the same is true of psychiatric disorders in the mentally retarded. Hence, the fourth principle focuses on maximizing developmental potential and involves a different type of goal setting from the usual treatment plan, addressing what the individual *can do* rather than the anticipation of cure. The goal then becomes one of maximally and, at the same time, realistically helping to rehabilitate the patient. This goal requires a delicate balance between reality-based expectations, on the one hand, and the avoidance of therapeutic nihilism, consequent less-than-

optimal treatment, and self-fulfilling prophecy, on the other. Herein lie both the "art" and the "science" of the key treatment approaches to this group.

5. *Normalization.* The principle of normalization[82] has literally revolutionized the field of mental retardation. Normalization implies that services will be provided within the communities; it stresses that the overwhelming majority of retarded persons are able to enjoy and profit from the rich variety of human experiences that are found there. These considerations include the opportunity to enjoy life experiences in a family setting or a small-group home, to have a work or school experience in a location separate from their dwelling, and to have developmentally appropriate activities within the context of the larger community. This trend became federally mandated in the United States via the deinstitutionalization policy of 1971, and as a result, a tremendous number of community support services, including mental health services, are necessary. The concept of normalization requires that such services be available to the dually diagnosed individual in her or his community, and it involves psychiatric and other mental health consultation to group homes, schools, and other educational and vocational settings. A relatively small percentage of retarded–mentally ill individuals will require short- or long-term inpatient mental-health placement for behavioral management because they are dangerous to themselves or to others. These individuals should be treated in mental health facilities in or near their home communities when their special needs exceed the capabilities and the expertise of most community-based programs. *Rarely,* some retarded individuals will require long-term care when they present with intractable psychiatric disorders (psychosis, affective disorder, severe personality disorder); these, too, should optimally be cared for in mental health facilities in their area rather than institutional settings for the retarded with limited or no psychiatric consultation.

6. *Coordination of services.* Coordination of the many services needed for individuals with dual diagnoses requires awareness of the various services available in a given community and a professional attitude that permits active collaboration. It necessitates sharing the overall treatment plan with the retarded individual (when appropriate), with the family, and with community resources (for example, teachers and group home personnel). Close attention to the clarity and the continuity of communication is essential, and the clinician must be able to flow smoothly through the roles of primary therapist, treatment consultant, and coordinator of multiple services.

In summary, it is necessary to remember that *combined* or balanced treatment approaches (see Table 5) are frequently indicated when one attempts to provide modern treatment intervention for these dually diagnosed individuals. The balanced treatment approach noted in Table 5 quickly reveals that a number of these approaches may need to be utilized simultaneously. Indeed, failure to use such balanced treatment approaches (because of the specialist's lack of interest or knowledge, or because of fixed professional-ideological blind spots to certain techniques) is one of the most commonly noted reasons for treatment failures in this clinical area. Thus, this is a rather large expectation of and from

Table 5. Balanced Treatment Approaches

1. Counseling, guidance, individual/group psychotherapy
2. Behavior modification
3. Psychoactive drugs
4. Parent counseling
5. Social ecology → residential
6. Vocational habilitation → work
7. Social → recreation
8. Follow-along services

the professional. Yet, less elaborate or less balanced treatment interventions too often miss the goals of the needed combined approaches to these complex individuals.

2.9. Current Mental-Health Approaches to Serving the Mentally Retarded

The last 30 years have been characterized by renewed interest in, involvement in, and commitment to the care and treatment of persons with mental retardation. These changes have been a result, in part, of *three* major events reflecting American society's reexamination of the lives of these individuals. The first of these events was the founding in 1951 of the National Association for Retarded Citizens (NARC). This citizens' advocacy group, largely made up of parents of retarded citizens, has been instrumental in publicizing the special needs of their family members, and in improving treatment and services for all retarded persons. Most of the recent changes in our country can be traced to the hard work and the dedication of this nationally and locally organized movement.

The second major event was the report of President Kennedy's Panel on Mental Retardation, which led to his benchmark legislation on behalf of the mentally retarded in 1963. The panel's report was translated into action (with the support of the NARC) through increased resources for research efforts, strong public-policy actions at the federal and state levels, the initiation and support of alternative community-based service programs, and greater public education efforts. As a result, 12 mental retardation research centers were established to further basic research, and a number of university-affiliated programs were initiated to provide education and training for the professionals who would provide service for the mentally retarded.

Finally, several important federal programs and legislative acts[89] have emphasized the legal mandate of providing the mentally retarded with the same rights, liberties, economic programs, and opportunities as are available to the nonretarded. Important among these is PL 94-142,[90] which states that local school systems must provide appropriate educational opportunities for all handicapped children. As a result, many special programs are already functioning in most communities.

Since the very place for delivery of professional services to the mentally retarded has changed (i.e., from the monolithic institution of the past to the dispersed community-based system of services of today), the psychiatrist or other mental health professional has had to adjust, adapt, and expand the roles or points of entry through which she or he can interact with mentally retarded individuals, with or without psychiatric disorders. Generally included within these roles are the following:

1. *Direct therapist.* As previously noted, many retarded people with psychiatric disorders can and do benefit from a traditional, insight-oriented psychotherapeutic approach. However, many others will benefit from a more direct, supportive, or behavioral approach, requiring the mental health professional as primary therapist to assume a more active, more concrete, and generally more flexible role than is usually necessary.

2. *Family therapist.* Nearly all families (or surrogates) of mentally retarded individuals require some psychotherapeutic services, either supportive or insight-oriented, at some point in their development. The community approach to the care of mentally retarded individuals, especially those with psychiatric disorders, may be likened to that associated with any "dependent" population, and it is quite similar in many ways to that of child or geriatric psychiatry. Thus, the families are best helped through the development of long-term supportive relationships with the professional, who can help them to acquire specific information, can make recommendations, and can work through developmental crises or illness exacerbation in their family members.

3. *Coordination of services.* The last 20 years have brought about great changes (deinstitutionalization, normalization, renewed interest) in the provision of services for the retarded, and the mental health professional must of necessity be aware of these if she or he is to adequately coordinate them for her or his patients. The very newness of some of these community-based programs, as well as their diversity in terms of the programs provided, the staffing ratios, and medical-surgical supervision, demands that the mental health professional keep abreast so as to maximize the services available to the individual with whom she or he works.

4. *Consultant.* The mental health professional can also function as an individual or programmatic consultant in several areas in which mentally retarded persons live and work. These include day-care centers for younger children, school programs for older children, residential and vocational settings or institutions for adults, or elected and appointed volunteer agencies that are mental retardation advocates. Failure to understand aspects of the services provided in these settings will limit the clinician's positive impact in these areas, for example:

   a. Mentally retarded children in day-care centers reveal significant variability of developmental skills within a single child; failure to recognize this variability will limit staff recognition and response in this area.
   b. Mentally retarded individuals with concurrent psychiatric disorders may have their emotional needs addressed by a mental health profes-

sional, but unless the clinician is sensitive to the individual's ongoing developmental needs, critical developmental periods may pass and lead to other psychiatric disorders in the future. This professional sensitivity requires special training and education (see Chapter 14) of mental health professionals who function as consultants to programs that serve the retarded.

c. Mental health consultants to institutions for the retarded fulfill a variety of purposes and must often differentiate between overt and covert reasons for consultation requests, if the needs of the individual, and not necessarily the institution, are to be foremost.

In summary, the last 30 years have seen progress made in several areas of improved functioning for mentally retarded persons, including those previously additionally limited by disabling psychiatric disorders. With this progress has come expanded involvement for the mental health professional in the care and treatment of the retarded, as new roles and expectations have formed in response to recent research, education, and commitment to realizing the full developmental potential of these citizens.

References

1. Gardner WF, Cole CL: Meeting the mental health needs of the mentally retarded. *Forum* 1;1–3, 1981.
2. Chess S, Hassibi M: *Principles and Practices of Child Psychiatry.* New York, Plenum Press, 1978.
3. American Psychiatric Association. *Diagnostic and Statistical Manual of Mental Disorders,* ed 3. Washington, D.C., Author, 1980.
4. Kanner L: *A History of the Care and Study of the Mentally Retarded.* Springfield, IL, C. C. Thomas, 1964.
5. Menolascino FJ: Psychiatry's past, current and future role, in Menolascino F (ed): *Psychiatric Approaches to Mental Retardation.* New York, Basic Books, 1970.
6. Itard J: *The Wild Boy of Aveyron* (original title: *De l'education d'un homme sauvage*). New York, Century, 1932.
7. Seguin E: *The Moral Treatment, Hygiene, and Education of Idiots and Other Backward Children.* New York, Columbia University Press, 1864.
8. Goddard HH: *The Kallikak Family.* New York, Arno Press, 1973.
9. Goddard HH: *Feeblemindedness: Its Causes and Consequences.* New York, Macmillan, 1914.
10. Vail D: *Dehumanization and the Institutional Career.* Springfield, IL, C. C. Thomas, 1966.
11. Wolfensberger W: The origin and nature of our institutional models, in Kugel R, Wolfensberger W (eds): *Changing Patterns in Residential Services for the Mentally Retarded.* Washington, D.C., Government Printing Office, 1969.
12. Blatt B, Kaplan F: *Christmas in Purgatory: A Photographic Essay in Mental Retardation.* Syracuse, Human Policy Press, 1974.
13. President's Committee on Mental Retardation. *Mental Retardation: Century of Decision.* Washington, D.C., Government Printing Office, 1976.
14. President's Committee on Mental Retardation. *Islands of Excellence.* Washington, D.C., Government Printing Office, 1977.
15. President's Committee on Mental Retardation. *Report of the Liaison Task Panel on Mental Retardation,* vol 4. Washington, D.C., Government Printing Office, 1978.
16. President's Committee on Mental Retardation. *Historical Overview.* Washington, D.C., Government Printing Office, 1979.

17. President's Committee on Mental Retardation. *Mental Retardation: The Leading Edge. Service Programs that Work*. Washington, D.C., Government Printing Office, 1978.
18. Potter H: The needs of mentally retarded children for child psychiatry services. *J Am Acad Psychoanal* 3;352, 1964.
19. Tarjan G: Cinderella and the prince: Mental retardation and community psychiatry. *Am J Psychiatr* 122;1057–1059, 1966.
20. Menolascino FJ: The facade of mental retardation: Its challenges to child psychiatry. *Am J Psychiatr* 12;1227–1235, 1976.
21. Beier D: Behavioral disturbances in the mentally retarded, in Stevens H, Heber R (eds): *Mental Retardation: A Review of Research*. Chicago, Chicago University Press, 1964.
22. Garfield S: Abnormal behavior and mental deficiency, in Ellis N (ed): *Handbook of Mental Deficiency: Psychological Theory and Research*. New York, McGraw-Hill, 1963.
23. Balthazar E, Stevens H, Gardner W: *International Bibliography of Literature of the Emotionally and Behaviorally Disturbed Mentally Retarded: 1914–1969*. Madison, State of Wisconsin Department of Health and Social Services, 1969.
24. Bernstein N: *Diminished People: Problems and Care of the Mentally Retarded*. Boston, Little-Brown, 1970.
25. Menolascino FJ: *Challenges in Mental Retardation: Progressive Ideologies and Services*. New York, Human Sciences Press, 1977.
26. Syzmanski LS, Tanguay PE (eds): *Emotional Disorders of Mentally Retarded Persons*. Baltimore, University Park Press, 1980.
27. Chess S; *An Introduction to Child Psychiatry*, ed 2. New York, Grune and Stratton, 1969.
28. Chess S, Horn S, Fernandez P: *Psychiatric Disorders of Children with Congenital Rubella*. New York, Brunner/Mazel, 1971.
29. Webster T: Unique aspects of emotional development in mentally retarded children, in Menolascino F (ed): *Psychiatric Approaches to Mental Retardation*. New York, Basic Books, 1970.
30. Hunt N: *The World of Nigel Hunt*. New York, Taplinger, 1967.
31. Penrose L: The contribution of mental deficiency research to psychiatry. *Br J Psychiatr* 112;747–755, 1966.
32. Pollack H: Brain damage, mental retardation and childhood schizophrenia. *Am J Psychiatr* 115;422–427, 1958.
33. Menolascino FJ: Emotional disturbances in institutionalized retardates: Primitive, atypical and abnormal behaviors. *Ment Retard* 10(6);3–8, 1972.
34. Menolascino FJ: Community psychiatry and mental retardation, in Bellack L, Barten H (eds): *Progress in Community Mental Health*. New York, Brunner/Mazel, 1975.
35. Balthazar E, Stevens H: *The Emotionally Disturbed Mentally Retarded: A Historical Contemporary Perspective*. Englewood Cliffs, NJ, Pretence-Hall, 1975.
36. May J, May J: *Overview of Emotional Disturbances in Mentally Retarded Individuals*. Presented at the Annual Convention of the National Association for Retarded Citizens, Atlanta, 1979.
37. Scheerenberger RC: *A History of Mental Retardation*. Baltimore, Brookes, 1983.
38. Menolascino FJ: Emotional disturbance in mentally retarded children: Diagnostic and treatment aspects. *Arch Gen Psychiatr* 19;456–464, 1967.
39. Dewan J: Intelligence and emotional stability. *Am J Psychiatr* 104;548–554, 1948.
40. O'Connor N: Neuroticism and emotional instability in high-grade male defectives. *J Neurol Neurosurg Psychiatr* 14;226–230, 1951.
41. Webster T: Problems of emotional development in young retarded children, in Menolascino FJ (ed): *Psychiatric Aspects of the Diagnosis and Treatment of Mental Retardation*. Seattle, Special Child Publications, 1971.
42. Chess S: Psychiatric treatment of the mentally retarded child with behavioral problems. *Am J Orthopsychiatr* 32;863–869, 1962.
43. Chess S: Emotional problems in mentally retarded children, in Menolascino FJ (ed): *Psychiatric Approaches to Mental Retardation*. New York, Basic Books, 1970.
44. Berman M: Mental retardation and depression. *Ment Retard* 5(6);19–21, 1977.

45. Menolascino FJ: Psychiatric aspects of mental retardation in children under eight. *Am J Orthopsychiatr* 35;852–861, 1965.
46. Menolascino FJ: Emotional disturbances in mentally retarded children. *Am J Psychiatr* 126(2);54–62, 1969.
47. Eaton LF, Menolascino FJ: Psychotic reactions of childhood: Experiences of a mental retardation pilot project. *J Nerv Ment Dis* 43;55–67, 1966.
48. Eaton LF, Menolascino FJ: Psychoses of childhood: A five-year follow-up of experiences in a mental retardation clinic. *Am J Ment Defic* 72(3);370–380, 1967.
49. Eaton LF, Menolascino FJ: Psychiatric disorders in the mentally retarded: Types, problems and challenges. *Am J Psychiatr*, 139(10),1297–1303, 1982.
50. Philips I, Williams N: Psychopathology: A study of one-hundred children. *Am J Psychiatr* 32;1265–1273, 1975.
51. Bender L: The life course of children with autism and mental retardation, in Menolascino FJ (ed): *Psychiatric Approaches to Mental Retardation.* New York, Basic Books, 1970.
52. Webster T: Problems of emotional development in young retarded children, in Menolascino FJ (ed): *Psychiatric Aspects of the Diagnosis and Treatment of Mental Retardation.* Seattle, Special Child Publications, 1971.
53. Menolascino FJ, Egger ML: *Medical Dimensions of Mental Retardation.* Lincoln, University of Nebraska Press, 1978.
54. Woodward K, Jaffee N, Brown D: Early psychiatric intervention for young mentally retarded children, in Menolascino FJ (ed): *Psychiatric Approaches to Mental Retardation.* New York, Basic Books, 1970.
55. Sumner W: *Folkways: A Study of the Sociological Importance of Usages, Manners, Customs, Mores and Morals.* Boston, Ginn, 1906.
56. Allen R: Toward an exceptional offenders court. *Ment Retard* 4;1, 1966.
57. Brown BS, Courtless TF: The mentally retarded in penal and correctional institutions. *Am J Psychiatr* 124(9);1164–1170, 1968.
58. Allen R: The law and the mentally retarded, in Menolascino FJ (ed): *Psychiatric Approaches to Mental Retardation.* New York, Basic Books, 1970.
59. Brown BS, Courtless TF: *The Mentally Retarded Offender.* Washington, D.C., The President's Commission on Law Enforcement and Administration of Justice, 1967.
60. Saenger G: *Factors in Influencing the Institutionalization of Mentally Retarded Individuals in New York City.* Albany, New York State Interdependent Health Resources Board, 1960.
61. Kugel R, Trembath J, Sagor S: Some characteristics of patients legally committed to a state institution for the mentally retarded. *Ment Retard* 2;8, 1968.
62. Eisenberg L: Emotional determinants of mental deficiency. *Arch Neurol Psychiatr* 80;114–121, 1958.
63. Benda C, Squires N, Ogonok J, et al: The relationships between intellectual inadequacy and emotional socio-cultural deprivation. *Compr Psychiatr* 5;294, 1964.
64. Eisenberg L: Caste, class and intelligence, in Murry R, Rossner P (eds): *The Genetic, Metabolic, and Developmental Aspects of Mental Retardation.* Springfield, IL, C. C. Thomas, 1972.
65. Beitenman E: The psychiatric consultant in a residential facility for mentally retarded, in Menolascino FJ (ed): *Psychiatric Approaches to Mental Retardation.* New York, Basic Books, 1970.
66. Slivkin S, Bernstein N: Group approaches to treating retarded adolescents, in Menolascino FJ (ed): *Psychiatric Approaches to Mental Retardation.* New York, Basic Books, 1970.
67. Rogers C, Dymond R: *Psychotherapy and Personality Change.* Chicago, University of Chicago Press, 1954.
68. Bailer I: Psychotherapy and adjustment techniques with the mentally retarded, in Baumeister A (ed): *Mental Retardation: Appraisal, Education, Rehabilitation.* Chicago, Aldine, 1957.
69. Bailer I: Emotional disturbances and mental retardation: Etiologic and conceptual relationships, in Menolascino FJ (ed): *Psychiatric Approaches to Mental Retardation.* New York, Basic Books, 1970.

70. Lott G: Psychotherapy of the mentally retarded, in Menolascino FJ (ed): *Psychiatric Approaches to Mental Retardation*. New York, Basic Books, 1970.
71. Katz E: *Mental Health Services for the Mentally Retarded*. Springfield, IL, C. C. Thomas, 1972.
72. Mowatt M: Group therapy approach to emotional conflicts of the mentally retarded and their parents, in Menolascino FJ (ed): *Psychiatric Approaches to Mental Retardation*. New York, Basic Books, 1970.
73. Zisfein L, Rosen M: Effects of a personality adjustment training group counseling program. *Ment Retard* 12(3);50–53, 1974.
74. Wolfensberger W: Diagnosis diagnosed. *J Ment Subnorm* 11;62–70, 1965.
75. Snyder S, Benerjee S, Yamamura H, et al: Drugs, neurotransmitters, and schizophrenia. *Science* 184, 1243, 1974.
76. Cohen DJ: The diagnostic process in child psychiatry. *Psychiatr Ann* 6;29–35, 1976.
77. Freeman R: Drug effects on learning in children: A selective review of the past thirty years. *J Spec Ed* 1;17–44, 1966.
78. Freeman R: Review of medicine in special education: Medical-behavioral pseudorelations. *J Spec Ed* 5(9);93–100, 1970.
79. Freeman R: *Role of Psychoactive Medications in the Retarded*. (*The Education and Rehabilitation of the Mentally Retarded Adolescent and Adult*.) New York, Aldine-Atherton, 1978.
80. Lipman R: The use of psychopharmacological agents in residential facilities for the retarded, in Menolascino FJ (ed): *Psychiatric Approaches to Mental Retardation*. New York, Basic Books, 1970.
81. Colodny D, Kurlander L: Psychopharmacology as a treatment adjunct for the mentally retarded; Problems and issues, in Menolascino FJ (ed): *Psychiatric Approaches to Mental Retardation*. New York, Basic Books, 1970.
82. Nirje B: The normalization principle and its human management implications, in Kugel R, Wolfensberger W (eds): *Changing Patterns in Residental Services for the Mentally Retarded*. Washington, D.C., Government Printing Office, 1969.
83. Lanzkron J: The concept of profschizophrenia and its prognosis. *Am J Ment Def* 61, 544–547, 1957.
84. Strider FD, Menolascino FJ: Treatment of the antisocial personality in the mentally retarded, in Reid W (ed): *The Treatment of Antisocial Syndromes*. New York, Van Nostrand, Rheinhold, 1981.
85. Pueschel SM, Rynder RT (eds): *Down's Syndrome: Advances in Biomedicine and the Behavioral Sciences*. Cambridge, Ware Press, 1982.
86. Monfils MJ, Menolascino FJ: Mental illness in the mentally retarded: Challenges for social work. *J of Soc Work in Health Care*, 9(1), 296–308, 1983.
87. Batshaw ML, Perret YM: *Children with Handicaps: A Medical Primer*. Baltimore, Paul Books, 1981.
88. Michaelis C: *Home and School Partnership in Exceptional Education*. Rockville, Md., Aspen, 1980.
89. Herr SS: *Rights and Advocacy for Retarded People*. Toronto: Lexington Books, 1983.
90. Goldsberg SS: *Special Education Law: A Guide for Parents, Advocates, and Educators*. New York, Plenum Press, 1982.

Need Assessment and Service Planning for Mentally Retarded-Mentally Ill Persons

Ruth Parkhurst

3.1. Introduction

This chapter reviews the establishment, function, and results of a special needs assessment and plan to develop services for persons who have been identified and diagnosed as *both* mentally retarded and emotionally disturbed. Because the findings and the plan of services developed by the project have been applied in other areas of the country, a community may wish to establish a similar approach to meet the needs of this special dual-diagnosis population.

3.2. Overview

This program, known as the Mental Retardation and Emotional Disturbance (MR/ED) Project came into being as a result of discussions in early 1978 among the nine community services boards in eastern Virginia, the Eastern State Hospital, the Southeastern Virginia Training Center, and the Community Services Division of the Virginia Department of Mental Health and Mental Retardation. This was a period during which the deinstitutionalization movement was returning the more severely handicapped population, including mentally retarded persons who were also mentally ill, to often unprepared communities in Virginia. The mentally retarded individual with emotional or psychiatric problems has consistently posed service delivery problems for all jurisdictions within the eastern Virginia region. The recurring problem of lack of adequate services often results in inappropriate or short-term placement. Many individuals were placed in any community-based service that would accept them even if that service did not meet the individual's needs. Others are forced on the institutional community, only to be released after a short assessment period. Those that were retained in the institution often received treatment that consisted solely of medication, room, and board. It appeared that each MH/MR service board within the eastern Virginia region had five or six cases annually that posed such significant problems that they demanded an inordinate proportion of staff time, and most staff felt that the eventual solutions

---

Ruth Parkhurst • North Dorchester Health Services, Hurlock, Maryland 21643.

for the problems were inadequate or, at best, temporary. Reports from other areas of the country suggest that Virginia was not unique in this dilemma of deinstitutionalization to unprepared communities. Clearly, there are many problems and issues to be resolved prior to the development of a service model that will ultimately provide service options for mentally retarded individuals with emotional problems.

The time frame for this project did not permit the resolution of all of the allied problems and issues; instead, simple articulation rather than resolution of some of the problems and issues affecting the service delivery system was a necessary step in the planning process. Problems relating to legislative issues and legislative barriers to services for mentally retarded individuals with emotional problems continued to be cited by community services boards, consultants, agencies, and others attempting to address such problems and to provide services. Those problems and issues are not detailed in this chapter.

The immediate focus of the project was to define the target population. The designation "mentally retarded–emotionally disturbed person," is a diagnostically hetergeneous description because the "dual diagnosis" covers a wide range of mental deficits coupled with a wide range of behavioral maladies. After extensive discussion of the population to be targeted for services, the MR/ED Project Management Committee devised a working definition of dual diagnosis. The committee did not agree unanimously on the definition but accepted it by consensus as a tool that agencies could use in documenting their experience with dually diagnosed clients.

The working definition utilized by the project referred to "A mentally retarded person with behavioral or emotional disturbances which were so severe that the individual could not be served in existing community programs." Further, the *dual* mental disabilities precluded admission to a mental retardation or a state mental-health institution. For example, the individual's past service history typically included expulsion from generic services, attempted service through generic mental-health and mental-retardation facilities, repeated instances of physical aggression that made the person dangerous to self and/or others, behaviors that had led to formal involvements with the courts, and psychiatric problems that are usually associated with mental illness rather than mental retardation.

Using this working definition, the project pragmatically began to address the major objectives, which, stated in simplified form, were to (1) develop a survey instrument to document the MR/ED population in eastern Virginia who have sought, but not received appropriate services; (2) conduct a regionwide needs assessment using the instrument; (3) survey existing service components that might be expanded to provide services to the dually diagnosed population; (4) survey programs for the dually diagnosed population nationwide, and assess the applicability of such models to eastern Virginia; (5) develop a service system model for the dually diagnosed population in eastern Virginia, coordinating services at the community and institutional levels for accessibility to both rural and urban populations; (6) include in the model cost estimates, personnel requirement strategies, location, and potential funding sources; (7) develop legislative and policy recommendations for the delivery of services to MR/ED individuals; and (8) gather data and service information to develop a public-education and prevention package.

Because the targeted population according to the working definition, had to meet the criterion of having attempted unsuccessfully to recieve services from agencies in the area, a survey instrument was designed to assess the experience of agencies with the dual diagnosis population. No attempt was made to document dually diagnosed individuals in the community who were unknown to service providers. Fifty-eight agencies responded to the survey, almost all of those that were contacted. Exceptions included several generic agencies that felt that labeling a client in this category was outside their purview and could possibly violate their clients' civil rights.

The survey instrument consisted of two major components. The first was a questionnaire, which was divided into several sections. In addition to general and staffing information, the questionnaire sought to enumerate separately requests for information on services, applications for services, and actual admissions during calendar year 1978. It then attempted to aggregate and categorize individuals served during that 12-month period on the basis of level of mental retardation, age, sex, and so on. The questionnaire also asked for an inventory of the services that were being provided for those clients being served, but who had not necessarily been dually diagnosed. Another section afforded an opportunity for agency staff to express their personal opinions regarding service delivery policy. The final section consisted of open-ended and multiple-choice questions on recommendations for appropriate planning for the targeted population.

The second major component of the survey instrument was a "special profile" form, which the 58 responding agencies were asked to complete for each person identified as MR/ED, based on their interpretation of the project's working definition. All of the participating agencies indicated that they had had contact with such persons during calendar year 1978. The special profiles constituted documentation of the targeted population in the area. They called for a client name in a coding system that is widely accepted as being nearly impossible to "break." The client name code assured confidentiality, yet made it possible to identify duplicate profiles received from two or more agencies. Each special profile incorporated demographic information, service history, services needed, time devoted to typical clients, diagnoses, descriptions of maladaptive behaviors, and the specific needs of the prospective client for habilitation or rehabilitation.

The project's problem statement projected that perhaps five or six MR/ED individuals were known to each of the nine community services boards. Of the special profiles returned, 31 were actually eliminated because the information reported did not include the dual diagnosis as described in the working definition. An additional 39 were eliminated as duplicates; 394 validated profiles remained.

Although most of the targeted population resided in the community, the Southeastern Virginia Training Center (SEVTC) returned 50 profiles. Because

Table 1. Sex-by-Age Grouping of MR/ED Population Reported in Eastern Virginia

	Age group					Age unknown	Total	%
	0–10	11–21	22–35	36–64	65+			
Number of males	17	86	76	33	3	1	216	55%
Number of females	13	51	62	47	5	0	178	45%
Total in age group	30	137	138	80	8	1	394	
Percentage of cases in age group	7.61%	34.77%	35.03%	20.3%	2.3%	.26%	100%	100%

the center operates as a transitional residence between more and less restrictive environments, these profiles were included in the count, unless duplicated by another agency. Eastern State Hospital did not return any special profiles.

Table 1 shows the age and sex distributions of the 394 cases identified, by percentage of males and females in various age ranges. The age range reported was from 3 to 88 years. Birth dates were not recorded for 17 individuals, and an "estimated age" was reported for 16 of these persons. The 1978 Census data for Virginia indicate that 24% of the general population were 14 years of age or younger, as compared to less than 19% of the MR/ED population. This underrepresentation may indicate that MR/ED individuals are not identified sufficiently early.

A review of Table 1 tends to confirm some preconceived ideas about this population. For example, nearly 70% of all reported cases were between ages 11 and 35, and approximately 35% were in the 11- to 21-year age range. The high rate in the latter group may be attributed partially to the expected higher frequency of adjustment difficulties associated with adolescence.

Approximately 55% of the cases reported were male and some 45% female. A larger population of males had been anticipated. However, the sex distribution closely approximates that in the general population: more MR/ED persons are male up to age 45, after which, more mentally retarded/emotionally disturbed persons are female.

Because the project focused on the MR/ED population, the survey was not designed to provide a good estimate of the prevalence of mental retardation in the region. However, those agencies responding were asked to indicate the mentally retarded population in their program as of December 31, 1978. Their responses became particularly interesting when it was noted that the number of dually diagnosed persons enumerated by the agencies represented approximately 10% of the mentally retarded clients enrolled for their services. Also, the number of dually diagnosed persons reported to be living in the Southeastern Virginia Training Center was approximately 25% of that facility's total population. The SEVTC, with a total of 198 residents on December 31, 1978,

Table 2. Primary Diagnosis by Age Grouping Indicating Level of Retardation

	Age group					Age unknown	Total	% of primary diagnosis
	3–10	11–21	22–31	32–45	46–88			
Mild MR	7	40	23	19	15		104	24.02
Moderate MR	9	30	37	13	8		97	22.40
Severe MR	10	21	11	6	4	1	53	12.24
Profound MR	3	4	1	1			9	2.08
Unspecified MR	1	9	9	1	1		21	4.85
Schizophrenia		17	12	7	8		44	10.16
Affective-depressive disorder		2	5	1	1		9	2.08
Other psychosis		4	8	1	3		16	3.70
Behavior disorder	3	18	7	1	2		31	7.16
Alcoholism				1	1		2	.46
Oher developmental disabilities	4	3	3	3	1		14	3.23
Other physical disorders		1	1				2	.46
Other	4	9	6	4	5		28	6.47
Not reported		2		1			3	.69
Total							433[a]	100%

[a] Total includes 39 duplicates.

provided 50 special profiles on dually diagnosed persons, or roughly 25% of their resident population. Fifty-seven other agencies reported an end-of-year enrollment of 3,503 mentally retarded persons, 394 of whom (11%) were classified as emotionally disturbed. The combined total of 3,701 MR/ED persons living at SEVTC and being served in the community constituted 10.6% of the total mentally retarded population reportedly enrolled in the eastern Virginia demographic area. These rates are similar to those reported in other studies. For example, several full-scale epidemiological studies[1,2] have noted that 12%–15% of the general population may need mental health service at some time in their lives. Institutional studies have indicated that up to 33% or 35% of the population may be dually diagnosed in state hospitals and in state facilities for retarded persons.

Table 2 presents the data on primary diagnosis and age range. As anticipated, most of the dually diagnosed persons were classified as mildly and moderately retarded.

We would anticipate that most of those individuals who were reported to have alcoholism or an affective-depressive disorder as a primary diagnosis to be in the higher functioning levels of mental retardation, and 2% were diagnosed as profoundly retarded. A graphic description of these rates would be an inverted triangle, but less flattened than projected from the four levels of mental retardation among the general population as defined by the American Association on Mental Deficiency.[3] Projections based on the AAMD definition of mental retardation and its four levels have resulted in the following approxi-

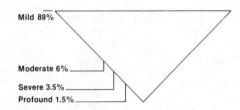

Figure 1. Projected distribution of the symptom of mental retardation.

mations among the general population based on the Wechsler scale: (1) mild mental retardation: 55–69; 89% of total mentally retarded population; (2) moderate retardation: 40–54; 6% of total mentally retarded population; (3) severe mental retardation: 25–39; 3.5% of total mentally retarded population; and (4) profound mental retardation: 0–25; 1.5% of total mentally retarded population. The resulting graphic symmetrical statement is a flattened inverted triangle such as that shown in Figure 1.

Projections based on the cases of mental retardation in eastern Virginia reported as a primary diagnosis result in the approximations noted in Table 3.

The resulting graphic symmetrical statement is an inverted triangle, less flattened than for the general population, as noted in Figure 2. If the data reported to the project were reviewed in such a way as to correlate mental retardation with *another* diagnosis, not distinguishing between primary and secondary diagnosis, then the triangle depicting the levels of mental retardation reported in eastern Virginia would approach the flatness of the classic triangle. For completeness, the data concerning the primary and secondary diagnoses in this sample (before adjustment for duplicated profiles) are presented in Table 4.

The rationale for an extended discussion of the data collected by the MR/ED project is twofold. First, precious little information has apparently been collected and published on this population, whether descriptive or for statistical analysis. The second reason follows from the first: although the data collected are mainly descriptive, they were found to have validity on the basis of census data and other limited but recent studies.

Table 3. Mental Retardation as the Primary Diagnosis

Level	% of primary diagnosis		% of total MR primary diagnosis
Mild and unspecified	28.87	=	44.02
Moderate	22.41	=	34.17
Severe	12.24	=	18.67
Profound	2.08	=	3.17
	65.59%		100%
	of primary diagnosis		of MR as primary diagnosis

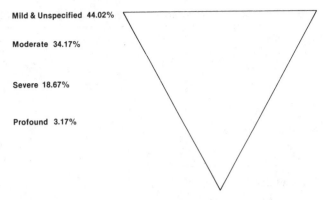

Mild & Unspecified 44.02%

Moderate 34.17%

Severe 18.67%

Profound 3.17%

Figure 2. Graphic depiction of mental retardation as primary diagnosis.

After documenting the MR/ED population who were in need of services in the region, the focus of the project turned to identifying program models that might be adapted to meet the existing needs in this area of human services.

3.3. Developing a Plan of Service for the Identified MR/ED Citizen

A search fo model programs serving the MR/ED population was made by the project through a nationwide national survey of each state's department of mental health and mental retardation. Thirty of these agencies responded. Twelve indicated that they knew of no programs for dually diagnosed persons. Several indicated they were under mandated deinstitutionalization but had made no plans for MR/ED clients, and they asked that the project provide information on its findings.

Each of the programs identified by the state agencies was then contacted by the project. Several responded that, contrary to the information received from the state, they did not provide services to MR/ED persons but were in need of such resources to which to refer clients. Often, they, too, asked to be informed on the progress of the project. Responses to this survey provided information on programs in mental retardation institutions, mental health institutions, day activities in community settings serving both institutionalized and community residents, and community residential programs—all designed specifically for persons dually diagnosed as mentally retarded and emotionally disturbed. The programs that responded affirmatively were screened by mail and phone. After information was obtained on services, staffing, costs, and details of programming, visits were made to programs in a variety of settings that had distinctive service features. These programs are described in detail in the final report of the project. Representatives from the programs visited were invited as consultants to a workshop setting in the eastern Virginia area. The response of those associated with effective programs for dually diagnosed persons was highly gratifying. Without fail, program administrators were willing

Table 4. Rank Order of Primary and Secondary Diagnoses Reported for the MR/ED Population

Primary diagnosis	*Frequency*
Mild MR	104
Moderate MR	97
Severe MR	53
Schizophrenia	44
Behavior disorder	31
Other	28
Unspecified MR	21
Other psychosis	16
Developmental disability	14
Profound MR	9
Affective-depressive disorder	9
Alcoholism	2
Other physical disability	2
Not reported	3
Total	433[a]

Secondary diagnosis	*Frequency*
Behavior disorder	107
Mild MR	68
Other	40
Schizophrenia	37
Moderate MR	31
Other psychosis	29
Affective-depressive disorder	21
Other physical disability	15
Developmental disability	12
Unspecified MR	11
Severe MR	10
Alcoholism	7
Drug abuse	3
Profound MR	2
Deafness	2
Not reported	38
Total	433[a]

[a] Totals include 39 duplicates.

to share their experiences and expertise in helping the eastern Virginia areas to initiate their own local programs.

To further aid project staff in developing recommendations following the workshop, each community services board examined its continuum of services to determine how the gap in services for the MR/ED client could be filled most expeditiously. As the Project Management Committee considered the aggregate of the community services boards' continua of services, the program models reviewed, and the earlier documentation of need, they came to a consensus in naming and prioritizing the following recommendations.

The first recommendation called for the establishment of *crisis center(s)* accessible throughout eastern Virginia for MR/ED persons. The second recommendation dealt with *special staff training* for the treatment of MR/ED persons in the community and in institutions. This recommendation was based on a finding of the project not detailed above: staff serving MR/ED clients in other areas had developed their own training programs, or the respective state had designed a specific training program. No generally accepted course of study was found to exist to train staff for such programs. The third recommendation addressed the *lack of community living arrangements* for the targeted population, particularly adults, and called for the development of community-based residences. How soon these and other recommendations of the project can be implemented will depend on a variety of factors, including funding sources, staffing, and innovation by those who carry other primary responsibilities but remain concerned about this population.

As an aside, the relatively few programs designed specifically to serve MR/ED persons might well benefit by developing a network; a newsletter for this purpose is under consideration. The need for such networking became evident during the course of the project as program staff facing similar service-delivery problems contacted the project with increasing frequency.

3.4. Summary

The Commonwealth of Virginia has actively advocated and promulgated its policy of attempting to provide services for all of its mentally handicapped citizens, whether that diagnosis refers to mental retardation or to mental illness. The method of delivery of these services in the state has been, either directly or indirectly, the subject of several recent studies. Certainly, the desire to provide appropriate services meshed with recent documentation of need can be the cornerstone of an effective service-delivery system that must include access for persons dually diagnosed as experiencing both mental retardation and mental illness.

References

1. Strolle J: *Mental Health in the Metropolis*. New York, McGraw-Hill, 1962.
2. Leighton A: *My Name is Legion*. New York, Basic Books, 1959.
3. Grossman H (ed): *Manual on Terminology and Classification in Mental Retardation*. Washington, D.C., American Association on Mental Deficiency, 1983.

II

Treatment and Management Interventions

Introduction

In Part I, we provided an overview of dual diagnosis, and numerous "why" questions were posed and analyzed regarding the nature, the incidence, and needs assessment for mentally ill/mentally retarded individuals. In Part II, the authors focus their attention on treatment strategies and management interventions for this population. In trying to answer the "how" question of treating and managing this population, we are faced with a particularly difficult challenge because the combined impairment of mental illness and mental retardation compounds the problem in such a way that traditionally proven techniques are not always effective. Treatment approaches for mentally ill individuals have basically required verbal techniques with a relatively sophisticated language basis. However, when we try to apply these same types of techniques with cognitively impaired individuals, we need to alter the approach and modify the process in such a way that we can communicate effectively.

These five chapters are comprehensive in their approach and focus on two major areas. The first area involves treatment and management techniques ranging from behavior therapy and multimodel therapy to individual and group treatment approaches. The second area focuses on age groups, with one chapter analyzing psychopharmacological approaches with children and the other chapter focusing on vocational habilitation techniques with adolescents and adults.

Chapter 4 is a scholarly piece of work by two individuals at the Waisman Center, which has a long history as one of the outstanding research centers in the country for the dually diagnosed population. Dr. Gardner has an international reputation in the area of behavior modification and its application to mentally retarded individuals, particularly in teaching this group the necessary skills for living in community-based settings. With the able contributions of his young colleague, Dr. Cole, this chapter describes the various behavioral therapy procedures available to professionals who want to provide services to mentally retarded individuals in various agencies and community settings.

Dr. Gardner compares the changes that have taken place since his 1970 chapter on behavior therapy with mentally retarded individuals in Dr. Menolascino's seminal work on the *Psychiatric Aspects of Mental Retardation*. In this current chapter, Gardner and Cole delineate the technological improvements that behavioral techniques have undergone during these last 14 years. Of major significance is the importance of reducing aversive conditioning as a way of modifying and changing the mentally retarded individuals's behavior. Indeed, Dr. Gardner and Dr. Cole offer techniques and strategies that are effective in alleviating serious self-injurious behaviors without resorting to punitive techniques, which result in adverse side effects. This chapter may well be the most comprehensive of its kind in treating the topic of behavior therapy with mentally retarded individuals, particularly in community-based settings.

In addition to focusing on various age levels and the different techniques to use with the mentally retarded-mentally ill, different chapters also focus on different cognitive levels of the mentally retarded population. In Chapter 5, we see a description of individual and group therapeutic approaches to mild and moderately retarded individuals. Although mentally retarded individuals were once thought incapable of benefiting from psychotherapy on an individual or group basis, they are indeed today participating in a wide range of therapeutic programs. The authors of this chapter, a psychiatric social worker and a psychiatrist, have had an extensive amount of applied experience with this population.

Most professionals in the field of mental health have had very little course work or experience in treating the mentally retarded. As a result, they lack the knowledge and the technique to alter their verbal techniques and approaches in working with mentally retarded individuals. Often, the same is true of those trained in mental retardation: They lack a basic understanding and knowledge of individual and group psychotherapeutic techniques and those variables that are important in achieving successful outcomes. Thus, the readers of Chapter 5 will find it quite helpful in understanding what counselor and client variables are important to a successful outcome as well as which therapeutic techniques are essential in treating specific problems in individual or group settings. These techniques are applied to specific problems exhibited by this population. Included is a review of the research findings in this area, which, we might add, are disappointingly few.

Chapter 6 is authored by Dr. Donaldson, a child psychiatrist who also has extensive experience in providing services and conducting research with mentally retarded children with emotional disorders. This chapter specifically focuses on behavioral disorders and the use of psychopharmacological approaches in the treatment of these disorders. In treating children with mental retardation and mental illness, it is important for the practitioner to be able to identify what abnormalities can and cannot be remedied with medication, what the pharmacological actions of medications are, what are the most common side effects of medication, and finally what are some of the typical problems that occur when providing psychotropic medication to this particular population. The reader should also find it extremely helpful to read the section on dietary and nutritional considerations, which provides additional alternatives to medications, particularly when drugs are not effective or cannot be used. In addition, Dr. Donaldson provides an important chapter for the understanding of which medications are no longer appropriate, particularly in terms of using them simply to control behavior. Rather, he feels the more accurate and important function of medications is to correct brain physiology and/or biochemistry in order to improve learning, interpersonal relationships, and productive behavior.

Numerous clinicians and researchers feel that the mentally ill-mentally retarded population is the most underserved population in the United States. If this is true, surely the severest of the severe are the most difficult, perplexing, challenging population, particularly if we are to be successful in providing deinstitutionalization for these neglected persons.

The questions that are most frequently asked by those individuals who work with this most severely affected population, particularly at the adolescent and adult level, are who they are, why we should provide services to them, what can be done to help them, and how can one best go about meeting their needs. The authors of Chapter 7 have had a combined experience of over 60 years in research, training, and clinical services with this population. Operating through a psychiatric institute and a university-affiliated program, they first provide the reader with insight into the parameters of this population via client profiles. Second, they dispel some of the mythology surrounding the traditional approaches in treatment to working with this population, such as utilizing diagnostic testing procedures, inappropriately packaged curriculum programs, and philosophical beliefs and values that have resulted in the construction of diversive techniques producing less than successful outcomes for this most difficult population.

The authors of this chapter provide the reader with teaching strategies for working with the mentally ill-mentally retarded and in conclusion discuss the content or the curriculum established in running programs to best meet the needs of this dually diagnosed population.

Finally, in Chapter 8, Dr. Bates pulls together all the techniques and treatment strategies in a multimodality approach in working with this population. Dr. Bates analyzes the efficacy of psychotherapy, psychopharmacological treatment, and finally the emerging role of biofeedback and relaxation training techniques. Dr. Bates provides a structural framework in which all of these approaches and techniques can be combined to provide a powerful, multidimensional approach to improving this population's skills and abilities.

Use of Behavior Therapy with the Mentally Retarded in Community Settings

William I. Gardner and Christine L. Cole

4.1. Introduction

As noted earlier in Chapter 2, the mentally retarded have an increased susceptibility to the development of various behavioral and emotional difficulties. Surveys of community clinics serving mentally retarded children suggest a high prevalence of mental health difficulties.[1,2] Other studies of mentally retarded individuals living in the community have reported a 20%–35% and higher frequency of behavioral and emotional disturbances.[3,4] Recent reports also suggest that a wide range of problems are present in the mentally retarded served by community developmental disability and mental health services.[5,6]

The presence of behavioral and emotional difficulties represents one of the major reasons for institutional placement of the mentally retarded. These difficulties also assume a significant role in the continued institutionalization[7] and in the majority of adjustment failures and reinstitutionalization of those placed in the community.[8,9] Maladaptive behaviors are frequently cited as a major factor contributing to community vocational failure.[10,11] Recent findings also indicate that community residential facilities not only are less likely to admit the mentally retarded with maladaptive behaviors but also are more likely to dismiss them for reinstitutionalization in public facilities.[12]

Recent legislation and litigations have increased the need for adequate attention to the mental health problems presented by the mentally retarded in the community. The deinstitutionalization movement has resulted in the return to community living arrangements of numerous individuals with severe personal adjustment problems. The very process followed in many states of quickly accomplishing deinstitutionalization and other normalizing service-delivery programs, such as mainstreaming, has exacerbated rather than reduced personal adjustment difficulties in many individuals. PL 94-142 (the Education of All Handicapped Children Act), passed and signed into law in 1975, mandated that every school system in the nation make provision for a free, appropriate public education for every child between the ages of 3 and 21, regardless of how, or how seriously, he or she may be handicapped. Thus, mentally retarded

William I. Gardner and Christine L. Cole • Waisman Center on Mental Retardation and Human Development, University of Wisconsin, Madison, Wisconsin 53706.

children, adolescents, and young adults with severe problems of adjustment can no longer be denied placement in community educational programs because of their difficulties in adapting to the requirements of the setting. Vocational rehabilitation agencies are mandated by PL 93-112 and the comprehensive Rehabilitation Services Amendments of 1978 to serve the more severely disabled. Numerous mentally retarded adults with severe mental health problems who previously had been categorically rejected as nonfeasible for vocational rehabilitation services must now be provided suitable rehabilitation programs. In summary, community living, educational, and rehabilitation agencies have no choice but to provide adequate services to the mentally retarded in the community.

The present chapter describes various behavior therapy procedures available to professionals providing services to the mentally retarded in community mental health, educational, developmental disabilities, and rehabilitation agencies. In our opinion, professionals in any agency providing services to the mentally retarded and their families should have basic clinical skills in identifying and providing effective treatment for behavioral and emotional difficulties in the setting in which these occur. Minor adjustment problems should not go unattended in non-mental health agencies until these develop into major difficulties. Educators, social workers, and rehabilitation personnel, for example, who provide services to the mentally retarded should be skillful in dealing with problems of development and adjustment *at the time* these occur in the community agency and home settings. Consultation from mental health specialists and/or referral to mental health agencies can then be reserved for those more difficult and chronic problems that do not respond sufficiently to services provided by generic staff within the more natural program settings of homes, schools, and recreational, vocational, and related agencies. The behavior therapy procedures are quite applicable for use in such settings by skillful agency staff of various professional disciplines.

The behavioral therapies to be described become especially significant in light of the difficulties associated with the use of various psychological and psychiatric treatment procedures with the mentally retarded. Although of obvious value in the treatment of some specific emotional and behavioral difficulties, the current limitations of psychotropic drug therapy in the effective and comprehensive treatment of many of the behavioral and emotional disorders of the mentally retarded are well documented.[13,14] The efficacy and practicality of various psychotherapy approaches, as typically defined and practiced, has been questioned by a number of writers.[15,16] Additionally, shortage of mental health professionals with both the skills for and the interest in serving the mentally retarded contributes to the necessity that available school, developmental disabilities, and rehabilitation agency personnel be knowledgeable about and proficient in the use of a variety of effective treatment approaches, including behavioral ones.[17]

Thirteen years have passed since the following observations were made by Gardner[18] in Menolascino's significant book, *Psychiatric Approaches to Mental Retardation*:

Recent results of the application of behavior modification techniques described in the clinical and research literature provide illustration of behavior change of a range, degree, and rate which most psychiatric, psychological, and educational personnel had not thought possible due to the inherent limitations of the mentally retarded. . . . It has been demonstrated that at least a significant degree of behavioral limitations of many mentally retarded individuals resides in an inappropriate or limited learning environment, rather than being an unalterable manifestation of the individual's retardation. Severely and profoundly involved mentally retarded persons who for years were beyond help or hope have, as a result of treatment programs using the systematic application of behavior modification procedures, developed language, motor, perceptual, cognitive, affective, and social skills that have rendered them more independent and more able to experience a meaningful personal and social existence. Additionally, other less disabled persons exhibiting an array of maladaptive behavior patterns have responded favorably to behavior modification efforts. (pp. 250–251)

In the years since these observations were made, behavior therapy approaches have continued to develop and to gain acceptance in a variety of settings, including the community mental health, education, vocational, and developmental disabilities agency programs providing services to the mentally retarded. The major advances in behavior therapy application to the mentally retarded that have occurred during the 1970s and the early 1980s are highlighted throughout the chapter. Additionally, the limitations and potential misuses of behavior therapy procedures are recognized.

An initial presentation of major assumptions and behavior principles that underlie the therapy procedures used with a variety of problem behaviors will provide a perspective for the reader who is not trained in the theory and practice of behavior therapy. Reference should be made to such resources as Gardner[19]; Hersen and Bellack[20]; Hersen, Eisler, and Miller[21]; Rimm and Masters[22]; and Walker *et al.*,[23] for more extensive descriptions of the nature of the current behavior therapies, as well as to recent works of Jansen[24]; Johnson and Baumeister[25]; Karan and Gardner[26]; Matson and McCartney[27]; and Schroeder, Mulick, and Schroeder,[28] for comprehensive critical reviews of the use of various behavior therapy procedures with the mentally retarded. Although the following discussion focuses on problem areas typically viewed as clinical or mental health problems (e.g., the treatment of phobias[29] and the treatment of an emotionally disturbed young adult[30]), reference is provided to the treatment of developmental, educational, and vocational difficulties to illustrate both the range of application and the basic similarities among the behavior therapy procedures employed regardless of the type of problems addressed or the settings in which the problems occur.

4.2. Basic Concepts

4.2.1. Definition of Behavior Therapy

The behavior therapy approach to the assessment, management, and treatment of difficulties of personal development and adjustment of the mentally retarded involves a variety of therapeutic procedures that have been found useful in influencing behavior in a beneficial manner. Groups of procedures are identified by such terms as *behavior modification, behavior therapy, social learning, respondent (emotional) learning, applied behavior analysis, cognitive behavior therapy, contingency management,* and *behavior management.* Although each term is used by various writers to refer to specific groups of procedures and to the major conceptual foundations underlying these, the term *behavior therapy* is used in a generic sense in the present chapter to refer to the variety of therapeutic procedures typically viewed as "behavioral." Kazdin[31] and Bellack, Hersen, and Kazdin[32] should be consulted by readers interested in the historical development and the contemporary status of specific groups of procedures.

4.2.2. Concepts of Etiology

The behavioral approach describes various chronic difficulties of adjustment or adaptation as *exceptional learning and behavior characteristics* and seeks to understand these by making use of principles and concepts of learning and related "theories" of behavior development, maintenance, and change.[19] Behavior characteristics are viewed as resulting from a biologically and experientially unique person as he or she has and does interact with social and physical environments. It is assumed that the person's behavioral capabilities—and difficulties—at any time represent the end result of a most complex learning history, whose effects have accumulated to provide both the form of current behaviors and the "meanings" or influences that certain environmental events have on the person's behaviors.[33]

A chronic excessive fear of social contact by a mentally retarded adult, in illustration, would be viewed as representing "the end point of the interaction of genetic constitutional factors, the current physiological state of the individual, his current environmental conditions, and past learning which, in turn, was a function of a similar interaction" (p. 6).[34] The physiological components of this cluster of influencing events refer to the person's total physical characteristics. As noted by Bijou,[35] atypical biological factors may limit a person's response equipment—his or her sensory, motor, and/or neurological connecting systems—and thus interfere with or reduce his or her normal response potential. Or these may provide an abnormal internal environment, so that the stimulation usually present is either absent or occurs with higher than usual intensity or duration. Under these conditions, atypical reactions may occur, as when a person is overreactive to minor distractions. In the case of sensory and muscular handicaps, the person may be limited in the types and intensities of stimulation to which she or he may be receptive and to the type of responses that she or he can make. Again, the mentally retarded person's current behavior, typical or exceptional, reflects the influence of these individually unique physical states or conditions. In view of the frequent occurrence of physical abnormalities in the mentally retarded, such factors must be considered in attempts to understand problem behaviors. However, it is recognized that problem behavior patterns that appear to be a direct result of physical factors may respond positively to behavior therapy approaches. In illustration, some mentally retarded individuals with CNS impairment may be prone to exhibit hyperactivity, impulsivity, and attentional problems. Nonetheless, it may be possible to obtain improvement in these problem areas through the use of behavior therapy procedures.[36] As a second example, mentally retarded persons with various medical disorders, such as the Lesch-Nyhan syndrome or the Cornelia de Lange syndrome, have a tendency to demonstrate severe and chronic episodes of self-injurious behaviors, such as biting the tongue, lips, and fingers; face slapping; and head banging. Various behavior therapy procedures have been found effective in reducing the severity and chronicity of severe self-mutilation in some instances, even though there appears to be a physical basis for the aberrant behavior.[37]

4.2.3. Common Set of Concepts

Exceptional characteristics are viewed as reflecting the same learning and related principles that are involved in the development and maintenance of appropriate characteristics. Thus, the behavioral features of the mentally retarded described by various psychopathological explanatory models as inadequate, inappropriate, symptomatic, neurotic, disordered, pathological, or maladaptive are viewed as resulting from the person's previous and current experiences. (As noted previously, the potential influence of physical factors is recognized. The physical factors obviously must be identified and treated by medical procedures when possible.) There is no assumption that there is a discontinuity between desirable and exceptional characteristics, that is, that normal behavior is caused by one set of factors and that "abnormal" or "pathological" behavior is caused by a different set of factors. A mentally retarded adolescent who engages in highly aggressive and disruptive behaviors at home and in school would not be viewed by the behavioral model as demonstrating a "conduct disorder" or a "disturbance of impulse control," nor would she or he be otherwise labeled with diagnostic constructs that reflect some internal deviancy. Rather, these behavioral characteristics would be viewed as reflecting a set of previous learning experiences and the effects of the current interactions between the adolescent and the social environment(s).

In a real sense, the social environments in which the exceptional behavior characteristics developed have provided inappropriate or "abnormal" experiences for the retarded adolescent. Such undesired learning or behavior characteristics frequently represent the *normal outcome* of the effects of an "abnormal" environment. The environmental experiences are viewed as abnormal, as these create or contribute to the person's difficulties. Abnormal features of the environment thus are defined relative to the response characteristics and capabilities of the mentally retarded person at a specific time. If a mentally retarded child is provided academic instruction in the classroom that assumes both prerequisite visual discrimination and memory skills that are not present, the child may not learn what is expected. The excessive failure and the resulting frustration may contribute to the range of disruptive emotional and social behaviors. The learning and related behavior difficulties reflect a mismatch between the child's characteristics and those assumed by the instructional program. As a second example, if a severely retarded child is exposed to frequent and intense abusive outbursts from an ill-tempered adult, intensive and pervasive negative emotional reactions may result. The behavioral model would not view the child as abnormal. The negative emotionality that the child displays would not be viewed as abnormal. The environmental experiences to which the child has been exposed, however, would represent the abnormal variable in the development of the debilitating emotional reactions.

The implication of this view of abnormality is both obvious and of considerable importance to the behavior therapist. Efforts to understand or to change such exceptional learning and behavior characteristics must focus on the previous and present abnormal experiences, instead of on any assumed abnormality residing in the child.

To emphasize, the particular experiences that are abnormal for any mentally retarded person are quite relative. For example, a given set of learning experiences may be quite successful in promoting appropriate behavior development for individuals who do not exhibit developmental difficulties. However, these same experiences may result in numerous problems for those who do demonstrate various exceptional difficulties. Many children may learn and behave quite well in an environment in which they are permitted to move freely from one activity to another. Other children with chronic difficulties in focusing and maintaining attention may find this a disastrous environment. A more highly structured situation, in which irrelevant stimuli are reduced, may result in more appropriate behaviors. As a second illustration, an open classroom environment may be excellent for many children, but for others with various peer relationship difficulties, such an unstructured environment may serve only to increase their disorganized, disruptive, and emotionally disquieting characteristics. This discussion emphasizes the necessity of tailoring the therapeutic experiences to an individual person's current characteristics. As the person develops more adaptive competency behaviors, the types of experiences provided can become more normalized.

4.2.4. Explanation of Behavior

The behavioral model approaches the question of explanation (e.g., "Why does my mentally retarded daughter have such intense temper outbursts?") from both the *developmental* (historical) and the *functional* (contemporary) viewpoints. A *developmental* viewpoint emphasizes that consistently occurring behavior patterns, whether appropriate or inappropriate, are frequently the end result of literally hundreds of previous experiences. At any given time, any specific experience may exert only a minute influence on the development, maintenance, or modification of various complex behavior patterns. But 25, 100, 200, 500, or 1,000 or more such experiences could, on the one hand, gradually result in an obnoxious, argumentative, highly anxious, aggressive person, whereas other, more appropriate experiences could result in a cooperative, attentive, enthusiastic individual. Thus, although the behavioral approach focuses on exceptional characteristics as these occur in a present social and physical environment, the approach recognizes that these behaviors are rooted in earlier experiences of the person. In fact, to the extent that present exceptional characteristics can be viewed as learned behavior, prior learning is a given.

In seeking an explanation for, or an understanding of, a person's current exceptional characteristics, the primary concern of the behavior therapist is to identify the current external and internal conditions that contribute to the occurrence of these behaviors, that is, to develop a *functional* explanation. If an adolescent engages in excessive verbal and physical aggression, the therapist is careful not to confuse description with explanation. It might be noticed that the adolescent who displays frequent aggressive outbursts is angry a majority of the time while attending his prevocational training program. It might be tempting to suggest, "John fights because he is angry," thus using a description of one of his characteristics as an explanation for another of his characteristics. Being angry may well be one of the conditions that increases the likelihood of fighting, but anger would not be viewed as an adequate explanation of the behavior. It would be necessary to identify other *preceding environmental conditions* (e.g., when teased by a peer who is smaller than he is), *consequences* (e.g., his verbal aggression terminates the teasing), and *personal features* (e.g., he has limited alternative skills in expressing his anger) of John as a basis for developing a more meaningful (useful) complex of interrelated functional hypotheses.

4.2.5. Focus of Behavior Therapy

The behavior therapy approach focuses primarily on the development of appropriate behaviors and not merely on reducing or eliminating excessive exceptional characteristics. A problem behavior or cluster of problems is not viewed as a *symptom* of some hypothetical internal deviancy or pathology. Rather, the *problem behaviors* are the primary focus of intervention. As a primary intervention strategy, the behavior therapy program is designed to teach prosocial behaviors to replace inappropriate ways of behaving. If the mentally retarded adult is displaying excessive temper tantrums in his home, he is taught not merely to "control his temper" but also to express his emotions in a more acceptable fashion. If a child is physically aggressive when she becomes "jealous" of the attention provided her peers and, as a result, has been isolated by her peers, the behavior therapy goals would consist of teaching the child appropriate means of actively relating to her feelings and her peers in a more socially appropriate and personally enhancing manner.

Mary, a 14-year-old moderately retarded adolescent, illustrates this therapy focus. She was engaging in numerous episodes of physical and verbal aggression in her school program and at home. During clinical behavioral assessment, a number of events, such as teasing by peers, teaching instructions, and lack of immediate availability of desired consequences, were identified as resulting in a heightened state of negative emotional arousal. When she was upset, any minor provocation resulted in aggressive outbursts. It thus appeared that a variety of experiences produced such emotional reactions as anger, sadness, loneliness, disappointment, or embarrassment, that, in turn, resulted in a common reaction of aggression. Mary had not learned to respond differently to different emotions. Rather, any state of negative emotional arousal resulted in the single reaction of aggression. Instead of attempting to suppress her aggression, the behavior therapy program was designed to teach Mary (1) to recognize and label different emotions; (2) to relate these different emotions to the differing precipitating conditions; and (3) to use a variety of self-managed socially appropriate behaviors to replace the undifferentiated aggressive reaction.

The behavioral approach thus does not attempt to "cure" the mentally retarded client, as no assumption is made that there are some central internal psychic factors that, if changed or eliminated, would reciprocally alleviate the person's symptomatic behavior problems. Rather a *direct* attempt is made to change those behavioral and environmental factors that are involved in or that comprise the person's difficulties. As noted, this viewpoint assumes that all consistent psychological characteristics of a mentally retarded person, appropriate and inappropriate, are the end results (symptoms, if you wish) of a history of experiences and of a contemporary set of conditions as these have and do interact with specific physical and psychological characteristics of the individual.

The behavior therapy model recognizes, of course, the interrelationships of various patterns or clusters of behavior difficulties. Some problem behaviors may have a functional relationship with other problem behaviors and thus, by their presence, influence the likelihood of the occurrence of other inappropriate behaviors. In illustration, a mentally retarded adult may become highly emotional and disruptive in a range of situations in which he does not "have his way." This behavior pattern, with a high probability of occurrence under the described conditions, may effectively block the occurence of other, prosocial behaviors that are available in his repertoire. Additionally, such disruptive outbursts may interfere with participation in various prosocial experiences with peers, so that, in turn, the acquisition of new or more complex and appropriate modes of behavior is impeded. The behavior therapy program thus may focus on a reduction of the strong, disruptive emotional outbursts as an integral component of teaching alternative skills of emotional expression and social interaction.

A practical basis for focusing on the development of prosocial replacement behaviors as an alternative to merely attempting to eliminate specific inappropriate behavior relates to the observation that the elimination or the suppression of behavior provides no guarantee that appropriate behaviors will, in fact, begin to occur. As emphasized by Jansen[24] and Touchette,[38] a mentally retarded person may have no other appropriate behavior in his or her repertoire to replace the one eliminated. Touchette[38] noted:

> Drugs, punishment, and restraint may solve the immediate problem of those who must care for the child, but they do not alleviate the problem of the child. The problem

is, and will continue to be, behavioral insufficiency. There is a real danger that procedures which suppress undesirable behavior and accomplish nothing else, will delay or prevent any constructive solution to the child's problems. (p. 199)

Additionally, as noted by Jansen[24]:

If one attempts to reduce or eliminate a retarded client's maladaptive behavior without developing a functional substitute for that behavior, it is likely that the maladaptive behavior will reappear in a very short time. (p. 226)

4.2.6. Location of Therapy

As behavior difficulties are viewed as reflecting the interactions between the individual and his or her social environments, the focus of therapy is on the problem behaviors as these occur in the person's everyday environments (e.g., the workshop, the home, and the classroom). Further, specific situations and relationships within these settings may become the major focus of interest. If, for example, the mentally retarded adolescent is highly disruptive during academic classes, the behavior therapy program is designed to treat the problem in these settings. If the adolescent becomes self-abusive in the prevocational training program, therapy is provided in that setting. If the child soils his clothing only in the school environment, the therapy for encopresis would occur within the school setting. Recall the previously described position that any excessively occurring behavior is best understood and influenced by viewing it as a function of the person *in interaction with* current social and physical settings. Changes must occur in the social experiences provided the person, in most instances, in order to ensure that the person will develop new adaptive behaviors.

4.2.7. Role of the Behavior Therapist

The behavior therapist frequently does not work directly with the mentally retarded client, in contrast to more traditional approaches to psychological treatment of emotional and behavioral difficulties in which the therapist assumes a central role in interacting with the client in a therapist—client relationship. The major emphasis in such therapy systems is on frequent close personal contact through play, verbal, or related modes of interaction.

As the behavioral approach views difficulties as reflecting the effects of current experiences within the client's physical and social environments, the major therapist role typically becomes that of changing the environmental experiences. If a child is having difficulty in the home, the child-in-the-family becomes the focus of treatment, with the therapist providing programmatic direction to rearranging various relationships. If an adolescent is having difficulties in *school and home*, family and school members as they interact with the adolescent become the focus of treatment. If an adult has difficulties relating to peers in her vocational training program because of her shy and passive demeanor, the work supervisor, the counselor, and her peers assume the therapeutic roles. In essence, the therapeutic role typically is assumed by parents, teachers, counselors, siblings, and others in the person's daily living environments. As a result, both the mentally retarded person and the relevant social environments change in a mutually beneficial manner.

4.2.8. Status of Diagnosis

The behavioral approach to diagnosis differs from the more traditional internal deviancy model, which uses assessment as a means of diagnosing some presumed internal mental deviancy, disorder, or illness. As noted earlier, the internal deviancy model views behavior difficulties as symptom manifestations of some underlying disorder(s) and thus focuses diagnostic and therapeutic attention on these more basic conditions.

In contrast, the diagnostic activities of the behavior therapist focus on identifying current problems, on describing them as objectively as possible and on relating them (1) to aspects of the person's external and internal environments and (2) to other behavioral features of the person.

Problem areas are viewed either as reflecting classes of *deficit* or *excessive* behaviors. Some exceptional characteristics create problems of learning and of personal adaptation because of their excessive nature. Excessive behaviors (e.g., temper outbursts, phobias, self-injurious acts, and rumination) are those behaviors that actively interfere with the occurrence of desired behaviors or with the acquisition of new appropriate ways of behaving, and that are viewed as undesirable by the person and/or by others in the person's social environments. Problem areas also may reflect the absence, the limited development, or the inconsistent occurrence of the behaviors or related personal characteristics required for adaptation to various situations, that is, *deficit* behavior areas (e.g., limited social skills, limited self-management skills, and poorly developed toileting skills).

Again, the diagnostic activities of the behavior therapist become those of describing and measuring the strength of the person's excessive and deficit behavior areas as these occur in designated social settings, and of developing hunches about the historical and current experiential conditions that influence these problem areas. Additionally, hunches are developed about the possible relationships between various excessive and deficit problem areas as a basis for deciding on the initial focus of therapy. An adolescent may consistently react with excessive withdrawal when criticized by adults or when teased by peers. These excessive reactions must be viewed in the context of deficit social and emotional skills of relating to such behavior of others. If alternative prosocial skills of expressing one's feelings and of resolving interpersonal conflict are not in the person's repertoire, the therapy program may focus initially on developing these skills and on encouraging their use in the context of adult and peer relationships. Merely attempting to control the withdrawal reactions through various suppressive procedures would have only temporary, if any, benefits, as the client would have no effective social and emotional skills of relating to the emotional agitation associated with criticism or teasing.

4.2.9. Development of Intervention Programs

As problem behaviors are viewed as resulting from an interaction of the mentally retarded person and his or her physical and social environments, *client-specific* assessment is undertaken. The purpose of such behavioral assessment is twofold. First, the therapist attempts to identify current internal and external factors that may contribute to the problem behaviors. Assessment data are used by the therapist to understand the problem, that is, to develop a series of hunches about *current* factors that contribute to the problem behaviors. Even though the therapist may attempt to reconstruct a previous history in an effort to understand how the current problem areas developed over time, this "understanding" is not viewed as a critical aspect of program development or as crucial to the realization of therapeutic goals. This assessment strategy is based on the assumption that there is no necessary relationship between those historical factors involved in the initial development of problem behaviors (etiology) and those contemporary factors that are currently functional in instigating and maintaining the problem behaviors.

Again, hunches are developed about current events or conditions that increase the likelihood that problem behaviors will occur (e.g., negative emotional arousal), as well as about the function served by the behaviors once they do occur (e.g., aggression produces social attention). Hunches are developed about such factors as these, which represent potential targets of behavioral intervention. The second purpose of behavioral assessment, therefore, is to select behavior therapy procedures. For example, a hunch may be developed that at least one function served by the highly disruptive behaviors of a mentally retarded adolescent toward his high school teacher is that they result in a negative reaction by the teacher. This hypothesis could then be translated into a set of intervention procedures aimed at removing or reducing the negative reactions, increasing the positive reinforcement value of the teacher, and teaching the adolescent other social skills that could be used to more appropriately exert personal influence over his teacher and other adults in authority roles. Thus, the behavior therapy program developed is *client-specific*.

A major assessment approach used by the behavior therapist is direct observation of the mentally retarded person in the various natural settings in which problems occur.[39] This observation may be by the therapist, by the client himself or herself, or by social agents in the client's environment. This direct observation assessment approach is of especial utility for those mentally retarded clients who are unable, because of limited verbal skills, to provide information about the problem behaviors and characteristics that might relate to the problems. As emphasized, behavior difficulties that occur in specific settings (e.g., home, school, or social group) in relation to specific persons or requirements must be assessed in these contexts. This approach, again, is based on the supposition that behavior is a function not solely of the person, but of a person in interaction with various social and physical environments. The problem behaviors can best be understood only in these contexts.

With this view, it would seldom make sense to remove the person from the natural environment and place him or her in another for evaluation.

Menolascino[3] has emphasized the difficulties inherent in observing a person in a variety of settings that are alien to the person, such as is done when the retarded child is placed in a diagnostic center for study. All too frequently, the characteristics observed in such settings are not those used as the basis for the referral or the diagnosis.

This situation is illustrated by a recent experience with a mildly retarded young man who had been dismissed from a vocational training program following frequent episodes of physical aggression toward peers, staff, and property. He was placed in a diagnostic work training center and remained there for three months without one single episode of aggression. During this diagnostic experience, he was provided a series of counseling sessions designed to facilitate insight into his aggressive tendencies.

Within two weeks of returning to the vocational training program, the client was again dismissed following the reoccurrence of aggressive outbursts. It was evident that the physical, social, and work-requirement conditions of the two settings were quite different. Assessment of these aggressive outbursts in the context of the vocational training program would have provided the needed insights into the client and the environmental factors that contributed to these outbursts.

4.2.10. Use of "Intrusive" Behavior Therapy Procedures

Although much of the applied behavior therapy literature relating to the treatment of excessive behaviors in the mentally retarded (e.g., aggression, disruption, and pica) focuses on suppression of such difficulties through various negative contingencies,[40] the present writers view these approaches used in isolation as categorically unacceptable. Although research does support the relative efficacy of various behavior-suppression procedures (e.g., punishment, time-out, response cost, and overcorrection)[25,27] the goals of behavior therapy are never met when such procedures are used in isolation. These procedures, especially when used with the severely mentally retarded, who, by definition, have a more limited repertoire of behaviors that may serve to replace the suppressed excessive behaviors, typically have only temporary effects. Thus, it is essential that the development and maintenance of replacement behaviors be the major goal of behavior therapy programs.[41,37]

Even though the particular effects of any type of procedure involving "negative" consequences are person-specific and may produce uncomfortable (aversive) physical or psychological reactions in a specific person, there is general consensus that a variety of behavior therapy procedures such as overcorrection, time-out (especially isolation), response cost, required relaxation, and presentation of aversive consequences (ranging from personal reprimand to electrical stimulation) do represent potentially intrusive procedures. Therefore, whenever any of these are used in a behavior therapy program with the mentally retarded, safeguards must be taken to ensure protection of the client from undue aversive experiences and also to ensure that the procedures will be embedded in a comprehensive approach designed to teach the client prosocial behaviors to replace those that are suppressed or eliminated.

The following are suggested as minimal guidelines for the use of intrusive procedures in behavior therapy programs:

1. *The use of intrusive procedures to suppress or eliminate excessive behaviors must be based on hunches concerning factors that are currently influencing the inappropriate behaviors. These hunches should be based on client-specific assessment data.* Excessive behaviors, especially those that create disturbance or difficulty for others, too frequently are treated with an "automatic application" approach. For example, if a person is being aggressive or otherwise noncompliant with classroom, work environment, or home routine, the therapy program may consist of a time-out procedure without client-specific assessment data that produce hunches about the function served by the behavior.

Two examples will illustrate such unacceptable practice. A young adult had been placed in a community group home facility following a series of verbally and physically aggressive outbursts in his home. The consulting staff of the facility recommended time-out and response cost procedures contingent on any verbal or physical outbursts. This decision was made without any client-specific assessment relative to the factors contributing to the outbursts. The program was effective in suppressing the aggressive behaviors for a short period of time. However, the threat-of-punishment contingency soon lost its effectiveness, with the result that the outbursts reappeared, and the young adult was placed in a residential facility. A second example involved a profoundly retarded adolescent who engaged in frequent stereotypical self-abusive outbursts (face slapping) and frequent episodes of throwing his food tray. The behavior program consisted of an overcorrection procedure for the self-abuse and a time-out for the food throwing. These were initiated without client-specific assessment data or related hypotheses concerning factors contributing to the occurrence and maintenance of the inappropriate behaviors. Although this program produced short-term suppressive effects, the gains were soon lost when the punishment program was removed. To repeat, the treatment procedures comprising a behavior program, especially those of a potentially intrusive nature, must be related to client-specific assessment data that provide support for their use.

2. *More intrusive procedures should be used only after less intrusive procedures have been found to be ineffective.*

3. *Intrusive procedures should never be used in isolation.* In every case, there must be equally or more powerful procedures designed to teach those alternative prosocial behaviors that will be functional to the individual in meeting his or her personal and developmental needs. The emphasis should be on "equally or more powerful" procedures. If, for example, a time-out procedure is being used in combination with a reinforcement procedure, there must be some basis for assuming that specific replacement behaviors will occur and will receive sufficient reinforcement to become predominant over the behavior being suppressed by time-out.

4. *Although any behavior program should be data-based, it is essential that programs using aversive procedures be closely monitored through a frequent analysis of objective behavioral data.* Both specific positive effects and potential negative side effects should be monitored. Procedures using intrusive stimulation may well be effective in producing short-term suppressive effects, but the result may be other negative consequences. These negative consequences can be minimized—or eliminated completely in most cases—by setting client-appropriate therapy goals, by providing a program for developing and/ or strengthening prosocial replacement behaviors, and by careful data-based monitoring of effects.

5. *The aversive components of behavior therapy programs should be phased out of the program as soon as possible.* In some instances, it may be desirable to initiate intrusive contingencies because of the critical nature of the behavior difficulties. In illustration, a family may be at a crisis point and feel that, unless something is done immediately to reduce the tantrums of their child, placement outside the home will have to be made. Aversive procedures may be used initially in combination with positive procedures to produce a rapid deceleration in the intensity, duration, or frequency of the tantrum behavior. However, once this crisis point has been passed, the intrusive procedures should be replaced with procedures designed to teach more appropriate reactions to the conditions that provoke the temper tantrums.

4.3. Major Forms of Behavior Therapy

Behavior therapy procedures have been used successfully with a wide range of psychological problems of development and adjustment and with individuals ranging from profound to mild levels of mental retardation. As suggested earlier, behavior therapy represents a constellation of clinical procedures derived from various learning and related theories of conceptual models of human behavior. An impressive array of empirically validated therapeutic techniques has evolved from these models. The behavior therapist selects those specific procedures that hold promise of meeting the therapy goals set for a specific client or group of clients. Various models and related behavior therapy procedures are described briefly as a background for the following discussion of specific applications to the mentally retarded.

4.3.1. Reinforcement and Related Procedures

The behavior therapy procedures used most frequently with the mentally retarded are based on concepts and principles of operant learning.[31] The basic premise of this model is that most of a person's behavior is influenced by the consequences produced by the behavior. Such behavior alters the physical and social environments, thus producing positive or negative consequences that have the effect of either increasing or decreasing the strength of that behavior. Procedures are available to weaken or remove maladaptive behaviors, to teach and strengthen new adaptive behaviors, and to strengthen adaptive behaviors already present in the person's repertoire. Additionally, procedures are available to ensure that behaviors will become appropriately discriminating, that is, will occur at the correct time and place to ensure the best adaptability. Finally, therapy procedures are available to encourage generalization of behavior gains across settings and their maintenance over time. The major procedures, examples of application, and the resulting behavioral effects are summarized in Table 1.

4.3.2. Modeling Procedures

Various modeling procedures, also known as *vicarious* or *observational learning*, have significant implications for the mentally retarded, especially those with limited verbal skills. There is considerable evidence that the mere observation of the behavior of others under certain prompting and reinforcing conditions produces predictable effects on the behavior of the observer.[33] Observation of the behavior of others has three possible effects. First, the observer may acquire new response patterns that were not in his or her repertoire prior to exposure to the model. Second, observation of the behavior of a model and the resulting environmental consequences may exert either an inhibitory or a disinhibitory effect on the behavior of the observer. The specific nature of the effect depends on the positive or aversive consequences produced by the model's behavior. Finally, exposure to a model may result in response facilitation. The behavior of the person observed serves as a discriminative event for similar behavior on the part of the observer. Observer behaviors that are neutral or socially acceptable have an increased likelihood of occurrence following exposure to a model who engages in these behaviors. Prompted rehearsal of the observed behavior adds to the effectiveness of the observation of a model. Following prompted behavior rehearsal, the model can demonstrate the behavior again, with emphasis on those components or features that the observer is missing. Immediate reinforcement can be provided desired behavior during the prompted rehearsal, thus increasing the strength of such behavior.

4.3.3. Emotional Retraining Procedures

Systematic desensitization is a behavior therapy technique used to reduce or eliminate maladaptive levels of anxiety. The technique, developed by Wolpe,[42] typically involves teaching the client deep muscle relaxation and then pairing this state of relaxation with imagined scenes depicting events or situations that cause anxiety in the client. The scenes are developed in a hierarchy from least to most anxiety-arousing and are presented to the client in a gradual manner to ensure a continued state of relaxation. The assumption is made that if the client is relaxed instead of anxious while imagining such scenes, then the real-life situations will be less anxiety-producing.

In working with the mentally retarded client with minimal verbal skills or minimal skills of imaginal representation of anxiety-provoking situations, other

Table 1. Influencing the Strength of Behavior: Reinforcement and Related Procedures

Therapy procedure	Example of procedure	Effects on behavior
Positive reinforcement: Specific behavior is followed by a positive event (reward).	Susan, an excessively shy adult, is praised for being assertive.	Susan's assertive behavior will increase in strength.
Negative reinforcement: A current aversive condition is removed following a specific behavior.	Timothy, a severely retarded child, engages in a temper outburst whenever teased by his peers, with the result that the teasing is terminated.	Timothy's temper-tantrum behavior will increase in frequency of occurrence following being teased by peers.
Shaping: Reinforcement is provided the successive approximations of a desired behavior.	Kay, a child with severe language deficits, is reinforced immediately after saying "au" when requested to say "ball." The teacher will gradually require closer approximations of "ball" prior to reinforcement.	Kay will learn to repeat the word "ball" when provided a model.
Discrimination training: Specific behavior is provided reinforcement when it occurs under specific stimulus conditions but not under other conditions.	Leroy, a severely retarded adult, is reinforced for initiating conversations during break periods but not for such verbal behaviors during work periods.	Leroy learns to discriminate between the settings in which his conversational behavior is and is not appropriate.
Behavior rehearsal and role playing: Desired behavior is practiced in situations that closely approximate those in which the behavior is to occur.	A shy, passive adolescent is provided guided practice in being assertive.	The adolescent is more likely to behave in an appropriate assertive manner when a situation requires such adaptive behavior.
Differential reinforcement of alternative behaviors to replace inappropriate behaviors: Incompatible Behaviors (DRI): Reinforcement is provided specific incompatible behaviors to replace inappropriate behaviors.	Tim, who typically is late for work, is praised for arriving on time.	Tim is more likely to arrive on time.

Other Behaviors (DRO): Reinforcement is provided any appropriate behaviors following a period in which the inappropriate behaviors have not occurred. A range of other behaviors may be strengthened.	Ralph, who has not yelled at his peers for 15 minutes, is praised for sitting quietly, or for working, or for talking appropriately.	Ralph is more likely to engage in these other behaviors than to yell at his peers.
Extinction of: *Behavior maintained by positive reinforcement:* Behavior is not followed by the positive event associated with previous occurrences.	Robert's chronic complaining is ignored by his teachers. They act as if the complaining has not occurred.	Robert is less likely to complain to his teachers.
Behavior maintained by negative reinforcement: Behavior is not followed by the removal of the aversive event associated with previous occurrence.	Helen is not permitted to ignore her math assignment, which she does not like, and leave the classroom following a temper outburst.	Helen is less likely to display temper outbursts in the classroom.
Stimulus Change (external and internal discriminative events that instigate and/or inhibit behaviors are presented, removed, or modified): *Physical events:* Physical stimulation that produces problem behavior is removed.	Troy, who begins to be self-abusive when in a noisy environment, is moved to a quiet living setting.	Troy's self-abusive behavior is reduced significantly.
Physical stimulation that produces desired behavior is presented.	The group home in which Tracy, a highly anxious adult, lives plays soft music each evening before dinner.	Tracy is more relaxed and sociable during dinner.
Program structure: Program structure that produces problem behavior is changed, or program structure that produces desired behavior is presented.	Performance standards are reduced to ensure reduction in failure.	Clients exhibit fewer temper outbursts.

(Continued)

Table 1. (*Continued*)

Therapy procedure	Example of procedure	Effects on behavior
Social events: Source and quality of social stimulation that produces/influences problem behaviors is changed, or social stimulation that produces desired behavior is presented.	Work supervisor who typically presents direction in a gruff manner provides instructions to Chris in a calm personable manner.	Chris is more likely to comply with requests.
Internal events: Mediating thinking and/or affective events that cue inappropriate behaviors are changed.	June, who dwells on how much she dislikes her peers, is taught to think about positive features of peers.	June is more likely to interact appropriately with peers instead of arguing with them.
Punishment: *Presentation of aversive events (PAC):* Behavior is followed by an aversive consequence.	Jim, who engages in tantrum behavior is reprimanded by his teacher.	Jim is less likely to engage in tantrum behavior.
Time-out (TO): Behavior results in the removal of possible reinforcing events for a designated period of time.	Ms. Jakes escorts Ralph to a time-out room and leaves him there for ten minutes following his breaking a window.	Ralph is less likely to break another window.
Response cost (RC): Behavior results in the loss of reinforcing events.	Mary loses her privilege of attending a movie following her throwing a tray in the dining room.	Mary is less likely to throw a tray in the dining room.
Overcorrection: *Restitution:* Following inappropriate behavior, the person is required to restore the environment to an improved state.	Kathy, after throwing reading materials on the floor in the dayroom, is required to straighten and dust the entire room.	Kathy is less likely to throw reading materials on the floor in the dayroom.
Positive practice: Following inappropriate behavior, the person is provided an opportunity to practice the appropriate behavior regularly.	Edward, following his pushing his way into a peer's room without knocking, is required to approach the room, knock, receive an invitation, and then enter. Practiced 10 times.	Edward is more likely to knock prior to entering the peer's room.

more direct procedures would be needed. It may be necessary to present various concrete representations of the anxiety-provoking objects, activities, or situations. If, in illustration, a mentally retarded adolescent is fearful of fire engine sirens and is unable to develop images of approximations of the feared stimuli, visual and auditory representations of these stimuli could be presented in a graduated series under conditions of relaxation.

Many fears and anxieties are acquired by the mentally retarded who have not had actual physically or psychologically injurious experiences with the feared object or situation. Such negative emotional reactions are influenced by the observation of others responding fearfully toward objects or situations or of talking about these in an emotionally aroused manner. Additionally, there is evidence that emotional response patterns can be reduced or eliminated vicariously, by having the mentally retarded client observe models engaging in the feared behavior (e.g., climbing stairs that produce considerable anxiety in the observer, or approaching a feared social situation) without experiencing aversive consequences.[43,44] This vicarious extinction of emotionality may be enhanced by evoking an antagonistic positive affective response in the observer. An important feature of the modeling procedures designed to facilitate the extinction of negative emotionality and related avoidance behavior is the manner in which the model relates to the feared object or activity. The modeled approach behavior and the interactions with the feared object are typically presented gradually over a series of exposures, as the model becomes more intimate and is directly involved in positive interactions toward the end of the therapy.

A variation of modeling is that termed *contact desensitization*, also referred to as *participant modeling* or *guided participation*.[45] In this therapy procedure, approach responses to the feared object or activity are modeled, and then the client is verbally and physically guided by the therapist in interacting with the phobic object or situation in graduated steps. Contact desensitization involves physical contact with both the therapist and the phobic object or activity.

A final emotional retraining procedure is that of *graduated extinction* or *counterconditioning*. This involves both the presentation of those events or situations that provoke fear and avoidance behavior and the added feature of presenting other events that simultaneously result in more favorable reactions. The "fear reaction" and the resulting avoidance behavior exhibited toward a new work supervisor by a young retarded adult whose previous supervisor had been quite negative could be reduced or eliminated by using this procedure *in vivo*. The new supervisor would initially present himself under pleasurable circumstances, such as when the client is having lunch, during break period, during "cigarette break" time, and/or during recreation activities. Through such graduated exposure, the supervisor will gradually lose his anxiety-provoking qualities and, with frequent association with situations that provoke competing positive emotional experiences, will become a cue for this positive emotionality.

4.3.4. Cognitive and Self-Control Procedures

Although many of the behavior therapy procedures used with the mentally retarded involve changing the external environmental experiences of the client, there has been a recent emphasis on influencing internal cognitive events as a means of increasing the client's self-management (control) skills.[46,47] The cognitive procedures teach the mentally retarded person to use cognitive behaviors in a deliberate manner to influence others of his or her thoughts or feelings as well as overt behaviors. The client may be taught to self-instruct as a means of initiating activity, and to anticipate future consequences as a means of continuing an activity until the goal and the resulting consequences are attained. Or he or she may be taught to covertly consider possible negative consequences and thus avoid selecting certain courses of action. Further, the client may be taught to influence the future likelihood of certain of his or her behaviors (1) through self-administered positive or negative reinforcement (self-delivery of external or internal positive reinforcers or self-removal of external or internal aversive conditions) and (2) through self-administered punishment (self-presentation of external or internal unpleasant consequences or self-removal of external or internal pleasant consequences). These and a variety of other self-control procedures involving skills of self-monitoring, self-evaluation, self-consequation, self-instruction, standard setting, and self-selection of consequences, offer promise to the mentally retarded client, who typically is a victim of internal and external conditions over which he or she has little control.

4.3.5. Multicomponent Treatment Programs

In most instances, the behavior therapy program combines procedures from a variety of these models. *Social skills training programs* used to teach prosocial behaviors, in illustration, may combine instruction, modeling, behavior rehearsal, feedback, and reinforcement.[48,49] Turner et al.[30] successfully used a social skills training program to improve the interpersonal functioning of a severely emotionally disturbed, intellectually deficient young adult. Harvey et al.[50] used a comprehensive treatment program consisting of relaxation training, cue conditioning, cognitive procedures, time-out, and positive reinforcement to eliminate the violent temper outbursts of a moderately retarded woman. Cole et al.[46] and Gardner et al.[51] used a multicomponent self-management therapy program to successfully treat conduct disorders in emotionally disturbed mentally retarded adults. These programs, to be described later, provide illustration of the need for a variety of therapeutic procedures when serving the mentally retarded.

4.4. Application to Clinical Problems

As suggested, the development and the clinical assessment of behavior therapy procedures have provided the clinician with a range of useful approaches for treatment of the behavioral and emotional difficulties of individuals identified as mentally retarded. Evaluation of the clinical literature emphasizes the particular applicability of these treatment procedures to the retarded, as no particular characteristics, such as speech or a certain level of cognitive and language development, are necessary prerequisites for treatment effects. Even the most severely involved person is a potential candidate for behavior therapy.[27,52] Additionally, there is ample documentation in published reports that a variety of behavior therapy procedures can be used successfully by caretakers and other nonprofessional persons in the settings in which the retarded client resides, including *residential staff*,[53] *volunteers*,[54,55] *teachers*,[56] and *parents*.[57,58] The use of behavior therapy procedures by nonprofessionals is especially valuable in view of (1) the *in vivo* treatment emphasis of the behavioral approach and (2) the limited number of available mental health professionals who have the training, the interest, and the time to provide effective services to the mentally retarded with various mental health and related difficulties.[59]

The following sections describe behavior therapy procedures reported to produce positive and clinically significant changes in a range of clinical problems presented in living, educational, and vocational settings by clients ranging in level of functioning from mild to profound mental retardation. As a brief presentation permits neither a comprehensive review nor a critical evaluation of the behavior therapy procedures available, an attempt is made to include examples of a wide array of applications. This sampling should offset the seemingly isolated and circumscribed focus of some of the applications described.

The reader should exercise caution in assuming that any specific behavior therapy procedure described will produce similar results in other mentally retarded clients with similar problems. As emphasized earlier, any specific therapy procedure(s) used with a client or group of clients should be selected as the treatment of choice only after a careful and thorough clinical behavior analysis, and not merely on the basis of reports that the procedure has been successful with similar problems.

4.4.1. Anorexia Nervosa and Related Eating Difficulties

Anorexia nervosa is a rare condition characterized by refusal to eat adequate amounts of food, marked loss of body weight, and an absence of any known physical illness to account for the weight loss. This eating disturbance can be a serious problem, even to the point of being life-threatening if the food refusal is severe or if it persists over a long period of time. Although anorexia nervosa, as currently defined,[60] is only rarely reported among the mentally retarded, behavior therapy approaches that have produced promising results with the nonretarded are available for use with the mentally retarded.[61-63] These behavioral approaches typically use a combination of response cost and time-out for inappropriate eating and positive reinforcement for appropriate eating and weight gains.

In perhaps the first published report of anorexia nervosa in the mentally retarded, Hurley and Sovner[64] described the successful treatment of a 15-year-old mildly retarded female who presented the classic signs of amenorrhea, 25% loss of body weight, and distorted body image. Following placement in an infirmary in which access to all activities was contingent on weight gain, the adolescent began eating and gaining weight. The program was discontinued following discharge from the infirmary on Day 50. Follow-up at six months and again at two years revealed normal eating patterns and weight. Mohl and McMahon[65] reported a second case study of anorexia nervosa in a 20-year-old female with mental retardation and a "schizoaffective" disorder. A reinfocement program, which provided such items as cigarettes, coffee, and diet soda contingent on eating and weight gain, contributed to the reestablishment of appropriate eating habits.

Fox and Karan[66] described a 26-year-old woman who at age 18 had successfully adjusted to living at home with her parents after attending a residential training school for 12 years. However, during a subsequent 2-year period at home, her independent living skills slowly deteriorated until she had experienced such extreme and pervasive behavioral regression that institutionalization was viewed as the only viable living arrangement for her. The most critical problem at the time of intervention was the woman's deficit eating behaviors, which had produced a serious weight loss (her weight had gone from 115 to 75 pounds). Hospitalization for 10 weeks for treatment of this eating disorder resulted in no improvement. A trial placement in a semi-independent group home was arranged and a behavior therapy program was initiated during mealtimes across three different settings. The program included positive reinforcement contingent on completion of the entire meal within a designated time, and simply removing the food if she did not finish. In addition, her daily weight was graphed, and ¼-pound weight gains were reinforced by staff and peers. The treatment resulted in a weight gain of 14 pounds over six weeks of intensive daily intervention. A 15-month follow-up indicated an appropriate weight level as well as improvement in other behavioral areas.

4.4.2. Conduct Difficulties

One of the more prevalent and socially disruptive problems among the mentally retarded is aggressive behavior and related conduct difficulties.[67,68] Such excessive reactions as physical violence toward others and property, explosive outbursts, temper tantrums, excessive negativism, and other disruptive activities effectively interfere with the development and the occurrence of adaptive behaviors. Such actions often result in dismissal or exclusion from various educational, recreational, rehabilitative, community residential, and vocational training programs.[69,28]

4.4.2.1. Structuring Antecedent Stimulus Events

In one of the few studies that used stimulus change procedures to reduce conduct difficulties in the mentally retarded, Boe[70] hypothesized that limited space and limited availability of activities were contributing to high rates of aggression in an institutional facility. He found, however, that the mere availability of toys did not decrease aggression in 24 severely and profoundly retarded females (aged 8–19), whereas increased space did. Murphy and Zahm[71] and Rago, Parker, and Cleland[72] obtained similar results following improvement of the physical living environments of severely and profoundly retarded males. The results of both studies indicated significant reductions in the frequency and the intensity of aggressive behavior following an improvement or an increase in the physical living space.

4.4.2.2. Reinforcement of Alternative Behaviors

A variety of differential reinforcement procedures have been used in classroom settings to reduce the disruptive behaviors of mentally retarded students. Repp, Deitz, and Deitz[73] reinforced three mildly retarded children for periods of nonoccurrence of inappropriate talking in the classroom; a variety of behaviors other than the target disruptive ones were reinforced. Disruptive behaviors were significantly reduced for all three students. Drabman and Spitalnik[74] described a procedure in which a highly disruptive, moderately retarded 14-year-old male in a morning class earned the privilege of serving as a "behavioral teaching assistant" in an afternoon class. His responsibilities included reinforcing those children judged by him to be appropriate during 15-minute time intervals. This peer-administered reinforcement was as effective as teacher-administered reinforcement in reducing the disruptive behavior of two severely retarded boys (aged 9 and 10). Further, inappropriate behaviors exhibited by the "teaching assistant" in his own class also decreased as a result of the program.

Perline and Levinsky[75] used a more specific reinforcement procedure with a preschool class of four severely retarded students who engaged in aggressive outbursts. The children were provided tokens for specific appropriate classroom behaviors that were physically incompatible with the disruptive ones. There was a decrease in aggression and an increase in desired behaviors following initiation of the program. Broden et al.[76] used a similar procedure with a junior high special education class of 13 students who engaged in such behaviors as cursing the teacher, refusing to complete assignments, fighting with peers, and general classroom disruption. Initially, when the teacher systematically attended to study behavior and ignored all nonstudying, there was an overall increase in appropriate study behavior. More specific token reinforcement at random intervals for working quietly resulted in a further increase in the students' studying behavior. Finally, when a complex point system was used that specified the number of points earned or lost for each appropriate and inappropriate behavior, as well as the number of points required for each activity or privilege, study behavior was increased even more. This high level was maintained throughout the school year. The authors conceded that such an elaborate point system may not be necessary or desirable in many classrooms, but they noted that it was useful for a beginning teacher in establishing classroom contingencies.

Deitz and Repp[77] described the use of a differential reinforcement procedure in which an entire class of 10 moderately retarded students were reinforced at the end of the period if fewer than five "talk-out" behaviors had occurred. This procedure significantly reduced the frequency of inappropriate talking in the classroom.

Such differential reinforcement procedures frequently have been used in combination with other procedures to treat conduct problems in both school and residential settings. Sewell, McCoy, and Sewell[78] used differential reinforcement plus time-out to decrease disruptive and aggressive behavior in four moderately and mildly retarded adolescent males identified by residential staff as "unmanageable." During intervention, staff delivered tokens for periods of nonoccurrence of inappropriate behavior (e.g., no yelling, defacing walls, profanity, or throwing debris) and a 30-minute time-out for severe aggressive behavior (e.g., physical attacks or property destruction). There were immediate and dramatic reductions in the disruptive and aggressive behaviors over the baseline levels. Hall *et al.*[79] and Repp and Deitz[80] successfully reduced chronic and high-rate physical aggression toward self and others in young mentally retarded males using differential reinforcement plus other procedures. In addition to providing edible reinforcement for periods of no aggression, the treatment packages included time-out (e.g., removal from group activities), response cost (e.g., removal of stars earned), and verbal reprimand. Reductions in aggression were reported in both studies. Polvinale and Lutzker[81] used differential reinforcement plus social restitution to modify assaultive and inappropriate sexual behavior in a 13-year-old Down's syndrome male in a school setting. Descriptive verbal praise was provided for periods of nonoccurrence of inappropriate behavior, and on the occurrence of a target behavior, the student was required to apologize to his victim and five other people. Physical guidance was provided when necessary, and an "extra person" was added whenever he hesitated for more than five seconds. The procedures eliminated the target behaviors in both structured and unstructured settings.

4.4.2.3. Withholding or Removing Reinforcement

a. Extinction. When conduct problems appear to be maintained by the social feedback that they produce, they may be reduced or eliminated by removing these reinforcing consequences. An example is the "victim control" (extinction) procedure described by Martin and Foxx,[82] in which the victim attempted to ignore all aggressive physical attacks of a moderately retarded 22-year-old woman. Although the procedure successfully reduced physical aggression, the authors noted:

> It is not feasible, in cases similar to Gail, to arrange for the ward staff to withdraw social reinforcement for aggressive behavior. This treatment is much too dangerous for individuals functioning as victims because of the passive role they must assume during attacks. (p. 165)

An illustration of the use of an extinction procedure with a less severe form of aggression was provided by Forehand,[83] who extinguished high-rate spitting behavior in a mildly retarded 6-year-old boy in the classroom. The teacher hypothesized that the attention received for spitting was maintaining the behavior and instructed her aides to completely ignore it. The spitting behavior decreased and eventually was eliminated.

b. Time-Out. In studies with the mentally retarded demonstrating conduct difficulties, time-out typically has involved (1) placing the person in a restricted and presumably less reinforcing environment[84-88] or (2) discontinuing therapist-administered reinforcement.[89] The time-out is contingent on the occurrence of inappropriate behavior and continues for previously specified periods of time.

White *et al.*[88] investigated the differential effects of three time-out durations (1 minute, 15 minutes, and 30 minutes) on the aggressive-disruptive behavior of 20 moderately and severely retarded residents (aged 7–21). The 15-minute time-out was most effective and the 1-minute time-out least effective in decreasing deviant behavior, although all time-out durations produced some suppressive effects. Calhoun and Matherne[84] and Clark *et al.*[85] examined the effects of brief (2- or 3-minute) periods of isolation for aggression in two mentally retarded girls, aged 7 and 8. In addition, these authors investigated the effects of intermittent schedules of time-out on the total rate of inappropriate behavior. In both studies, time-out was effective in decreasing aggressive behavior, and the most effective time-out schedules were those that consequated the largest percentage of inappropriate behavior exhibited.

Foxx and Shapiro[89] used the procedure of discontinuing teacher reinforcement for aggressive-disruptive behavior (e.g., yelling, throwing objects, hitting others, or self-abuse) in a class of five severely retarded males (aged 8–18). Initially, each boy was provided a different colored ribbon, which hung around his neck, and was reinforced intermittently with praise and edibles for wearing the ribbon and engaging in appropriate behavior. Then, whenever a child engaged in disruptive-aggressive behavior, the ribbon was removed, signaling the discontinuation of teacher attention and child involvement in activities for three minutes, or until the behavior ceased. There was a significant decrease in aggression for all five students using the time-out ribbon. The authors concluded:

> The ribbon procedure appears to be a viable form of timeout, provided that disruptive behaviors during timeout can be tolerated within the setting, or a backup procedure such as exclusionary timeout is available when needed. (p. 125)

Although time-out procedures have been demonstrated to be effective in reducing a variety of conduct problems in the mentally retarded, they also, in some cases, have produced unacceptable negative reactions in clients. A clear example is provided by Pendergrass,[87] who reported the use of a time-out procedure designed to decrease the aggressive behavior of a 5-year-old girl. Whenever the child hit another person, the trainer stated, "No, don't hit," and removed the child to an isolation booth for a specified time interval. Although the time-out procedure was effective in reducing the girl's hitting behavior, the author reported that "*S* gradually developed strong emotional responses of trembling and crouching when *E* called 'Don't hit.'" Further, the child "consistently wet in the isolation chamber" and "spent long periods of time lying fact down on the floor when not in TO" (p. 79).

As is evident in this example, it cannot be assumed that a particular procedure will automatically produce the same effects in different individuals. The unique characteristics of each person must be carefully assessed prior to the selection and the implementation of any therapy procedure, especially a punishment procedure such as time-out.

Time-out has frequently been used in combination with other procedures to reduce conduct difficulties in the mentally retarded. Bostow and Bailey[90] used time-out and differential reinforcement procedures in a program designed to reduce the loud, aggressive behavior of a mentally retarded, institutionalized 58-year-old woman confined to a wheelchair. On each occurrence of inappropriate behavior, the resident was wheeled to a nearby corner of the dayroom, removed from her wheelchair, and placed on the floor for two minutes. An escalating schedule was used to reinforce her for periods of remaining quiet. Significant suppression effects were observed. Peniston[91] used time-out and response cost (i.e., token withdrawal) with 14 severely and profoundly retarded institutionalized adults to modify physical and verbal aggression. During the initial baseline phase, 35%–40% of the residents' time was spent engaging in aggressive behavior. This was reduced to infrequent occurrence on the introduction of the time-out plus a response cost contingency.

More recently, Foxx *et al.*[92] reported the effects of a multicomponent treatment program on the physically violent behavior of a severely retarded, institutionalized 23-year-old male. The package included 24-hour time-out, physical restraint, relaxation training, and overcorrection contingent on aggression plus differential reinforcement (token reinforcement) for appropriate behavior. Aggressive episodes were reduced to near-zero after one year.

c. *Response Cost.* Sulzbacher and Houser[93] were among the first to demonstrate the efficacy of response cost in reducing conduct difficulties in the mentally retarded. In a study with 14 students in a special education class, specific disruptive behaviors by any one student resulted in loss of priviledges for the entire class. An immediate reduction in the disruptive behaviors was observed. Greene and Pratt[94] used a similar response cost contingency to successfully reduce inappropriate behaviors (e.g., talking out, using obscenities, and refusing to follow directions) in 11 classes involving 100 students (mean age 15.4; mean IQ 65).

Axelrod[95] compared the effectiveness of individual versus group response cost contingencies in reducing the undesirable behaviors (e.g., being out of seat, hitting others, and throwing objects) of 31 educably mentally retarded students from two special education classrooms. With the group contingency procedure, the teacher listed the numbers 25, 24, . . . , 0 vertically on the blackboard. When inappropriate behavior occurred, the teacher crossed off one number and wrote on the board the name of the child who had misbehaved.

At the end of each session, the highest remaining number on the board represented the number of tokens that each child received. With the individual contingency, each child's name was listed on the chalkboard, and the number of tokens received was determined by individual performance. The more convenient and efficient group contingency was as effective as the individual contingency in reducing undesirable classroom behaviors.

4.4.2.4. Presentation of Aversive Consequences

a. Overcorrection. Foxx and Azrin[96] used restitutional overcorrection to modify aggressive-disruptive behavior in three profoundly retarded institutionalized females. On occurrence of a target behavior, the resident was required to engage in a functionally related activity for a designated period of time. For example, after overturning furniture, the resident was required to set the furniture upright, apologize to others, remake beds, and straighten the entire living area for 30 minutes. Significant reductions in all the target behaviors were observed following the introduction of the treatment.

Shapiro[97] used a similar overcorrection procedure with a highly aggressive, moderately retarded 5½-year-old girl enrolled in a day-school program. Initially, she spent much of her unstructured time tearing paper, thus destroying books and other educational materials. During intervention, if the child tore paper, she was instructed (1) to pick up all the torn paper and other toys in the area for two minutes, and (2) to look through a book without tearing for five minutes. Physical guidance was provided when necessary and no reinforcement was given. The paper tearing decreased by the use of overcorrection and had been eliminated at an 18-month follow-up check.

Davidson-Gooch[98] combined overcorrection and differential reinforcement in modifying the aggressive behavior of a severely retarded, institutionalized 17-year-old male. Reinforcement was provided for periods of nonoccurrence of aggression, and following each target response, the resident was required to repeat a forced-arm exercise 20 times. Following intervention, the rate of aggressive behavior decreased 88% from the initial baseline rate.

b. Aversive Electrical Stimulation. Birnbrauer[99] provided one of the first demonstrations of the use of aversive electrical stimulation to modify physical aggression in a profoundly retarded, institutionalized 14-year-old male. The target behaviors including biting peers' fingers, destroying property, and tearing clothing. Staff reported a "gradual decline in all offenses and a general increase in sociability and cooperation" following treatment. Brandsma and Stein[100] obtained similar, but more immediate and dramatic, results using aversive electrical stimulation with a moderately retarded, physically aggressive 24-year-old female. After the first day of treatment, the resident aggressed only once during the remainder of the study.

Ball et al.[101] described the use of an accelerometer-activated jacket that delivered aversive electrical stimulation on the occurrence of assaultive behavior with a severely retarded 13 ½-year-old girl who had not responded to other procedures. The high-rate aggression gradually decreased to zero after eight months of treatment and remained at near-zero levels for over one year.

Despite its demonstrated efficacy, aversive electrical stimulation, like time-out, may produce negative effects in clients. In the Birnbrauer[99] study, for example, the client began wetting himself and, "when shock was 'due,' Mike ran to a corner of the room, jumped in place, hit himself and yelled" (p. 206). Such reactions are unacceptable in the absence of client-specific behavioral assessment data and a prior evaluation of less intrusive procedures.

   c. Additional Punishment Procedures. Greene and Hoats[102] used aversive tickling to modify physical aggression in a mentally retarded, institutionalized 13-year-old girl. Staff approached her from the rear and tickled her under the arms "forcefully and somewhat aggressively" for three to five seconds contingent on each target behavior. A gradual reduction in the frequency of aggressive behavior was reported when this procedure was used.

   Schutz, Rusch, and Lamson[103] compared the effects of verbal warning and verbal warning plus suspension from work on the verbal aggression of three moderately retarded young adults in a vocational training setting. The results suggested that warning alone was ineffective, whereas warning plus suspension produced dramatic reductions in verbal abuse.

4.4.2.5. Multicomponent Treatment Programs

   Harvey *et al.*[50] described a multicomponent behavior therapy program created to teach the self-control of aggressive outbursts in a moderately retarded 38-year-old woman. The therapists hypothesized, following a clinical analysis of the client's difficulties, that the outbursts were being maintained both by positive reinforcement (social attention) and negative reinforcement (escape from frustrating interactions with others). In addition, they noted that the client had limited skills in behaving appropriately in provoking situations. Thus, the multicomponent treatment package included a self-managed token program to strengthen appropriate work behavior, a three-minute time-out for "complaining or blow-ups," and relaxation training to establish a coping skill. In addition, numerous cognitive procedures (e.g., positive self-statements during relaxation training, positive cue cards, and the self-recording of appropriate behavior) were utilized to replace the client's negative self-statements with more positive, appropriate statements about herself. Aggressive outbursts were virtually eliminated in work and residential settings. A one-year follow-up indicated maintenance of the therapeutic gains. The therapists suggested that, although the differential effectiveness of individual components was not assessed, the cognitive change procedures appeared to be important factors contributing to the maintenance of the positive behavior change.

   More recently, Gardner *et al.*[51] used a self-management intervention package to modify high-rate verbal aggression in two moderately retarded adults in a vocational training setting. Observation of these and other mentally retarded adults presenting conduct difficulties suggested that they most often reacted impulsively to sources of provocation. Thus, the clients were taught to self-manage (i.e., self-monitor, self-evaluate, and self-consequate) their own work-related behavior. The intervention resulted in immediate and significant reductions in the target aggressive behaviors, and the treatment gains were maintained at a six-month follow-up. Extensions of this study to a second class of inappropriate verbalizations (disruptive verbal ruminations[104]) and to severe and chronic forms of physical and verbal aggression[46] have been reported.

4.4.3. Encopresis and Enuresis

Since Ellis[105] outlined a reinforcement analysis of toilet-training procedures for severely retarded persons, there have been numerous demonstrations of the use of behavior therapy techniques in effectively teaching independent toileting skills to the retarded child and adult, and in treating difficulties in the use of these skills, once acquired.[106] The basic rationale for teaching toileting skills and eliminating toileting accidents is that these behaviors are responses that can be influenced by their consequences.

4.4.3.1. Positive Reinforcement and Presentation of Aversive Consequences

The typical reinforcement training procedure is illustrated by Waye and Melnyr[107] in their therapy program to toilet-train a nonverbal and blind retarded adolescent who had been incontinent since birth. During the initial week of the program, the frequency and the time of all eliminations were recorded. The time chart was used during treatment to schedule the periods during which the client was seated on the toilet. A behavioral assessment identified both effective reinforcers and client and environmental features that appeared to influence the toileting behavior. Further, it was noted that (1) wet or soiled cothing was removed by the adolescent and thus presumed to be aversive to him, and (2) elimination occurred in two favorite locations in his living area. During treatment, the client was placed on the toilet at times when he normally voided. Following elimination, reinforcement was provided immediately. In addition, he was kept from the two favorite spots for toileting accidents and was required to remain in his soiled clothing for 30 minutes following an accident. Elimination using conventional toileting facilities was established, with a decrease in accidents. A one-year follow-up revealed maintenance of the program effects.

Luiselli,[108] with a program consisting of reinforcement for voiding on the toilet and time-out and loss of privileges for having accidents, successfully treated the toileting problems of an adolescent who had toileting skills but did not use them. The client demonstrated phobiclike behavior toward the toilet and thus had numerous toileting accidents. Appropriate voiding resulted in a variety of tangible and activity reinforcers. Loss of privileges and a 40-minute period of being ignored followed a toileting accident. Following therapy, the number of accidents dropped from 15 per week to zero. A one-year follow-up revealed maintenance of these effects.

4.4.3.2. Multicomponent Treatment Programs

Foxx and Azrin[109] and Azrin, Sneed, and Foxx[110] have provided descriptions of a comprehensive behavior therapy program for training independent daytime and nighttime toileting skills that had been used to train self-initiated toileting to over 1,000 clients living in institutional settings. In addition to a component of training and reinforcement procedures to support and strengthen the desired toileting skills, the program includes full cleanliness training contingent on inappropriate wetting and soiling. Following an accident, clients are required to correct the results of their inappropriate behavior by cleaning themselves and their clothing. The rationale for this procedure is that (1) it teaches responsibility, in that the detrimental effects of inappropriate behavior must be corrected, and (2) it serves as a negative reaction to the accident, thereby motivating the clients to toilet themselves and to remain dry in order to avoid the nuisance of having to clean up their accidents.

Raborn[111] provided an example of use of the Foxx–Azrin toileting program with two moderately retarded boys (aged 8 and 10) attending a day-school program. Both were ambulatory and used expressive language. Prior to treatment, each boy averaged four accidents daily. Training was provided in a bathroom located next to the classroom. Each child was gradually reintegrated into the regular class schedule as appropriate toileting behavior was acquired. Additionally, the boys' parents continued training in the home setting, with positive results obtained for both daytime and nighttime cleanliness.

Doleys and Arnold[112] successfully used a modified version of the Foxx–Azrin program in the treatment of encopresis in a moderately retarded 8-year-old boy. The boy had repeatedly soiled his pants at home during the previous four years, but only rarely in school. The soiling behavior was complicated by the boy's refusal to sit on the toilet at home or at school, although he used it appropriately for urinating. It was hypothesized that his fear of the toilet was related to an early incident of painful defecation.

The toilet phobia was treated successfully through a combination of modeling and reinforcement of successive approximation of the desired behavior. Following his using the commode without hesitation, the boy was (1) reinforced for periods of time in which he had "dry and clean pants"; (2) reinforced on the toilet; (3) reinforced for successful use of the toilet; and (4) required to follow the full cleanliness training when it was detected that the boy had soiled his pants. Bowel control was obtained, with only infrequent accidents.

4.4.4. Hyperactivity

It has been estimated that 15%–20% of the mentally retarded exhibit the behavioral features of hyperactivity: overactivity, short attention span, impulsivity, and distractibility.[113] Hyperactivity is thus one of the most frequently occurring problems faced in educational and training settings. High rates of activity and related distractibility not only interfere with the hyperactive person's participation in and benefits from program experiences but also are often quite disturbing to others in the educational or vocational training environments.

4.4.4.1. Reinforcement of Alternative Behaviors

Doubros and Daniels[114] reduced the hyperactivity of moderately retarded boys in a playroom setting. During intervention, behaviors other than those defined as hyperactive were provided token reinforcers that were exchanged later for a variety of backup items. Hyperactivity was reduced, and the boys became more constructive in their play activities. These changes were maintained as the reinforcement contingency was withdrawn. Whitman, Caponigri, and Mercurio[115] demonstrated the value of reinforcing specific, incompatible, adaptive behavior to increase the sitting behavior of a severely retarded, hyperactive 6-year-old girl in a classroom setting. Prior to the behavior therapy program, the child had moved about the classroom excessively, being instructed to sit down 10 or more times within a 15-minute period. Although she typically complied with the teacher's instruction, she would remain seated for only short periods. Food items and praise for sitting on request and remaining seated for increasingly longer periods of time were used to teach the adaptive alternative behavior and thus reduce the child's hyperactivity in the class setting. In a similar demonstration, Twardosz and Sajwaj[116] used a prompting and a differential reinforcement procedure to increase sitting in a hyperactive retarded boy in a remedial preschool. This procedure not only increased sitting but had the additional effects of increasing the use of toys and the proximity to other children, all socially desirable effects.

Alabiso[117] demonstrated the usefulness of a behavior program in influencing other dimensions of hyperactivity: short attention span and distractibility. This therapist used token and social reinforcement to increase attention span, focus of attention, and selective attention of hyperactive, moderately retarded children attending a special education class.

4.4.5. Obesity

Obesity, a prevalent health problem for both the mentally retarded and the non-mentally retarded, is especially severe for the mentally retarded both because of the increased health problems created by being obese and because of the social stigma associated with being obese as well as with being mentally retarded. Although the behavior therapy literature addressed to the treatment of obesity in the mentally retarded is of recent origin, these reports do provide some encouraging results.[118]

4.4.5.1. Reinforcement of Alternative Behaviors

Foxx[119] presented a case report of an adolescent female who was mildly retarded and obese and who lost a significant amount of weight when systematically socially reinforced for a specified weight loss. The adolescent weighed

264 pounds when institutionalized six months prior to the study and had lost only 23 pounds during this period, despite a controlled diet and restricted canteen purchases. During intervention, a loss of 1 ½ pounds during the week was reinforced by a trip to the canteen with the therapist. In 42 weeks, she lost a total of 79 pounds. The therapist reported continued weight loss following completion of the treatment and speculated that her more appropriate eating behavior was not being reinforced by others in her environment. In another study, Joachim and Korboot[120] also found that a therapist's contact with 16 male and 16 female obese mentally retarded adults had a significant positive impact on their weight loss.

4.4.5.2. Multicomponent Treatment Programs

Foreyt and Parks[121] used a multicomponent weight-loss package with three severely retarded obese women who lived in the community and attended a day-care facility. The program consisted of (1) a weight loss manual for the parents; (2) colored tokens representing food groups for use by the clients in self-monitoring their daily food intake; (3) weekly payment of 50 cents for weekly weight loss of at least 1 pound; and (4) a public posting of the results of daily weighings. In addition, staff attention, verbal praise, and verbal encouragement were given generously for progress made. After the end of the 11-week program, all clients had lost weight (an average of 8 ½ pounds). At 29-week follow-up, the average loss exceeded 15 pounds, even though payment for weight loss had been discontinued.

Joachim and Korboot[120] and Joachim[122] reported the use of a multicomponent program that emphasized self-monitoring. The latter study involved a mildly retarded 32-year-old female, overweight since childhood, who weighed 234 pounds at intervention. The self-monitoring package required the client (1) to record her weight four times per day; (2) to monitor all her food and drink intake; and (3) to meet weekly with the therapist to discuss her goals and progress. The program resulted in a loss of 36 pounds. However, at 46-week follow-up, the woman had regained all but 7 of the pounds previously lost, a result suggesting a need for maintenance procedures in weight loss programs for the retarded.

Numerous other multicomponent weight-loss packages utilizing a variety of procedures have recently been developed for the mentally retarded.[123–128] In one study by Rotatori,[129] 10 mildly retarded adults participated in a seven-week multicomponent behavioral weight-reduction program. The package incorporated environmental control procedures (e.g., becoming aware of the relationship between food and weight gain or loss, eliminating food cues), external and self-reinforcement, self-monitoring, self-recording procedures (e.g., an eating diary and daily weight records), and energy expenditure procedures (e.g., regular exercise). In addition, a variety of instructional techniques were used during each session, including verbal description, videotape modeling, therapist modeling, client role-playing, therapist feedback, and individual counseling. A six-week maintenance phase followed intervention. The individuals involved in this program lost significantly more weight than eight other mildly retarded adults who were instructed to lose weight on their own. The weight loss was maintained at a follow-up check 10 weeks later. This multicomponent program has been successfully used with a number of additional groups of mildly and moderately retarded children, adolescents, and adults and is described in a recent treatment manual by Rotatori and Fox.[130]

4.4.6. Phobias and Fears

The presence of phobias and fears and related avoidance reactions is a clinically significant problem among the mentally retarded. Such difficulties may range from shyness or hesitation in specific social situations to severe emotional and related avoidance reactions that actively interfere with normal daily functioning. Although limited, the developing clinical and research literature illustrates the application of various behavior therapy procedures to the treatment of fears and phobias in the mentally retarded.

4.4.6.1. Systematic Desensitization

Systematic desensitization procedures typically have been modified to reflect the cognitive limitations of this clinical group. Rivenq,[131] for example, treated trichophobia (fear of hair) in a mildly retarded 13-year-old male using such a procedure. Rather than imagining fear-provoking scenes, the client was presented a graduated series of pictures of increasingly hairy men. At the same time, he was given candies and French pastries to create a state of positive emotional arousal that would compete with his fear response. The hair phobia was eliminated in four sessions.

In a second example, Guralnick[132] eliminated acrophobia (fear of heights) in a 21-year-old Down's syndrome male who was severely retarded. The client's fear of heights was termed a "constant source of anxiety" that "markedly restricted his participation" in program activities such as physical education class. Initially, an anxiety hierarchy was developed, beginning with the client's standing supported for brief periods at a low height and ending with his standing unsupported on a 20-inch-high ledge for three minutes and jumping to the floor (an exercise required in his physical-education class). Following four sessions of relaxation training, a three-component procedure—relaxation, verbal presentation, and *in vivo* practice—was implemented for each step in the hierarchy. In addition, increased duration and gross motor stability were reinforced with food, candy, and verbal praise. The client successfully completed the 31-item hierarchy in 42 sessions, and the reduction of fearful behavior generalized to the gym class.

4.4.6.2. Reinforced Practice

A more direct teaching approach is reinforced practice, also termed *shaping, successive approximation,* or *in vivo desensitization.* Here, clients are reinforced for practicing the desired behaviors *in vivo*, that is, in the presence of the actual feared object.

Freeman, Roy, and Hemmick[133] used this approach to eliminate fear of physical examination in a mildly retarded 7-year-old boy. The child had a retinal disorder that required frequent examinations by various physicians. His fear became so intense that it had become necessary to carry out the six-month ophthalmological examination under general anesthesia. An 11-step hierarchy of the ophthalmological examination was initially established, and each successive step was paired with an anxiety-free situation, that is, the presence of a nurse with whom he had a positive relationship. The steps of the examination were subsequently presented by a familiar physician accompanied by the nurse, and the nurse was then gradually faded from the situation. The fear was eliminated in 11 sessions, and the treatment gains generalized to unfamiliar physicians and to another type of physical examination (for plastic surgery).

Mansford[29] used reinforced practice with a moderately retarded 35-year-old woman who was fearful of riding in automobiles. Prior to intervention, the woman spent most of her time "confined to her room." Her extreme fear became most apparent when a vocational counselor suggested that she become involved in a workshop program requiring daily travel. A 19-item hierarchy dealing with the client's car-riding fear was constructed, and completion of each step was reinforced with tokens. Only 9 of the 19 items in the behavioral hierarchy from "talking to therapist in office about cars" through "talking to therapist with car door open and both inside," were completed before the behavioral objective of "taking ride to outside workshop all the way" was attained. At 10-month follow-up, the client continued to attend outside programs by car without fear.

4.4.6.3. Participant Modeling

Matson[43] used participant modeling to eliminate fear of participating in community-based activities in mildly and moderately retarded adults. Twenty-four clients, all identified as experiencing fear of approaching stores and as being unable to perform overall shopping skills, were matched on their degree of fear and their sex, and a member of each pair was randomly assigned to either a no-treatment control group or a participant modeling group.

The initial participant modeling sessions, held in a sheltered workshop, included a discussion of fears, the trainer's modeling entering stores and performing store-related activities, and the client's rehearsal of these activities. In the next phase, the trainer accompanied the clients to a community store, where they performed various shopping tasks (e.g., reading their shopping lists, locating the food they planned to buy, and carrying groceries from the store). When necessary, the trainer provided feedback and prompts to clarify and to assist the clients in successfully performing the desired shopping behaviors. Participant modeling was significantly more effective than no treatment in reducing overall fear.

A similar participant modeling procedure, with parents serving as trainers, was used by Matson[134] to reduce the clinically significant fears of three moderately retarded children (aged 8, 8, and 10). The intervention successfully taught the children to approach and talk to strange adults and decreased the children's ratings of overall fear. The gains were maintained at six-month follow-up.

4.4.6.4. Comparison of Procedures

Peck[44] evaluated the relative effectiveness of various procedures in the treatment of fear of animals and heights. In a study involving 20 mildly retarded adults (aged 19–61), comparison groups were provided contact desensitization, systematic desensitization, and vicarious symbolic desensitization, as well as placebo attention and no treatment. Hierarchies were developed for each fear and were applied to each of the three treatment groups. Contact desensitization, in which the therapist modeled approach responses and physically and verbally encouraged the subjects through the desired approach behavior, resulted in an overall fear reduction and appeared to be the only effective treatment procedure.

4.4.7. Pica and Coprophagy

Pica is the repeated ingestion of substances that have no nutritional value. Examples of these substances include garbage, strings, hair, grass, pebbles, cigarette butts, bugs, paper, cloth, and a variety of small objects. *Coprophagy* is a form of pica that involves the repeated ingestion of feces. The feces may be obtained through rectal digging or through eating the feces of others.[135,136]

Such behaviors have obvious adverse and potentially serious physical and psychological effects, as emphasized by Ausman, Ball, and Alexander[137] in a report of life-threatening pica in a severely retarded 14-year-old male. Lead poisoning may result from excessive ingestion of paint. Other physical conditions associated with pica behavior include nutritional anemia, encephalitis, frequent constipation, and intestinal obstruction. The ingestion of fecal matter may include such intestinal parasites as *Trichuris trichuria* and result in diarrhea, constipation, emaciation, and anemia. Additionally, pica behavior, especially the ingestion of feces, results in negative reactions of peers and staff. Interactions are minimized and tend to be of poor quality.[137,138]

Pica and coprophagy occur mostly among the severely and the profoundly mentally retarded. Although somewhat rare in occurrence, it is observed more frequently among those persons who have a limited behavioral repertoire, who are involved in minimally structured programming, who have a history of neglect, and who are poorly supervised. Pica is reported equally for both sexes.

4.4.7.1. Time-Out and Differential Reinforcement

Ausman *et al.*[137] used a time-out procedure following pica combined with consistent tangible and social reinforcement for periods of no pica behavior to treat the life-threatening pica behavior of a severely retarded 14-year-old male. The time-out procedure involved placing a helmet over the boy's head for 15 minutes following each occurrence of pica. Twenty-four-hour observation and treatment were required to accomplish generalized pica reduction in all settings.

4.4.7.2. Physical Restraint and Verbal Reprimand

Bucher *et al.*[136] used a 30-second physical restraint and a verbal reprimand to reduce the pica behavior of two profoundly retarded children. Extension of treatment across physical and social settings was necessary to ensure generalization. Elimination of pica in one of the children was accomplished only after the punishment contingency was applied to the earliest detectable response in the chain of behaviors resulting in the pica response.

4.4.7.3. Overcorrection

Foxx and Martin[138] demonstrated the use of various overcorrection procedures in successfully treating pica and coprophagy in four profoundly retarded persons. Following each occurrence of pica or coprophagy, an overcorrection program consisting of oral hygiene, personal hygiene, and restitutional procedures, combined with positive practice and graduated guidance, was implemented. It was reported that (1) pica behavior was reduced by 90% within four days of treatment and remained at near-zero levels throughout the intervention periods; (2) overcorrection was more effective than a physical restraint procedure; (3) long-standing *Trichuris trichuria* was eliminated from the three subjects who demonstrated coprophagy; (4) treatment effects were situation-specific and required the extension of treatment to other settings in which the clients functioned; and (5) positive side effects were reported, including increased awareness and responsiveness to the environment, the learning of new skills from the hygienic program, and increased appetites, resulting in a 30-pound weight gain for an individual who previously had been described as "gaunt and emaciated."

4.4.8. Seizure Disorders

Seizure disorders occur quite frequently among the mentally retarded.[139] Illingsworth[140] reported that up to 33% of any large group of the severely retarded will exhibit seizure disorders. A major motor seizure occurring in a community setting is not only physically and psychologically damaging to the person experiencing the seizure but is also often frightening to those who witness such occurrences.[141] Any procedures, medical or behavioral, that offer the possibility of decreasing the frequency of seizures thus contribute to the retarded client's rehabilitation and to his or her social acceptability in community programs.[142]

4.4.8.1. Reinforcement and Response Interruption

Zlutnick, Mayville, and Moffatt[143] described a program consisting of interruption of the behavioral chain that precedes seizure activity and differential reinforcement of other competing behavior. Seizures were conceptualized as the terminal link in a behavioral chain, resulting in a strategy aimed at identifying and modifying behaviors that reliably preceded the seizure climax. Seizure frequency was reduced in four of five children and adolescents. As an illustration of the procedures, the therapists observed that a mentally retarded 17-year-old female consistently raised her arms prior to a seizure. Whenever this occurred, her arms were lowered to her side or her lap, and following five seconds of no-seizure behavior, reinforcement was provided. Major motor seizures were reduced to a near-zero level and remained so at nine-month follow-up after program discontinuation.

4.4.8.2. Reinforcement and Time-Out

Similar results were obtained by Iwata and Lorentzson,[144] who used a differential reinforcement procedure, increased daily activities, and a contingent time-out program to decrease the seizurelike behavior of a retarded 41-year-old male. Seizures were markedly reduced by means of this combination of procedures. The effects were maintained during subsequent fading of the activities and the reinforcement.

4.4.8.3. Reinforcement and Extinction

Cautela and Flannery[145] reduced the seizure activities of a young adult male by providing social praise and food reinforcers from a teacher-therapist for the absence of seizures during the day and by removing attention whenever a seizure occurred.

4.4.8.4. Presentation of Aversive Consequences

Wright[146] described a case study of a mentally retarded 5-year-old boy who engaged in high-rate induced seizure behavior. Results from two separate three- to four-day aversive electrical-stimulation intervention periods indicated a significant decrease in the frequency of self-induced seizures that was maintained at seven-month follow-up. There was no evidence of negative side effects. Additionally, the child was described as being more alert and attentive, as displaying a higher level of cognitive functioning, and as being improved in his social interaction skills.

4.4.9. Self-Injurious Behavior

One of the most unusual, dangerous, and puzzling behavior difficulties observed in the mentally retarded is self-injurious behavior. Self-injurious behaviors (SIBs) are those repetitious and chronic self-stimulating acts that result in direct physical damage or that potentially endanger the physical well-being of the person displaying the behavior. Self-injurious behaviors include such acts as self-striking (e.g., head banging, face and head slapping); biting various body parts (e.g., biting hands, arms, and lips); and pulling or scratching various body parts (e.g., hair pulling, scratching and picking at sores, eye poking, rectal digging). Self-injurious behaviors such as head banging may take many forms, such as hitting the head on the floor, a wall, a chair, or other hard objects. In other persons, or even in the same person, this SIB may take such forms as hitting the chin with the fist or banging the head against the knees.[37]

Self-injurious behaviors are significant not only because these place the person in serious jeopardy of physical harm but also because frequent and intense episodes of self-injurious acts emphatically interfere with staff efforts at providing positive social and educational experiences for the person. In addition, the physical and chemical restraints used to manage and protect the person may interfere significantly with habilitative program efforts. Finally, the prolonged use of physical and/or chemical restraints may result in physical damage.

Although SIBs do occur among the mildly and the moderately retarded, the greatest frequency is observed among the severely and the profoundly mentally retarded with minimal communication skills and long histories of institutional living, and in those diagnosed as brain-injured or autistic. Typically, the lower the person's IQ level, the more frequent and severe the SIBs are likely to be. Most individuals who engage in some form of self-injury demonstrate other self-stimulatory behaviors, such as repetitive screaming and body rocking.

4.4.9.1. Structuring Antecedent Stimulus Events

Based on the observation that SIB is more prevalent in some situations than in others, Favell, McGimsey, and Schell[147] and Lockwood and Bourland[148] successfully reduced SIBs in profoundly retarded young adults by providing access to those conditions associated with little or no self-injury. When provided toys that could be manipulated and that provided preferred sensory stimulations, these adults with long histories of various SIBs replaced the self-injurious activities with more appropriate toy manipulation and play.

4.4.9.2. Reinforcement of Alternative Behaviors

The procedure of differential reinforcement involves providing more frequent and valuable consequences for appropriate behaviors and reducing or removing the reinforcement associated with SIB. Thus, an extinction procedure designed to weaken the behavior and a differential reinforcement procedure designed to strengthen alternative appropriate behaviors are combined. The differential reinforcement procedure may consist of DRO (reinforcement is provided immediately following periods of time in which no self-injury occurs) or DRI (reinforcement is provided for specific behavior that is appropriate and incompatible with self-injury).

Lovaas *et al.*[149] reduced to a near-zero level the high-rate self-hitting behavior of a 9-year-old boy after systematically reinforcing him with smiles and praise for clapping his hands to music. Weiher and Harman[150] reduced to near-zero the chronic head banging of a severely retarded 14-year-old boy by reinforcing him with applesauce at the end of various time intervals during which the SIB did not occur. Regain and Anson[151] used a DRO procedure with a severely retarded 12-year-old girl who, prior to intervention, spent much of her time engaging in self-scratching and head banging behaviors. Although not totally eliminated, these SIBs were significantly reduced. As a final illustration, Tarpley and Schroeder,[152] in treatment of three profoundly retarded adults, found a DRI procedure to be more useful than DRO in effectively reducing head banging.

Differential reinforcement has also been used in combination with other procedures to treat SIB. Azrin, Besalel, and Wisotzek[153] reduced the severe and chronic self-injurious behavior of severely and profoundly retarded adults to near-zero levels in both school and living settings. A DRI plus a physical interruption procedure was used that consisted of providing reinforcement following periods of no self-injury and the occurrence of play, social, or other appropriate behaviors, combined with interrupting each self-injurious episode and requiring the person's hands to rest in his or her lap for two minutes.

4.4.9.3. Withholding or Removing Reinforcement

a. Extinction. Rincover and Devany,[154] with young profoundly retarded children whose self-injury appeared to be self-stimulatory and thus maintained by the sensory stimulation that it produced, demonstrated the value of a *sensory extinction* procedure in immediately and substantially reducing the SIB behaviors. In sensory extinction, the sensory stimulation associated with the specific SIB of each child was removed. In illustration, one boy who engaged in head banging was provided a helmet that attenuated the tactile sensory consequences of the SIB. Another child, who engaged in self-injurious face scratching was required to wear thin rubber gloves—a procedure that prevented her from damaging her skin but, although significantly reducing the sensory stimulation, did not prevent her from scratching.

b. Time-Out. A time-out procedure, consisting of removing the person from the opportunity to obtain reinforcement immediately following each occurrence of SIB has been used successfully in reducing SIB in some individuals. An underlying assumption in use of this procedure is that the person, at the time of removal, is in an environment that is positively reinforcing. A report by Solnick, Rincover, and Peterson[155] highlighted this assumption. The self-injury of a severely retarded adolescent was not reduced significantly following the initiation of a time-out contingency until the environment from which the person was removed was enriched through increased stimulating and reinforcing activities and objects. Following enrichment, the time-out was effective in suppressing the SIB. Typically the time-out procedure is used under conditions of reinforcement of alternative behaviors.

Hamilton, Stephens, and Allen[86] demonstrated the effectiveness of a time-out in eliminating the head and back banging behaviors of severely retarded females. The SIB had not recurred at follow-up checks several months later. Similar results were reported by Wolf, Risley, and Mees,[156] who used time-out to eliminate the self-destructive behavior of a mentally retarded 3 ½-year-old male in both a hospital and a home setting. Wolf *et al.*[157] reported that three years later, the same child's SIB was again eliminated by means of time-out, this time in a school setting. The SIB was eliminated with only three time-out experiences in this second setting, a result suggesting that the child's prior experience with the time-out contingency had increased its effectiveness.

4.4.9.4. Presentation of Aversive Consequences

A final procedure of the behavioral treatment of SIB consists of presenting an aversive or punishing event contingent on each occurrence of self-injury.

a. Overcorrection. Several reports have demonstrated the usefulness of overcorrection procedures in reducing SIBs. The most common form of overcorrection used with SIB involves training in which the part of the client's body involved in the SIB is moved to a series of positions where it is held for several seconds. Harris and Romanczyk[158] applied this type of overcorrection to the chronic head and chin banging behavior of a moderately retarded 8-year-old boy at school and at home. The frequency of SIB dropped dramatically when overcorrection was used, and it remained at near-zero levels in both settings. Using a similar procedure of "forced arm exercise," deCatanzaro and Baldwin[159] eliminated the head hitting behaviors of young profoundly retarded boys. The overcorrection procedure produced an initial reduction in SIB and was subsequently combined with a DRO procedure that reduced the SIB to near-zero levels. The overcorrection effects were generalized by extending intervention to several different settings.

Overcorrection, used in combination with other procedures, is favored by a number of therapists. Measel and Alfieri[160] demonstrated the efficacy of a combination of DRI and overcorrection to eliminate the head slapping and head banging behaviors exhibited by two profoundly retarded boys. Johnson *et al.*[161] successfully reduced a variety of SIBs in profoundly retarded adults through overcorrection and differential reinforcement procedures. These therapists observed, however, that overcorrection alone produced most of the therapeutic effects. Azrin and colleagues[162] combined three overcorrection approaches (autism reversal, required relaxation, and hand-awareness training) to significantly decrease the SIBs of 11 clients, 10 of whom were severely or profoundly retarded. An analysis of benefits indicated that SIB was reduced by 99%. However, the therapists speculated that this multicomponent approach would be most effective (1) with a client who possessed a high level of outward-directed behavior prior to intervention or (2) if the social environment was one that strongly encouraged outward-directed activity.

b. Aversive Electrical Stimulation. Butterfield[163] described this technique as delivering a physically harmless but psychologically aversive electrical stimulus to the person's limb or back for a brief duration immediately following the occurrence of self-injury. This procedure is the most widely researched and the most generally effective method of initially suppressing self-injury. The only published exceptions to the effectiveness of shock are with persons presenting the Lesch–Nyhan syndrome.[37]

Tate and Baroff[164] virtually eliminated the high-rate SIB (head banging, self-hitting, and self-kicking) of a 9-year-old blind boy following the implementation of a shock contingency. These therapists reported the positive side effects of increased eating and decreased posturing, saliva-saving, and clinging behaviors. Similar results were obtained by Lovaas and Simmons[165] with severely retarded boys. The desirable side effects following the reduction of SIBs included a reduced avoidance of staff, less whining behavior, and increased exploration of the environment. Finally, Merbaum[166] described the use of electrical stimulation by a mother in the treatment of the SIBs of her 12-year-old son. SIBs were reduced in home and school settings. A one-year follow-up indicated maintenance of the SIBs at a near-zero level, and the mother reported that her son was "quieter, happier, and wonderful around the house."

c. Additional Punishment Procedures. Other procedures have been reported as effective in reducing self-injurious behavior. These include (1) *facial screening*—the person's face is briefly covered with a terry cloth bib following the SIB[167]; (2) *water mist*—water mist is sprayed in the person's face following SIB[168]; (3) *aromatic ammonia*—ammonia is held briefly under the person's nose following SIB[169]; (4) *aversive tickling*—the person is tickled for a prolonged period following SIB[102]; and (5) a *rage reduction technique*—the person is physically restrained and forced to hit the therapist's hand.[170]

4.4.10. Self-Stimulatory Behavior

Many mentally retarded and other developmentally disabled persons engage in chronic, excessive self-stimulatory (stereotypical) behaviors. These highly repetitive motor and posturing behaviors seemingly have no adaptive or positive environmental consequences. In both residential and community program settings, self-stimulatory behavior is one of the most frequently occurring problems among the severely and the profoundly retarded. Studies suggest that 60%–70% of the mentally retarded in residential facilities engage in repetitive self-stimulatory acts.[171] Similarly, Wehman and McLaughlin,[172] in a survey of teachers of severely delayed students, found self-stimulatory behavior to be one of the most frequently cited problems occurring in the classroom. These studies also reveal that the lower the intellectual level of the person, the greater is the likelihood of self-stimulatory behaviors. In some cases, the self-stimulatory activities fill most of the person's time and are incompatible both with learning new behaviors and with engaging in those appropriate actions that are currently in his or her repertoire.

Self-stimulatory behaviors include such repetitive actions as head rolling, toe walking, rubbing the fingers together, body rocking, trunk twisting, waving the hands in front of the eyes, weaving the hands from side to side, object spinning, rubbing objects, sucking and mouthing the fingers and/or objects, nonsocial vocalizations, and arm flapping. The common characteristics of these different behaviors are that (1) the behaviors are performed in the same mechanical, stereotypical manner each time they occur, and (2) the stereotyped behaviors are engaged in over and over again (e.g., the same posture, such as an arm entangled in a shirt, is maintained for a long period of time; the person sits on the floor and rocks back and forth rapidly for an extended period of time).

4.4.10.1. Reinforcement of Alternative Behaviors

Repp, Deitz, and Speir[173] demonstrated the value of providing positive reinforcement for increasingly longer periods of time in which self-stimulatory behaviors were absent in three severely retarded persons who exhibited high rates of various kinds of stereotypical responding. During treatment, a timer was set for a predetermined period of time. If self-stimulatory behavior did not occur during the interval, a bell rang and the teacher hugged and verbally praised the client for a few seconds. The self-stimulation was rapidly reduced to near-zero occurrence. Favell,[174] through reinforcing appropriate behavior (toy play) that physically competed with stereotypical behaviors, successfully reduced the high-rate self-stimulation of severely and profoundly retarded children.

4.4.10.2. Reinforcement and Physical Interruption

Azrin and Wesolowski[175] reduced to infrequent occurrence the self-stimulatory behaviors of seven profoundly retarded adults who, prior to treatment, had spent 40% or more of their time in stereotypical movements while in a group classroom training program. Each client initially was provided intensive individual training in the adaptive behaviors (e.g., table task, eye contact, and following instructions) included in the classroom program. Appropriate behaviors were reinforced by praise, stroking, and snack items. When self-stimulation occurred, the client was reprimanded verbally, the behavior was interrupted, and the client was required to place his or her hands in his or her lap or on the edge of the table for two minutes. Each client was returned to the group classroom setting, with the interruption procedure gradually faded as the stereotypical behaviors were reduced to infrequent occurrence.

4.4.10.3. Withholding or Removing Reinforcement

a. Sensory Extinction. Based on the notion that self-stimulation in some persons is intrinsically reinforced by the resulting auditory, visual, or proprioceptive sensory stimulation, Rincover *et al.*[176] eliminated the high-rate self-stimulatory behaviors of four developmentally disabled children by removing or minimizing the sensory consequences of such actions. These therapists then used the preferred sensory stimulation of each child to establish appropriate toy play by selecting toys that provided this reinforcing consequence. A music box and an autoharp were selected for the child whose self-stimulatory behaviors produced auditory stimulation, building blocks and stringing beads for proprioception, and a bubble-blowing kit for visual stimulation. After each child was trained to play with the toys until each spontaneously played correctly, the stereotypical behavior remained at a low level as appropriate toy play replaced it.

   b. Time-Out. Mattos[177] decreased facial tics and finger sucking by stopping music, which a child enjoyed, contingent on self-stimulation.

4.4.10.4. Presentation of Aversive Consequences

   a. Overcorrection. A number of reports have demonstrated the potential usefulness of an overcorrection procedure in suppressing stereotypical behavior in some mentally retarded clients. Foxx and Azrin[178] used the procedure to virtually eliminate the self-stimulatory behaviors displayed by four profoundly retarded children. To illustrate, for children who repetitively mouthed objects, a tooth brush immersed in an oral antiseptic was brushed in the child's mouth and the child's lips were wiped with a washcloth. To decrease head weaving, the therapist restrained the child's head and then instructed her to hold her head either up, down, or straight ahead for 15 seconds. The positions were randomly changed for 5 minutes, with manual guidance provided as necessary to ensure that the child performed as required. As a second example of the effectiveness of overcorrection, Matson and Stephens[179] used "hand overcorrection" to treat a variety of stereotyped behaviors of long standing in severely retarded adults. Such behaviors as wall patting, face patting, hair flipping, and head rubbing were followed by a 5-minute overcorrection procedure requiring the client to hold his or her hands either over his or her head, straight out, or at his or her side. Each position was held for 15 seconds before proceeding to the next position.

   b. Other Aversive Consequences. A number of other aversive consequences have been used in successful programs for reducing stereotypical behaviors. These include such events as *facial screening* for repetitive finger sucking, *depressing tongue with wooden blade* for recurring tongue protrusion,[180] and *distortion of the sound of music* contingent on body rocking.[181]

4.4.11. Social Skill Deficits

   A major concern in community integration of the mentally retarded is the limited ability of many individuals to interact with others in a socially acceptable manner across a variety of settings. As a result, there has been a growing interest in developing and evaluating social skills training programs using behavioral techniques in a wide range of deficit behavioral areas. Positive results have been reported with deficits in *conversational skills,*[182-186] *vocational adjustment,*[187-189] *recreational skills,*[190] *cooperation,*[191] *independent living skills,*[192,193] and *other interpersonal skills.*[194-197] Bates[198] and Matson[199] used social skills training procedures to facilitate the development of assertive behaviors and communication skills in mentally retarded adults within the context of training *shopping skills.* Such techniques have also been applied to improving the *job interview skills* of the retarded[200] and other skills necessary to acquire and maintain employment.[201] Finally, applications of social skills training procedures have been extended to lower functioning retarded individuals in teaching *appropriate mealtime behavior,*[193] *community pedestrian skills,*[192] and *interpersonal skills.*[202]

Social skills training, derived from social learning theory, involves a variety of techniques. The most salient components include verbal instruction, modeling, coaching, behavioral rehearsal, and feedback.[203] Other components—such as social reinforcement, prompting, token reinforcement, self-monitoring and self-reinforcement, *in vivo* practice, homework, booster sessions, and relaxation training—have also been included.[204] The training typically is provided in therapy settings, although rehearsal in the natural environment is occasionally employed. Role-play scenes typically are used both to assess and to train target skills.

4.4.11.1. Multicomponent Treatment Programs

Turner *et al.*[30] described a social skills training package that is representative of the type of multicomponent program frequently used with the mentally retarded. This package combined behavior rehearsal, modeling, instruction, feedback, and reinforcement procedures in teaching a mentally retarded 19-year-old male such prosocial behaviors as eye contact and smiling. Consistent with the social skills training model, role-play scenes depicting interpersonal situations that were a problem for the client were presented during training sessions. Following is an example of the type of scene presented:

> *Narrator:* You are walking into the cafeteria. After you get your food, you see an empty seat at a table where several patients who you know from your group are seated. As you place your tray on the table and begin to be seated, another patient walks up to you and asks you to find another seat as she would like to join this group. She says . . .
> *Role Model:* "Bill, I'd like to sit here. I know you wouldn't mind moving to another table." (p. 255)

The client then was instructed to respond as if he were actually in that situation. Although the client's target behaviors improved initially with this social skills training package, his skill performance had declined at six-month follow-up. Booster sessions implemented at this time again increased his skill level. The authors suggested that the availability of a therapeutic environment in which the client had frequent opportunities to practice and be reinforced for his newly acquired skills appeared to be an important factor contributing to the maintenance and the generalization of the behaviors.

Kelly et al.[200] reported more immediate and spontaneous generalization of behavior change in a study designed to teach job interview skills to four mentally retarded adolescents. The skills learned in the natural setting not only transferred to a posttreatment *in vivo* setting (McDonald's) but also resulted in competitive employment for two of the clients within six months following training.

4.4.11.2. Comparison of Procedures

A few studies have compared the differential effectiveness of various social skills training components. Gibson et al.[191] compared the efficacy of (1) modeling, (2) instructions and feedback, and (3) modeling, instructions, and feedback in teaching three mildly retarded adults three social responses: verbalization, recreation, and cooperation. All three training procedures increased all three responses, but the most effective procedure was the use of modeling, instructions, and feedback. Matson and Andrasik[184] compared the effectiveness of (1) social skills training and (2) social skills training, self-monitoring, and self-reinforcement in teaching conversational skills to eight mentally retarded adults. Social skills training, self-monitoring, and self-reinforcement were shown to be more effective than social skills training alone.

4.4.12. Vomiting and Rumination

Problems of chronic vomiting (self-induced emesis or regurgitation of previously ingested food) and rumination (reingestion of vomitus) may pose serious dangers to a person's health because of malnutrition, severe weight loss, dehydration, and decreased resistance to disease. In some cases, the problem can cause a life-threatening condition.[205] Such activity also creates general caretaker problems and contributes to the person's interpersonal difficulties. In some cases, chronic vomiting may occur in the absence of organic antecedents and thus may offer the possibility of various behavioral treatment approaches.

4.4.12.1. Structuring Antecedent Stimulus Events

a. Food Satiation. Based on the hypothesis that vomiting behaviors in two profoundly retarded adults were being maintained by the reinforcing qualities of the reconsumption of the vomitus because of a state of food deprivation, Jackson et al.[206] provided the adults with as much food as they would eat at each meal. In addition, the adults were provided a milk shake between each meal to maintain the effect of satiation throughout the day. A 94% reduction in the frequency of vomiting was obtained with one adult and a 50% improvement in the other. Success with this procedure of food satiation was also reported by Libby and Phillips[207] in treatment of a 17-year-old and by Rast *et al.*[208] with severely and profoundly retarded adults.

   b. Food Satiation and Aversive Consequences. Foxx, Snyder, and Schroeder[209] used the food satiation in combination with an oral-hygiene overcorrection procedure.

   Finally, the chronic rumination of a profoundly retarded male was treated successfully by use of a combined procedure of food satiation and time-out from tactile stimulation provided by the therapist. The combination of the procedures was more effective than either used in isolation.[210]

4.4.12.2. Reinforcement of Alternative Behaviors

   Barmann[205] successfully eliminated life-threatening ruminative vomiting in a blind, profoundly retarded 6-year-old boy through a procedure of providing positive reinforcement for periods of time in which hand mouthing, a prevomiting response, was not occurring. Vibratory stimulation, an experience that the child enjoyed, was provided during therapy sessions for having "dry hands." The treatment gains generalized to nontreatment settings and were maintained over a one-year follow-up period.

4.4.12.3. Withholding or Removing Reinforcement

   a. Extinction and Positive Reinforcement. Wolf *et al.*[211] provided one of the initial examples of the successful use of behavior therapy with a clinical problem presented by a nonverbal 9-year-old child diagnosed as "suffering from mental retardation, cerebral palsy, aphasia, hyperirritability, and brain damage." Within three months of the child's being enrolled in a school program, vomiting had become practically an everyday occurrence. Drug therapy had no effect in treatment of the problem. Further, medical staff did not view the vomiting as being due to physical factors.

   As the child was removed to the living area following a vomiting episode in the classroom, the therapists hypothesized that such consequences were reinforcing and thus maintaining the vomiting behavior. The behavior therapy program consisted of keeping the child in the classroom for the scheduled period regardless of her vomiting. This extinction procedure removed the possible sources of positive and/or negative reinforcement that the vomiting had previously produced. Additionally, the teacher provided the child with tangible and social reinforcers following a variety of appropriate classroom behaviors. The vomiting behavior was eliminated within a month. Other behaviors that occurred with virtually every vomiting episode—screaming, clothes tearing, and destruction of property—also disappeared. The therapists noted that productive classroom behavior and responsiveness to the teacher's requests improved markedly. These rather severe "emotional" problems were dealt with by developing hunches about the environmental factors contributing to the problems and by restructuring the child's experiences in the natural settings in which the problems were occurring.

b. Extinction and Response Cost. Smeets[212] also demonstrated the possible usefulness of an extinction procedure in a program for a profoundly retarded 18-year-old male. Contingent withdrawal of social attention and the remainder of the meal following vomiting behavior resulted in a reduction of vomiting and rumination.

c. Time-Out from Positive Reinforcement. Davis, Wieseler, and Hanzel[213] eliminated rumination in a profoundly mentally retarded 26-year-old male through the contingent removal of music. Music was played continuously throughout the treatment. Rumination resulted in a loud sharp "No" from the therapist and the absence of the music for short periods of time. In this manner, a long-standing pattern of ruminatory behavior was controlled.

4.4.12.4. Presentation of Aversive Consequences

a. Overcorrection. Azrin and Wesolowski[214] and Duker and Seys[215] demonstrated the usefulness of behavioral programs using positive practice, self-correction, and restitutional overcorrection combined with a procedure of differentially reinforcing appropriate behavior in eliminating vomiting in profoundly retarded adults.

b. Aversive Electrical Stimulation. Luckey, Watson, and Musick[216] and Kohlenberg[217] used a punishment procedure involving aversive electrical stimulation to significantly reduce persistent vomiting in severely retarded clients. Luckey *et al.*[216] provided the electrical stimulation immediately following the observation of vomiting or ruminating behavior. A marked reduction in these behaviors were evident by the fifth day of treatment. A general improvement in overall behavior was also noted. Similar results were reported by Gilbraith, Byrick, and Rutledge[218] and by Bright and Whaley.[219] Kohlenberg,[217] in the treatment of a severely retarded woman whose progressive weight loss due to vomiting after every meal had become a serious medical problem, reasoned that the vomiting behavior was the last response in a chain of behaviors. Contingent aversive electrical stimulation was provided following the occurrence of stomach tensions, a prevomiting response that consisted of an overt abdominal movement. A rapid reduction in vomiting was obtained, with resulting weight gain.

c. Lemon Juice Therapy. Becker, Turner, and Sajwaj[220] reported the successful reduction of chronic and high-rate rumination in a profoundly retarded 36-month-old child following the initiation of a procedure that involved the injection of lemon juice into the child's mouth contingent on rumination. Also noted following the reduction in the rumination was an increase in the child's social behaviors and language, along with a greater interest in manipulating objects.

4.5. Application to Developmental Problems

Behavior therapy procedures have been used successfully with a variety of developmental problems, including *academic*,[221] *dressing*,[222,223] *feeding*,[224,225] *grooming*,[226] *imitative behavior*,[227,228] *language*,[229,230] *leisure skills*,[231] *locomotion*,[232] and *nonspeech communication*.[233] As indicated earlier, even the young and the more severely retarded are suitable clients for programming, as therapy procedures are designed to begin at each person's current skill level and to teach new skills step-by-step. Typically, behavior shaping procedures are used in which positive reinforcement is provided for behaviors that represent closer approximations of the desired goal. Additionally, a variety of other procedures described earlier are used to ensure the maintenance and the generalization of newly acquired functional skills. The interested reader should refer to the suggested references for detailed descriptions of the specific procedures used.

4.6. Conclusions

The behavior therapy procedures described represent possible treatment resources for professionals serving those mentally retarded children, adolescents, and adults who may present a variety of emotional and behavioral difficulties in living, educational, and vocational settings. As emphasized, the development of an appropriate therapy program for any specific client should be based on a thorough clinical assessment of that client in the settings in which the difficulties occur. The major focus of the behavior therapy program should be on the development and the strengthening of the skills of personal competency, and not merely on the suppression or elimination of behaviors viewed as inappropriate. As noted, the assumption cannot be made that, once excessive inappropriate characteristics have been suppressed or extinguished, the mentally retarded client will automatically begin to function appropriately.

References

1. Philips I, Williams N: Psychopathology and mental retardation: I. Psychopathology. *Am J Psychiatr* 132;1265–1271, 1975.
2. Reid, AH: Psychiatric disorders in mentally handicapped children: A clinical and follow-up study. *J Ment Defic Res* 24;287–298, 1980.
3. Menolascino FJ: *Challenges in Mental Retardation.* New York, Human Sciences Press, 1977.
4. Szymanski LS, Tanguay PE (eds): *Emotional Disorders of Mentally Retarded Persons.* Baltimore, University Park Press, 1980.

5. Jacobson JW: Problem behavior and psychiatric impairment within a developmentally disabled population I: Behavior frequency. *Appl Res Ment Retard* 3;121–139, 1982.

6. Reiss S: Psychopathology and mental retardation: Survey of a developmental disabilities mental health program. *Ment Retard* 20;128–132, 1982.

7. Eyman RK, Borthwick SA, Miller C: Trends in maladaptive behavior of mentally retarded persons placed in community and institutional settings. *Am J Ment Defic* 85;473–477, 1981.

8. Eyman RK, Call T: Maladaptive behavior and community placement of mentally retarded persons. *Am J Ment Defic* 82;137–144, 1977.

9. Schalock RL, Harper RS, Carver G: Independent living placement: Five years later. *Am J Ment Defic* 86;170–177, 1981.

10. Seltzer MM, Seltzer G: *Context for Competence.* Cambridge, Mass, Educational Projects, 1978.

11. Schalock RL, Harper RS: Placement from community-based mental retardation programs: How well do clients do? *Am J Ment Defic* 83;240–247, 1978.

12. Hill BK, Bruiniks RH: *Physical and Behavioral Characteristics and Maladaptive Behavior of Mentally Retarded People in Residential Facilities.* Minneapolis, University of Minnesota, Department of Psychoeducational Studies, 1981.

13. Breuning SE, Davis VJ, Poling AD: Pharmacotherapy with the mentally retarded: Implications for clinical psychologists. *Clin Psychol Rev* 2;79–114, 1982.

14. Sprague RL, Baxley GB: Drugs for behavior management with comment on some legal aspects, in Wortis J (ed): *Mental Retardation,* vol 10. New York, Brunner/Mazel, 1978.

15. Robinson NM, Robinson HB: *The Mentally Retarded Child,* ed 2. New York, McGraw-Hill, 1976.

16. Sternlicht M: Issues in counseling and psychotherapy with mentally retarded individuals, in Bialer I, Sternlicht M (eds): *The Psychology of Mental Retardation: Issues and Approaches.* New York, Psychological Dimensions, 1977.

17. Gardner WI, Cole CL: Meeting the mental health needs of the mentally retarded. *Community Services Forum* 1(3);1–3, 1981.

18. Gardner WI: Use of behavior therapy with the mentally retarded, in Menolascino FJ (ed): *Psychiatric Approaches to Mental Retardation.* New York, Basic Books, 1970.

19. Gardner WI: *Learning and Behavior Characteristics of Exceptional Children and Youth.* Boston, Allyn and Bacon, 1977.

20. Hersen M, Bellack AS: *Behavior Therapy in the Psychiatric Setting.* Baltimore, Williams and Wilkins, 1978.

21. Hersen M, Eisler RM, Miller PM (eds): *Progress in Behavior Modification,* vol 12. New York, Academic Press, 1981.

22. Rimm DC, Masters JC: *Behavior Therapy,* ed 2. New York, Academic Press, 1979.

23. Walker CE, Clement PW, Hedberg A, *et al*: *Clinical Procedures for Behavior Therapy.* Englewood Cliffs, NJ, Prentice-Hall, 1981.

24. Jansen PE: Basic principles of behavior therapy with retarded persons, in Szymanski LS, Tanguay PE (eds): *Emotional Disorders of Mentally Retarded Persons.* Baltimore, University Park Press, 1980.

25. Johnson WL, Baumeister AA: Behavioral techniques for decreasing aberrant behaviors of retarded and autistic persons, in Hersen M, Eisler RM, Miller PM (eds): *Progress in Behavior Modification,* vol 12. New York, Academic Press, 1981.

26. Karan OC, Gardner WI (eds): *Habilitation Practices with the Developmentally Disabled who Present Behavioral and Emotional Disorders.* Madison, WI, Rehabilitation Research and Training Center in Mental Retardation, 1983.

27. Matson JL, McCartney JR: *Handbook of Behavior Modification with the Mentally Retarded.* New York, Plenum Press, 1981.

28. Schroeder S, Mulick JA, Schroeder CS: Management of severe behavior problems of the retarded, in Ellis NR (ed): *Handbook of Mental Deficiency, Psychological Theory and Research,* ed 2. Hillsdale, NJ, Lawrence Erlbaum, 1979.

29. Mansdorf IJ: Eliminating fear in a mentally retarded adult by behavioral hierarchies and operant techniques. *J Behav Ther Exp Psychiatr* 7;189–190, 1976.

30. Turner SM, Hersen M, Bellack AS: Social skills training to teach prosocial behaviors in an organically impaired and retarded patient. *J Behav Ther Exp Psychiatr* 9;253–258, 1978.
31. Kazdin AE: *History of Behavior Modification.* Baltimore, University Park Press, 1978.
32. Bellack AS, Hersen M, Kazdin AE (eds): *International Handbook of Behavior Modification and Therapy.* New York, Macmillan, 1982.
33. Bandura A: *Social Learning Theory.* Engelwood Cliffs, NJ, Prentice-Hall, 1977.
34. Ross AO: *Psychological disorders of children.* New York, McGraw-Hill, 1974.
35. Bijou SW: Behavior modification in teaching the retarded child, in Thoresen CE (ed): *The Seventy-Second Yearbook of the National Society for the Study of Education, Part I—Behavior Modification in Education.* Chicago, University of Chicago Press, 1972.
36. Ross DM, Ross SA: *Hyperactivity,* ed 2. New York, Wiley, 1982.
37. Flavell JE (Task Force Chairperson): The treatment of self-injurious behavior. *Behav Ther* 13;529–554, 1982.
38. Touchette PE: Mental retardation: An introduction to the analysis and remediation of behavioral deficiency, in Marholin D II (ed): *Child Behavior Therapy.* New York, Gardner Press, 1978.
39. Hersen M, Bellack AS: *Behavioral Assessment: A Practical Handbook,* ed 2. New York, Pergamon Press, 1981.
40. Ellis NR: The Parlow case: A reply to Dr. Roos. *Law Psychol Rev* 5;15–49, 1979.
41. May JG, Risley TR, Twardosz S, et al: *Guidelines for the Use of Behavioral Procedures in State Programs for Retarded Persons.* Arlington, TX, NARC Monograph MR Research, 1976.
42. Wolpe J: *The Practice of Behavior Therapy.* Oxford, Pergamon Press, 1973.
43. Matson JL: A controlled outcome study of phobias in mentally retarded adults. *Behav Res Ther* 19;101–107, 1981.
44. Peck CL: Desensitization for the treatment of fear in the high level adult retardate. *Behav Res Ther* 15;137–148, 1977.
45. Ritter B: The group desensitization of children's snake phobias using vicarious and contact desensitization procedures. *Behav Res Ther* 6;1–6, 1968.
46. Cole CL, Gardner WI, Karan OC: *Self-Management Training of Mentally Retarded Adults with Chronic Conduct Difficulties.* Madison, WI, Rehabilitation Research and Training Center in Mental Retardation, 1983.
47. Shapiro ES: Self-control procedures with the mentally retarded, in Hersen M, Eisler RM, Miller PM (eds): *Progress in Behavior Modification,* vol 12. New York, Academic Press, 1981.
48. Berger C, Markos P, Gardner WI: *Social Skills Training with the Mentally Retarded: Research Needs.* Madison, WI, Rehabilitation Research and Training Center in Mental Retardation, 1983.
49. Gresham PM: Social skills training with handicapped children: A review. *Rev Educ Res* 51;139–176, 1981.
50. Harvey JR, Karan OC, Bhargava D, et al: Relaxation training and cognitive behavioral procedures to reduce violent temper outbursts in a moderately retarded woman. *J Behav Ther Exp Psychiatr* 9;347–351, 1978.
51. Gardner WI, Cole CL, Berry DL, et al: Reduction of disruptive behaviors in mentally retarded adults: A self-management approach. *Behav Modif* 7;76–96, 1983.
52. Whitman TL, Scibak JW: Behavior modification research with the severely and profoundly retarded, in Ellis NR (ed): *Handbook of Mental Deficiency, Psychological Theory and Research,* ed 2. Hillsdale, NJ, Lawrence Erlbaum, 1979.
53. Watson LS: *A Management System Approach to Teaching Independent Living Skills and Managing Disruptive Behavior.* Tuscaloosa, AL, Behavior Modification Technology, 1979.
54. Gladstone BW, Sherman JA: Developing generalized behavior modification skills in high school students working with retarded children. *J Appl Behav Anal* 8;169–180, 1975.
55. Gladstone BW, Spencer CJ: The effects of modelling on the contingent praise of mental retardation counsellors. *J Appl Behav Anal* 10;75–84, 1977.
56. Parsonson BS, Baer AM, Baer DM: The application of generalized correct social contingencies: An evaluation of a training program. *J Appl Behav Anal* 7;427–437, 1974.

57. Fowler SA, Johnson MR, Whitman TL, *et al*: Programming a parent's behavior for establishing self-help skills and reducing aggression and noncompliance in a profoundly retarded adult. *AAESPH Rev* 3(3);151–161, 1978.
58. Forehand R, McMahon RJ: *Helping the Noncompliant Child*. New York, Guildford Press, 1981.
59. Cushna B, Szymanski LS, Tanguay PE: Professional roles and unmet manpower needs, in Szymanski LS, Tanguay PE (eds): *Emotional Disorders of Mentally Retarded Persons*. Baltimore, University Park Press, 1980.
60. American Psychiatric Association: *Diagnostic and Statistical Manual of Mental Disorders* (DSM-III). Washington, DC, Author, 1980.
61. Agras WS, Barlow DH, Chapin HN, *et al*: Behavior modification of anorexia nervosa. *Arch Gen Psychiatr* 30;279–286, 1974.
62. Claggett MS: Anorexia nervosa: A behavioral approach. *Am J Nurs* 8;1471–1472, 1980.
63. Ollendick TH: Behavioral treatment of anorexia nervosa: A five year study. *Behav Modif* 3;124–135, 1979.
64. Hurley AD, Sovner R: Anorexia nervosa and mental retardation: A case report. *J Clin Psychiatr* 49;480–482, 1979.
65. Mohl PC, McMahon T: Anorexia nervosa associated with mental retardation and schizoaffective disorder. *Psychosomatics* 21;602–606, 1980.
66. Fox R, Karan O: Deinstitutionalization as a function of inter-agency planning: A case study. *Educ Tr Ment Retard* 11;255–260, 1976.
67. Forehand R, Baumeister AA: Deceleration of aberrant behavior among retarded individuals, in Hersen M, Eisler RM, Miller PM (eds): *Progress in Behavior Modification*, vol 2. New York, Academic Press, 1976.
68. Repp AC, Brulle AR: Reducing aggressive behavior of mentally retarded persons, in Matson JL, McCartney JR (eds), *Handbook of Behavior Modification with the Mentally Retarded*. New York, Plenum Press, 1981.
69. Plaska T, Ragee G: The intensive training project: A program to prepare aggressive and disruptive residents for community placement, in Hamerlynck LA (ed): *Behavioral Systems for the Developmentally Disabled: II. Institutional Clinic and Community Environments*. New York, Brunner/Mazel, 1979.
70. Boe RB: Economical procedures for the reduction of aggression in a residential setting. *Ment Retard* 15;25–28, 1977.
71. Murphy MJ, Zahm D: Effects of improved physical and social environments on self-help and problem behaviors of institutionalized retarded males. *Behav Modif* 2;193–210, 1978.
72. Rago WV, Parker RM, Cleland CC: Effects of increased space on the social behavior of institutionalized profoundly retarded male adults. *Am J Ment Defic* 82;554–558, 1978.
73. Repp AC, Deitz SM, Deitz DED: Reducing inappropriate behaviors in classrooms and in individual sessions through DRO schedules of reinforcement. *Ment Retad* 14(1);11–15, 1976.
74. Drabman R, Spitalnik R: Training a retarded child as a behavioral teaching assistant. *J Behav Ther Exp Psychiatr* 4;269–272, 1973.
75. Perline IH, Levinsky D: Controlling maladaptive classroom behavior in the severely retarded. *Am J Ment Defic* 73;74–78, 1968.
76. Broden M, Hall R, Dunlap A, *et al*: Effects of teacher attention and a token reinforcement system in a junior high school special education class. *Except Child* 36;341–349, 1970.
77. Deitz SM, Repp AC: Decreasing classroom misbehavior through the use of DRL schedules of reinforcement. *J Appl Behav Anal* 6;457–463, 1973.
78. Sewell E, McCoy JF, Sewell WR: Modification of an antagonistic social behavior using positive reinforcement for other behavior. *Psychol Rec* 23;499–504, 1973.
79. Hall HV, Price AB, Shinedling M, *et al*: Control of aggressive behavior in a group of retardates using positive and negative reinforcement procedures. *Trng Sch Bull* 70;179–186, 1973.
80. Repp AC, Deitz SM: Reducing aggressive and self-injurious behavior of institutionalized retarded children through reinforcement of other behaviors. *J Appl Behav Anal* 7;313–325, 1974.
81. Polvinale RA, Lutzker JR: Elimination of assaultive and inappropriate sexual behavior by reinforcement and social restitution. *Ment Retard* 18;27–30, 1980.

82. Martin PL, Foxx RM: Victim control of the aggression of an institutionalized retardate. *J Behav Ther Exp Psychiatr* 4;161–165, 1973.
83. Forehand R: Teacher recording of deviant behavior: A stimulus for behavior change. *J Behav Ther Exp Psychiatr* 4;39–40, 1973.
84. Calhoun KS, Matherne P: The effects of varying schedules of time-out on aggressive behavior of a retarded girl. *J Behav Ther Exp Psychiatr* 6;139–143, 1975.
85. Clark HB, Rowbury T, Baer AM, *et al*: Timeout as a punishing stimulus in continuous and intermittent schedules. *J Appl Behav Anal* 6;443–455, 1973.
86. Hamilton J, Stephens L, Allen P: Controlling aggressive and destructive behavior in severely retarded institutionalized residents. *Am J Ment defic* 71;852–856, 1967.
87. Pendergrass VE: Effects of length of time-out from positive reinforcement and schedule of application in suppression of aggressive behavior. *Psychol Rec* 21;75–80, 1971.
88. White GD, Nielsen G, Johnson SM: Timeout duration and the suppression of deviant behavior in children. *J Appl Behav Anal* 5;111–120, 1972.
89. Foxx RM, Shapiro ST: The timeout ribbon: A nonexclusionary timeout procedure. *J Appl Behav Anal* 11;125–136, 1978.
90. Bostow DE, Bailey JB: Modification of severe disruptive and aggressive behavior using brief timeout and reinforcement procedures. *J Appl Behav Anal* 2;31–37, 1969.
91. Peniston E: Reducing problem behaviors in the severely and profoundly retarded. *J Behav Ther Exp Psychiatr* 6;295–299, 1975.
92. Foxx CL, Foxx RM, Jones JR, *et al*: Twenty-hour social isolation: A program for reducing aggressive behavior of a psychotic-like retarded adult. *Behav Modif* 4;130–144, 1980.
93. Sulzbacher S, Houser JE: A tactic to eliminate disruptive behaviors in the classroom: Group contingent consequences. *Am J Ment Defic* 73;88–90, 1968.
94. Greene RJ, Pratt JJ: A group contingency for individual misbehaviors in the classroom. *Ment Retard* 10(3);33–35, 1972.
95. Axelrod S: Comparison of individual and group contingencies in two special classes. *Behav Ther* 4;83–90, 1973.
96. Foxx RM, Azrin NH: Restitution: A method of eliminating aggressive disruptive behavior of retarded and brain damaged patients. *Behav Res Ther* 10;15–27, 1972.
97. Shapiro ES: Restitution and positive practice overcorrection in reducing aggressive-disruptive behavior: A long-term follow-up. *J Behav Ther Exp Psychiatry* 10;131–134, 1979.
98. Davidson-Gooch L: Autism reversal: A method for reducing aggressive-disruptive behavior. *Behav Ther* 3(2);21–23, 1980.
99. Birnbrauer JS: Generalization of punishment effects: A case study. *J Appl Behav Anal* 1;201–211, 1968.
100. Brandsma JM, Stein LI: The use of punishment as a treatment modality: A case report. *J Nerv Ment Dis* 156;30–37, 1973.
101. Ball TS, Sibbach L, Jones R, *et al*: An accelerometer-activated device to control assaultive and self-destructive behaviors in retardates. *J Behav Ther Exp Psychiatr* 6;223–228, 1975.
102. Greene RJ, Hoats DL: Aversive tickling: A simple conditioning technique. *Behav Ther* 2;389–393, 1971.
103. Schutz RP, Rusch FR, Lamson DS: Eliminating unacceptable behavior: Evaluation of an employer's procedure to eliminate unacceptable behavior on the job. *Community Services Forum* 1(1);4–5, 1979.
104. Gardner WI, Clees T, Cole CL: Self-management of disruptive verbal ruminations by a mentally retarded adult. *Appl Res Ment Retard* 4;41–58, 1983.
105. Ellis NR: Toilet training the severely defective patient: An S-R reinforcement analysis. *Am J Ment Defic* 68;98–103, 1963.
106. McCartney JR, Holden JC: Toilet training for the mentally retarded, in Matson JL, McCartney JR (eds): *Handbook of Behavior Modification with the Mentally Retarded*. New York, Plenum Press, 1981.
107. Waye MF, Melnyr WT: Toilet training of a blind retarded boy by operant conditioning. *J Behav Ther Exp Psychiatr* 4;267–268, 1973.

108. Luiselli, J: Case report: An attendant-administered contingency management programme for the treatment of a toilet phobia. *J Ment Defic Res* 21;283–288, 1977.

109. Foxx RM, Azrin NH: *Toilet Training the Retarded: A Rapid Program for Day and Nighttime Independent Toileting.* Champaign, IL, Research Press, 1973.

110. Azrin NH, Sneed TS, Foxx RM: Dry bed: A rapid method of eliminating bedwetting (enuresis) of the retarded. *Behav Res Ther* 11;427–434, 1973.

111. Raborn JD: Classroom applications of the Foxx-Azrin toileting program. *Ment Retard* 16(2);173–174, 1978.

112. Doleys DM, Arnold S: Treatment of childhood encopresis: Full cleanliness training. *Ment Retard* 13(6);14–16, 1975.

113. Payne D: Regional cooperation in mental retardation data collection. *Ment Retard* 6;52–53, 1968.

114. Doubros SG, Daniels GJ: An experimental approach to the reduction of overactive behavior. *Behav Res Ther* 4;251–258, 1966.

115. Whitman TL, Caponigri V, Mercurio J: Reducing hyperactive behavior in a severely retarded child. *Ment Retard* 9;17–19, 1971.

116. Twardosz S, Sajwaj T: Multiple effects of a procedure to increase sitting in a hyperactive, retarded boy. *J Appl Behav Anal* 5;73–78, 1972.

117. Alabiso F: Operant control of attention behavior: A treatment for hyperactivity. *Behav Ther* 6;39–42, 1975.

118. Rotatori AF, Switzky H, Fox R: Rehavioral weight reduction procedures for obese mentally retarded individuals: A review. *Ment Retard* 19;157–161, 1981.

119. Foxx RM: Social reinforcement of weight reduction: A case report on an obese retarded adolescent. *Ment Retard* 10(4);21–23, 1972.

120. Joachim R, Korboot P: Experimenter contact and self-monitoring of weight with the mentally retarded. *Aust J Ment Retard* 3;222–225, 1975.

121. Foreyt JP, Parks JT: Behavioral controls for achieving weight loss in the severely retarded. *J Behav Ther Exp Psychiatr* 6;27–29, 1975.

122. Joachim R: The use of self-monitoring to effect weight loss in a mildly retarded female. *J Behav Ther Exp Psychiatr* 8;213–215, 1977.

123. Altman K, Bondy A, Hirsch G: Behavioral treatment of obesity in patients with Prader-Willi Syndrome. *J Behav Med* 1(4);403–412, 1978.

124. Buford LM: Group education to reduce overweight: Classes for mentally handicapped children. *Am J Nurs* 75(11);1994–1995, 1975.

125. Heiman MF: The management of obesity in the post-adolescent developmentally disabled client with Prader-Willi syndrome. *Adolescence* 13(50);291–296, 1978.

126. Rotatori AF, Fox R: The effectiveness of a behavioral weight reduction program for moderately retarded adolescents. *Behav Ther* 11;410–416, 1980.

127. Rotatori AF, Fox R, Switzky H: A multicomponent behavioral program for achieving weight loss in the adult retarded person. *Ment Retard* 18;31–33, 1980.

128. Rotatori AF, Switzky H: Successful behavioral weight loss with moderately mentally retarded individuals. *Inter J Obesity* 3;223–228, 1979.

129. Rotatori AF: The effect of different reinforcement schedules in the maintenance of weight loss with retarded overweight adults. *Dissertation Abst Inter* 38;4738–N, 1978.

130. Rotatori AF, Fox R: *Behavioral Weight Reduction Program for Mentally Handicapped Persons.* Baltimore, University Park Press, 1981.

131. Rivenq B: Behavioral therapy of phobias: A case with gynecomastia and mental retardation. *Ment Retard* 12(1);44–45, 1974.

132. Guralnick MJ: Behavior therapy with an acrophobic mentally retarded young adult. *J Behav Ther Exp Psychiatr* 4;263–265, 1973.

133. Freeman BJ, Roy RR, Hemmick S: Extinction of a phobia of physical examination in a seven-year-old mentally retarded boy: A case study. *Behav Res Ther* 14;63–64, 1976.

134. Matson JL: Assessment and treatment of clinical fears in mentally retarded children. *J Appl Behav Anal* 14;287–294, 1981.

135. Albin JB: The treatment of pica (scavenging) behavior in the retarded: A critical analysis and implications for research. *Ment Retard* 15(4);14–17, 1977.
136. Bucher B, Reykdal B, Albin J: Brief physical restraint to control pica in retarded children. *J Behav Ther Exp Psychiatr* 7;137–140, 1976.
137. Ausman J, Ball TS, Alexander D: Behavior therapy of pica with a profoundly retarded adolescent. *Ment Retard* 12(6);16–18, 1974.
138. Foxx RM, Martin ED: Treatment of scavenging behavior (coprophogy and pica) by overcorrection. *Behav Res Ther* 13;153–162, 1975.
139. Corbett JA, Harris R, Robinson RC: Epilepsy, in Wortis J (ed): *Mental Retardation and Developmental Disabilities*. New York, Brunner/Mazel, 1975.
140. Illingsworth RS: Convulsions in mentally retarded children with and without cerebral palsy: Their frequency and age incidence. *J Ment Defic Res* 3;88–93, 1959.
141. Connaughton MC: Management of child health care, in Neisworth JT, Smith RM (eds): *Retardation: Issues, Assessment, and Intervention*. New York, McGraw-Hill, 1978.
142. Krafft KM, Poling AD: Behavioral treatments of epilepsy: Methodological characteristics and problems of published studies. *Appl Res Ment Retard* 3;151–162, 1982.
143. Zlutnick S, Mayville WJ, Moffatt S: Modification of seizure disorders. The interruption of behavior chains. *J Appl Behav Anal* 8;1–12, 1975.
144. Iwata BA, Lorentzson AM: Operant control of seizure-like behavior in an institutionalized retarded adult. *Behav Ther* 7;247–251, 1976.
145. Cautela J, Flannery R: Seizures: Controlling the uncontrollable. *J Rehab* 39;34–35, 1973.
146. Wright L: Aversive conditioning of self-induced seizures. *Behav Ther* 4;712–713, 1973.
147. Favell JE, McGimsey JF, Schell RM: Treatment of self-injury by providing alternate sensory activities. *Anal Intervention Dev Disab* 2;83–104, 1982.
148. Lockwood K, Bourland G: Reduction of self-injurious behaviors by reinforcement and toy use. *Ment Retard* 20;169–173, 1982.
149. Lovaas OI, Freitag G, Gold VJ, et al: Experimental studies in childhood schizophrenia: Analysis of self-destructive behavior. *J Exper Child Psychol* 2;67–84, 1965.
150. Weiher RG, Harman RE: The use of omission training to reduce self-injurious behavior in a retarded child. *Behav Ther* 6;261–268, 1975.
151. Regain RD, Anson JE: The control of self-mutilating behavior with positive reinforcement. *Ment Retard* 14(3);22–25, 1976.
152. Tarpley H, Schroeder S: Comparison of DRO and DRI on rate of suppression of self-injurious behavior. *Am J Ment Defic* 84;188–194, 1979.
153. Azrin NH, Besalel VA, Wisotzek IE: Treatment of self-injury by a reinforcement plus interruption procedure. *Anal Intervention Dev Disab* 2;105–113, 1982.
154. Rincover A, Devany J: The application of sensory extinction procedures to self-injury. *Anal Intervention Dev Disab* 2;67–81, 1982.
155. Solnick JV, Rincover A, Peterson CR: Some determinants of the reinforcing and punishing effects of timeout. *J Appl Behav Anal* 10;415–424, 1977.
156. Wolf M, Risley T, Mees H: Application of operant conditioning procedures to the behavior problems of an autistic child. *Behav Res Ther* 1;305–312, 1964.
157. Wolf M, Risley T, Johnston M, et al: Application of operant conditioning procedures to the behavior problems of an autistic child. A follow-up and extension. *Behav Res Ther* 5;103–111, 1967.
158. Harris SL, Romanczyk RG: Treating self-injurious behavior of a retarded child by overcorrection. *Behav Ther* 7;235–239, 1976.
159. deCatanzaro DA, Baldwin G: Effective treatment of self-injurious behavior through a forced arm exercise. *Am J Ment Defic* 82;433–439, 1978.
160. Measel CJ, Alfieri PA: Treatment of self-injurious behavior by a combination of reinforcement for incompatible behavior and overcorrection. *Am J Ment Defic* 81;147–153, 1976.
161. Johnson WL, Baumeister AA, Penland MJ, et al: Experimental analysis of self-injurious, stereotypic, and collateral behavior of retarded persons: Effects of overcorrection and reinforcement of alternative responding. *Anal Intervention Dev Disab* 2;41–66, 1982.

162. Azrin NH, Gottlieb L, Hughart L, *et al*: Eliminating self-injurious behavior by educative procedures. *Behav Res Ther* 13;101–111, 1975.
163. Butterfield WH: Electric shock—Safety factors when used for the aversive conditioning of humans. *Behav Ther* 6;98–110, 1975.
164. Tate BG, Baroff GS: Aversive control of self-injurious behavior in a psychotic boy. *Behav Res Ther* 4;281–287, 1966.
165. Lovaas OI, Simmons JQ: Manipulation of self-destruction in three retarded children. *J Appl Behav Anal* 2;143–157, 1969.
166. Merbaum M: The modification of self-destructive behavior by a mother-therapist using aversive stimulation. *Behav Ther* 4;442–447, 1973.
167. Lutzker JR: Reducing self-injurious behavior by facial screening. *Am J Ment Defic* 82;510–513, 1978.
168. Dorsey MF, Iwata BA, Ong P, *et al*: Treatment of self-injurious behavior using the water mist: Initial response suppression and generalization. *J Appl Behav Anal* 13;343–353, 1980.
169. Altman K, Haavik S, Cook J: Punishment of self-injurious behavior in natural settings using contingent aromatic ammonia. *Behav Res Ther* 16;85–96, 1978.
170. Saposnek DT, Watson LS Jr: The elimination of the self-destructive behavior of a psychotic child: A case study. *Behav Ther* 5;79–89, 1974.
171. O'Brien F: Treating self-stimulatory behavior, in Matson JL, McCartney JR (eds): *Handbook of Behavior Modification with the Mentally Retarded.* New York, Plenum Press, 1981.
172. Wehman P, McLaughlin PJ: Teachers' perceptions of behavior problems with severely and profoundly handicapped students. *Ment Retard* 17(1);20–21, 1979.
173. Repp AC, Deitz SM, Speir NC: Reducing stereotypic responding of retarded persons by the differential reinforcement of other behavior. *Am J Ment Defic* 79;279–284, 1974.
174. Favell JE: Reduction of stereotypes by reinforcement of toy play. *Ment Retard* 11;21–23, 1973.
175. Azrin NH, Wesolowski MD: A reinforcement plus interruption method of eliminating behavioral stereotypy of profoundly retarded persons. *Behav Res Ther* 18;113–119, 1980.
176. Rincover A, Cook R, Peoples A, *et al*: Sensory extinction and sensory reinforcement principles for programming multiple adaptive behavior change. *J Appl Behav Anal* 12;221–233, 1979.
177. Mattos RL: *Operant Control of Facial Ticking and Finger Sucking in a Severely Retarded Child.* Read before the Annual Convention of the American Association on Mental Deficiency, San Francisco, 1969.
178. Foxx RM, Azrin NH: The elimination of autistic self-stimulatory behavior by overcorrection. *J Appl Behav Anal* 6;1–14, 1973.
179. Matson JL, Stephens RM: Overcorrection treatment of stereotyped behaviors. *Behav Modif* 5;491–502, 1981.
180. Barrett RP, Matson JL, Shapiro ES, *et al*: A comparison of punishment and DRO procedures for treating stereotypic behavior of mentally retarded children. *Appl Res Ment Retard* 2;247–256, 1981.
181. Greene RJ, Hoats DL, Hornick AJ: Music distortion: A new technique for behavior modification. *Psychol Rec* 20;107–109, 1970.
182. Kelly JA, Furman W, Phillips J, *et al*: Teaching conversational skills to retarded adolescents. *Child Behav Ther* 1;85–97, 1979.
183. Kelly JA, Wildman BG, Urey JR, *et al*: Group skills training to increase the conversational repertoire of retarded adolescents. *Child Behav Ther* 1;323–336, 1979.
184. Matson JL, Andrasik F: Training leisure-time social interaction skills to mentally retarded adults. *Am J Ment Defic* 86;533–542, 1982.
185. Rychtarik RG, Bornstein PH: Training conversational skills in mentally retarded adults: A multiple baseline analysis. *Ment Retard* 17;289–293, 1979.
186. Tofte-Tipps S, Mendonca P, Peach RV: Training and generalization of social skills: A study with two developmentally handicapped, socially isolated children. *Behav Modif* 6;45–71, 1982.
187. Greenspan S, Shoultz B: Why mentally retarded adults lose their jobs: Social competence as a factor in work adjustment. *Appl Res Ment Retard* 2;23–38, 1981.

188. Greenspan S, Shoultz B, Weir MM: Social judgment and vocational adjustment of mentally retarded adults. *Appl Res Ment Retard* 2;335–346, 1981.
189. LaGreca AM, Stone WL, Bell CR: Assessing the problematic interpersonal skills of mentally retarded individuals in a vocational setting. *Appl Res Ment Retard* 3;37–53, 1982.
190. Lancioni GE: Normal children as tutors to teach social responses to withdrawn mentally retarded schoolmates: Training, maintenance, and generalization. *J Appl Behav Anal* 15;17–40, 1982.
191. Gibson FW Jr, Lawrence PS, Nelson RO: Comparison of three training procedures for teaching social responses to developmentally disabled adults. *Am J Ment Defic* 81;379–387, 1976.
192. Matson JL: A controlled group study of pedestrian-skill training for the mentally retarded. *Behav Res Ther* 18;99–106, 1980.
193. Matson JL, Ollendick TH, Adkins J: A comprehensive dining program for mentally retarded adults. *Behav Res Ther* 18;107–112, 1980.
194. Bornstein PH, Bach PJ, McFall ME, *et al*: Application of a social skills training program in the modification of interpersonal deficits among retarded adults: A clinical replication. *J Appl Behav Anal* 13;171–176, 1980.
195. Matson JL, Senatore V: A comparison of traditional psychotherapy and social skills training for improving interpersonal functioning of mentally retarded adults. *Behav Ther* 12;369–382, 1981.
196. Meredith RL, Saxon S, Doleys DM, *et al*: Social skills training with mildly retarded young adults. *J Clin Psychol* 36;1000–1009, 1980.
197. Stacy D, Doleys DM, Malcolm R: Effects of social-skills training in a community-based program. *Am J Ment Defic* 84;152–158, 1979.
198. Bates P: The effectiveness of interpersonal skills training on the social skill acquisition of moderately and mildly retarded adults. *J Appl Behav Anal* 13;237–248, 1980.
199. Matson JL: Use of independence training to teach shopping skills to mildly retarded adults. *Am J Ment Defic* 86;178–183, 1981.
200. Kelly JA, Wildman BG, Berler ES: Small group behavioral training to improve the job interview skills repertoire of mildly retarded adolescent. *J Appl Behav Anal* 13;461–471, 1980.
201. Rusch FR, Mithaug DE: *Vocational Training for Mentally Retarded Adults: A Behavior Analytic Approach.* Champaign IL, Research Press, 1980.
202. Matson JL, Earnhart T: Programming treatment effects to the natural environment: A procedure for training institutionalized retarded adults. *Behav Modif* 5;27–37, 1981.
203. Bornstein MR, Bellack AS, Hersen M: Social skills training for unassertive children: A multiple-baseline analysis. *J Appl Behav Anal* 10;183–195, 1977.
204. Curran JP: Social skills: Methodological issues and future directions, in Bellack AS, Hersen M (eds): *Research and Practice in Social Skills Training.* New York, Plenum Press, 1979.
205. Barman BC: Use of contingent vibration in the treatment of self-stimulatory hand-mouthing and ruminative vomiting behavior. *J Behav Ther Exp Psychiatry* 11;307–311, 1980.
206. Jackson GM, Johnson CR, Ackron GS, *et al*: Food satiation as a procedure to decelerate vomiting. *Am J Ment Defic* 80;223–227, 1975.
207. Libby DG, Phillips E: Eliminating rumination behavior in a profoundly retarded adolescent: An exploratory study. *Ment Retard* 17(2);94–95, 1979.
208. Rast J, Johnston JM, Drum C, *et al*: The relation of food quantity to rumination behavior. *J Appl Behav Anal* 14;121–130, 1981.
209. Foxx RM, Synder M, Schroeder F: A food satiation and hygiene punishment program to suppress chronic rumination by retarded persons. *J Autism Dev Disord* 9;399–412, 1979.
210. Borreson PM, Anderson JL: The elimination of chronic rumination through a combination of procedures. *Ment Retard* 20;34–38, 1982.
211. Wolf M, Birnbrauer J, Lawler J, *et al*: The operant extinction, reinstatement, and extinction of vomiting behavior in a retarded child, in Ulrich R, Stachnik T, Mabry J (eds): *Control of Human Behavior: From Cure to Prevention.* Glenview, IL, Scott, Foresman, 1970, vol 2.
212. Smeets PM: Withdrawal of social reinforcers as a means of controlling rumination and regurgitation in a profoundly retarded person. *Trng Sch Bull* 67;158–163, 1970.

213. Davis WB, Wieseler NA, Hanzel TE: Contingent music in management of rumination and out-of-seat behavior in a profoundly mentally retarded institutionalized male. *Ment Retard* 18;43–45, 1980.
214. Azrin NH, Wesolowski MD: Eliminating habitual vomiting in a retarded adult by positive practice and self-correction. *J Behav Ther Exp Psychiatry* 6;145–148, 1975.
215. Duker PC, Seys DM: Elimination of vomiting in a retarded female using restitutional over-correction. *Behav Ther* 8;255–257, 1977.
216. Luckey RE, Watson CM, Musick JK: Aversive conditioning as a means of inhibiting vomiting and rumination. *Am J Ment Defic* 73;139–142, 1968.
217. Kohlenberg R: The punishment of persistent vomiting: A case study. *J Appl Behav Anal* 3;241–245, 1970.
218. Gilbraith DA, Byrick RJ, Rutledge JT: An aversive conditioning approach to the inhibition of chronic vomiting. *Can Psychiatric Assoc J* 15;311–313, 1970.
219. Bright GO, Whaley DL: Suppression of regurgitation and rumination with aversive events. *Mich Ment Health Res Bull* 11;17–20, 1968.
220. Becker JV, Turner SM, Sajwaj T: Multiple behavioral effects of the use of lemon juice with a ruminating toddler-age child. *Behav Modif* 2;267–278, 1978.
221. Weisberg P, Packer PA, Weisberg RS: Academic training, in Matson JL, McCartney JR (eds): *Handbook of Behavior Modification with the Mentally Retarded*. New York, Plenum Press, 1981.
222. Azrin NH, Schaeffer RM, Wesolowski MD: A rapid method of teaching profoundly retarded persons to dress by a reinforcement-guidance method. *Ment Retard* 14(6);29–33, 1976.
223. Watson LS, Uzzell R: Teaching self-help skills to the mentally retarded, in Matson JL, McCartney JR (eds): *Handbook of Behavior Modification with the Mentally Retarded*. New York, Plenum Press, 1981.
224. Azrin NH, Armstrong PM: The "mini-meal"—A method of teaching eating skills to the profoundly retarded. *Ment Retard* 11(1);9–13, 1973.
225. Nelson GL, Cone JD, Hanson CR: Training correct utensil use in retarded children: Modeling vs. physical guidance. *Am J Ment Defic* 80;114–122, 1975.
226. Watson LS: *How to Teach Independent Living Skills and Manage Disruptive Behavior*. Tuscaloosa, AL, Behavior Modification Technology, 1978.
227. Bry PM, Nawas MM: Is reinforcement necessary for the development of a generalized imitation operant in severely and profoundly retarded children? *Am J Ment Defic* 76;658–667, 1972.
228. Butz RA, Hasazi JE: Developing verbal imitative behavior in a profoundly retarded girl. *J Behav Ther Exp Psychiatr* 4;389–393, 1973.
229. Jones A, Robson C: Language training the severely mentally handicapped, in Ellis NR (ed): *Handbook of Mental Deficiency, Psychological Theory and Research*, ed 2. Hillsdale, NJ, Lawrence Erlbaum, 1979.
230. McCoy JF, Buckhalt JA: Language acquisition, in Matson JL, McCartney JR (eds): *Handbook of Behavior Modification with the Mentally Retarded*. New York, Plenum Press, 1981.
231. Marchetti A, Matson JL: Training skills for community adjustment, in Matson JL, McCartney JR (eds): *Handbook of Behavior Modification with the Mentally Retarded*. New York, Plenum Press, 1981.
232. O'Brien F, Azrin NH, Bugle C: Training profoundly retarded children to stop crawling. *J Appl Behav Anal* 5;131–137, 1972.
233. Fristoe M, Lloyd LL: Nonspeech communication, in Ellis NR (ed): *Handbook of Mental Deficiency, Psychological Theory and Research*, ed 2. Hillsdale, NJ, Lawrence Erlbaum, 1979.

5

Modified Individual and Group Treatment Approaches for the Mentally Retarded-Mentally Ill

Michael J. Monfils and Frank J. Menolascino

Individual and group therapeutic approaches with the mentally retarded (mild to moderate range) have gained increased acceptance in recent years. Retarded individuals, who once were thought to be incapable of benefiting from psychotherapy,[1] are, in fact, participating in a wide range of therapies in various treatment settings. An assortment of innovative strategies, procedures, and techniques has been developed and refined for use with retarded citizens. The purpose of this chapter is to discuss and consider the role of individual and group psychotherapy with the retarded as important treatment procedures that can be used effectively by mental health professionals.

In examining individual therapy, attention is given here to the therapist and client variables that are indicative of successful outcomes. We also consider pathways to building a therapeutic relationship with the client, the development of specific treatment goals, and techniques of intervention. Common themes or areas of discussion in individual and group therapy with retarded persons are also examined. With regard to group approaches, the principles of group purpose and composition are scrutinized as they apply to the retarded. Specific group approaches and techniques, as well as leadership styles, are also reviewed.

5.1. Individual Approaches: Historical Context

Reports describing individual psychotherapy with mentally retarded persons can be found in the early 1940s.[2] Interestingly, there were also many articles written on this subject from 1950 to 1970, yet comparatively fewer in the 1970s. Sternlicht[3] and Lott[4] have provided comprehensive reviews of the literature of the 1950s and 1960s. Many of the early articles on this subject questioned the effectiveness of psychotherapy with the retarded, based on the

Michael J. Monfils • Department of Psychiatry, Nebraska Psychiatric Institute, University of Nebraska Medical Center, Omaha, Nebraska 68105.   Frank J. Menolascino • Departments of Psychiatry and Pediatrics, Nebraska Psychiatric Institute, University of Nebraska Medical Center, Omaha, Nebraska 68105.

contention that the clients lacked verbal skills and could not gain insight into their behaviors. These views have been refuted by the literature of the 1970s, and there is now a more widespread acceptance of individual treatment approaches.

Recent authors have stressed the diversity of approaches that may be adapted for use with the retarded. For example, Halpern and Berard[5] noted that the techniques used in individual therapy with the retarded have many similarities to approaches used with the nonretarded; they offered a series of recommendations concerning how these techniques may be adapted for use with the retarded. Selan[6] pointed out the importance of nonverbal techniques, such as role-play exercises and psychodrama, to the success of therapy. Rosen, Clark, and Kivitz[7] reviewed some of the more novel approaches that have been tried, such as hypnosis, and have developed a therapy choice model based on the amount of control and direction that the therapist assumes. Finally, Szymanski[8] provided a useful summary of both verbal and nonverbal techniques in individual therapy, including such activities as play therapy with children.

5.2. Therapist Variables

Much attention has been devoted in the literature to client factors in treatment and the suitability of mentally retarded persons for individual psychotherapy. Concomitantly, insufficient consideration has been given to the therapist variables that are necessary for effective therapy. As a starting point, professionals need to inspect their own feelings and attitudes about working with the retarded.[9] Often, the prejudices and the negative attitudes of the therapist toward the retarded client impede the development of a therapeutic relationship. The therapist thus needs to develop an acceptance of the client and positive attitudes toward mental retardation and the individual's developmental potential.

In addition, the professional should acquire knowledge regarding the medical dimensions of mental retardation, for example, information concerning general principles of genetics, the impact of epilepsy on retarded persons, and a basic understanding of the commonly used psychopharmacological agents. The therapist should feel comfortable in interpreting fundamental medical information for parents and family members. Finally, the professional should possess a sufficient storehouse of information regarding personality theory and normal and abnormal human development.

Therapists who work with retarded citizens have to be patient individuals who are able to tolerate a certain amount of frustration.[6] This frustration may result from working with clients who are handicapped in their verbal-expressive abilities, or it may be seen as a corollary of the slow progress toward goals that often occur. In these situations, therapists who are warm, flexible, and empathic are able to maintain the necessary commitment to their clients. These clients are often involved in some way with other community agencies or resources. Therefore, the therapist needs to be knowledgeable concerning the available community services and support systems. This approach calls for an ecological perspective on the part of professionals, in which broader environmental resources are utilized.

5.3. Client Variables

Mentally retarded persons are unique individuals, with a diversity and a variety equal to other segments of the population. It is a mistake to focus one's attention on individual deficits or on labels such as *mildly retarded* or *autistic*. Each client must be respected and must be viewed as possessing an inherent dignity as a person. This does not mean that the therapist overlooks or minimizes deficits in verbal development or abstract thinking, but rather that these deficits are to be viewed within the context of the total person.

This posture of respect for the dignity and uniqueness of the individual should lead the therapist to adopt a flexible, eclectic approach in individual therapy. A client-centered approach, therefore, is not necessarily the best approach for all mildly retarded clients, just as a behavioral approach should not always be perceived as optimum for the severely retarded. Each client should be considered individually in terms of developmental and social history, as well as personal strengths and weaknesses. The therapeutic approach and technique should thus be tailored to the specific needs of the client, rather than according to the philosophical school of the therapist.

Which retarded individuals can benefit the most from individual therapy? Level of intelligence cannot be used as the sole criterion in deciding this question. Rather, one must look at this factor in conjunction with other realities, such as motivation, amount of verbal expression, and degree of insight. Clients who are aware that they are experiencing distress or problems in daily functioning, and who possess at least a minimal desire to effect changes in their lives, are suitable candidates for therapy. Ideally, these should be individuals who are able to respond to a warm, supportive relationship with a helping professional.

Clients who are acutely paranoid or psychotic are poor candidates for therapy until the acute phase of their condition has been ameliorated through the use of psychotropic medications or behavioral intervention. Also, individuals who are prone to physical aggression or threatening behaviors toward the therapist are a poor risk. Severely or profoundly retarded persons should not be excluded from therapy simply on the basis of their intellectual deficits. Again, each case must be considered individually. Those clients who possess minimal verbal-expressive abilities are often able to benefit from a structured behavioral approach, focusing on instruction in basic social and living skills.

5.4. Building a Therapeutic Relationship

Beginning with the initial contact with the client, the human service professional begins to build and solidify a therapeutic relationship. This relationship is so fundamental to the success of therapy that it has been termed the "heart of helping people."[10] The therapist must communicate qualities such as concern, acceptance, empathy, and genuineness to the client as the basis for the relationship. Without the establishment and the maintenance of this working alliance, efforts at change in the individual will be inadequate. The rapport, communication, and commitment that are established early in therapy lay the groundwork for future effective intervention.

In the initial stage of therapy, the therapist's use of self and use of relationship are all-important. The therapist is the instrument of therapy, through which knowledge and understanding flow to the client. The desire to help and sensitivity on the therapist's part create the climate in which the client can feel free to disclose thoughts and feelings. In this type of "relationship therapy," the therapist becomes a role model by demonstrating to the client qualities such as emotional control, warmth, and respect.[11]

The ability to listen in an active and concerned manner to the concerns of the client is an often-overlooked factor in the beginning stage of therapy. This implies an active process of becoming aware of the meaning of the client's verbal and nonverbal communication. The temptation to take control of the session can be attractive to the therapist; this becomes an easy way to avoid uncomfortable silences and to structure the interaction. Doing so, however, interferes with the client's freedom of expression, which is an integral part of therapy. Therapists need, therefore, to cultivate the ability to listen to the client.

If as professionals we have failed in our attempts to develop a helping relationship with the mentally retarded client, perhaps it is because we have not developed the sensitivity to see the world through the eyes of the client. This type of "insight" means developing an ability to experience and comprehend the same daily frustrations and anxieties that the client experiences. Perhaps the greatest challenge to the therapist, then, is to cultivate this ability to "get inside the other's skin," to leave our own frame of reference behind and truly understand the client's situation. The use of this skill makes it possible for the therapist and the client to advance to the next stage of therapy: goal setting.

5.5. Goals of Treatment

As client and therapist jointly assess the client's situation and needs, goals for therapy should begin to emerge. Much ambiguity in the therapeutic process derives from a failure to develop clear treatment goals. Mentally retarded clients need to understand the reasons for their referral into therapy; often they are sent to work with a therapist without any clear perception of the purpose of the treatment. The goal-setting process in therapy should arrive at clear and specific objectives. The objectives should be concrete, well defined, practical, and measureable.[7] They should also be mutually agreed upon, rather than a unilateral perception on the therapist's part regarding the client's needs.

A contract between client and therapist is a useful tool in goal setting. The contract, which can be verbal or written, is a product of the joint input and planning of the client and the professional. It should spell out target problems and goals, as well as the strategies of intervention to be used and the roles of both participants. The contract can, of course, be renegotiated at a later date as the client's needs change or as treatment goals are reached, yet it remains the foundation for therapy. It can be particularly helpful in dealing with resistance and client defenses, as it can be reviewed at these times as a way of focusing once again on the specific goals of treatment.

In conceptualizing the goals of treatment it will be advantageous to both parties to distinguish whether treatment is to be short term or long term. Several useful models of brief, therapy-crisis intervention have been developed[12,13]; these models can readily be adapted for use with retarded citizens. In brief therapy, the treatment goal is more abbreviated, often revolving around an attempt to restore the individual to a former level of functioning by reconstructing healthy coping mechanisms. Techniques such as support, reassurance, reality testing, and clarification are important in this approach. Therapy, in these instances, is often targeted at changing very specific behaviors, such as problems in a work setting or aggressive acts toward others.

At the beginning of treatment, or once short-term goals have been realized, a decision must be made concerning possible long-term psychotherapy. This decision should be made based on many factors, including the client's motivation and the therapist's willingness to make a commitment to long-term involvement. Several kinds of client needs would indicate the desirability of longer treatment, for example, a wish to explore and understand the dynamics in one's family of origin, or the relationship of family characteristics to current problems. The client may express an aspiration to effect broad personal changes in motivation, attitudes, or social skills. Long-term therapy could also focus globally on personality traits and the development of insight into emotions and self-concept. Mildly retarded individuals are generally more able to benefit from this type of introspection than lower functioning clients.

5.6. Techniques

A variety of techniques have been developed and adapted for use with retarded citizens. The therapist needs to acquire a broad familiarity with these techniques and their application to both children and adults. Because the needs of clients are so diverse, professionals should not rely solely on any one technique or therapeutic school. Rather, a flexible, eclectic approach is indicated, in which the therapist possesses a multiplicity of skills and techniques.

In general, therapists will discover that they need to be active and directive in sessions with retarded clients. Within the framework of building a therapeutic relationship and allowing freedom of expression, there are always limits of acceptable behavior that must be enforced. For example, destructive or aggressive behavior toward the therapist or toward property cannot be tolerated.

The therapist must set limits and provide sufficient structure to permit therapy to proceed. A directive approach also means calling the client's attention back to the goals and the objectives of the therapy, thereby encouraging the client to express thoughts and feelings within reasonable boundaries.

Play therapy techniques (such as painting and the use of puppets) are nonverbal procedures that may be used effectively with retarded children possessing limited verbal repertoires. Such techniques allow children to express their physical energy and to experience a measure of control and success in their lives.[5] The therapist functions as an observer-participant in play exercises, structuring the play and interpreting its meaning to the child. Play can be used not only in building a relationship with the child, but also as a means of expressing conflicts and hostilities within the child and the family. It is important, therefore, to allow the child freedom and spontaneity of expression.

In using verbal techniques with the retarded, therapists should be acutely aware of the client's language development and comprehension. A common mistake made by therapists is to utilize terminology that is too complicated for clients to understand. Language should be clear and concise because verbal discussion and instruction are of primary importance. Such discussion is often focused on teaching the client appropriate adaptive behaviors and social skills.

Reeducation is often an integral part of verbal therapy. Clients have frequently acquired maladaptive behaviors as a way of managing stressful situations. Alternatives to these behaviors can be explored as the therapist suggests and teaches constructive patterns of behavior. One area in which retarded individuals frequently need reeducation is sexuality. The retarded person is often lacking fundamental knowledge concerning physiology and reproduction or has little sophistication regarding relationships and sexual identity. One-to-one education or reeducation in these facets of sexuality is instrumental in teaching clients acceptable means of expressing of their sexuality. Such instruction also assists the retarded in avoiding a lonely, isolated existence.

With many retarded clients, particularly those who are severely and profoundly handicapped, behavioral techniques are the most suitable approach. These techniques are often used to instruct clients in simple, concrete social-adaptive skills. Gardner[14] has recommended that a behavioral approach be used more extensively as a way to specify the goals and the behaviors that are the center of therapy. Behavioral techniques may be particularly helpful in individual therapy in teaching new behaviors and in decreasing destructive or self-injurious behaviors. Prominent techniques that may be used include observational learning (modeling), behavior rehearsal, relaxation training, and desensitization procedures. The advantage of these tactics is that clients can learn new, observable behaviors that can be transferred to other settings outside the therapy hour.

The client who is psychotic, primitive, or minimally verbal presents a unique challenge to therapists and requires modifications in traditional counseling techniques. These individuals seem to be out of touch not only with the exterior world, but also with their own feelings and behaviors. They need to develop an awareness of reality as a first step toward learning new techniques that will aid them in coping with that reality. In working with these persons, therapists need to continually reflect information about the clients' physical and emotional world back to them. This technique may include messages concerning the individual's environment, body posture, facial expression, or verbalizations. For example, when working with a client who will not express his or her feelings, the therapist should comment on the client's facial expression (e.g., "You look angry today") and then elicit feedback on this observation from the client. These types of reflections, as Prouty[15] has noted, will help the individual to reflect, to feel, and to begin to experience reality.

5.7. Common Themes

A number of common issues or themes recur in individual and group therapy with retarded persons. Therapists need to develop an awareness of these issues and should be prepared to assist clients in exploring and resolving them. For example, many clients possess a very inadequate self-image; they do not view themselves as capable of being loved.[6] This poor self-esteem may stem in part from the series of unsuccessful experiences (within the family and at school) that the client endures. Certainly, many individuals in society view retarded persons as failures, thereby reinforcing the client's negative self-perception. The challenge to the therapist is to structure therapy in such a way that the client experiences success, even in seemingly minor steps. These successes, as problems are solved and the client learns new behaviors, will begin to rebuild the individual's shattered self-concept.

Sexual problems have been briefly mentioned above as a frequent concern for the retarded. Counseling in this area must often be extended to family members as well, in order to instruct them in the management and education of the client. In working with clients, group discussions with peers regarding sexuality are often a helpful adjunct to individual therapy. Mentally retarded individuals have the right to receive in individual or group therapy a complete range of services, including information on reproduction, physiology, contraception, premarital counseling, and instructions concerning how to develop healthy friendships and relationships.

Interpersonal relationships are frequently a source of irritation and frustration for retarded persons. Clients may not have learned how to channel their emotions into constructive activities or outlets; as a result, they either lash out angrily toward others or withdraw into their own loneliness and isolation. Individual and group therapy can assist the individual in gaining a basic understanding of how emotions operate in influencing behavior. The professional functions once again in the role of educator and role model, in teaching the client acceptable social skills. Techniques in stress management, problem solving, and communication skills are useful in this endeavor. One ultimate goal in therapy with many clients is to enhance their ability to relate adaptively to peers and others by gaining increased emotional control.

Many handicapped persons, especially the mildly retarded, are acutely aware of the fact that they are different from others and unable to perform on an intellectual par with nonretarded peers or siblings. Therefore, the individual's feelings about being retarded are a frequent theme in therapy. Initially, the client should be encouraged to ventilate his or her feelings (anger, frustration) about this issue. Therapists can then assist the client in conducting a realistic self-appraisal, noting both personal strengths and personal weaknesses. This self-assessment should be used to enhance and bolster the individual's self-acceptance.[16] The client needs to formulate an accurate self-perception as the first step in setting realistic personal goals.

Finally, the mentally retarded young adult typically encounters adjustment problems when separating from the family and moving into community residences and vocational placement. These young-adult years are difficult for the client. Crucial issues that must be faced include the person's perspective of time, his or her structuring of the major themes of work and love, and changes in self-concept and identify.[17] Separation issues often indicate the need for a total family-therapy approach. Individual and group psychotherapy with the young person should allow the client to express and understand his or her ambivalent feelings about the situation. Support, reassurance, and reality testing are specific techniques that may be employed. Often, the therapist can assist with arranging concrete case-management services, such as housing, budgeting, and vocational plans. The encouragement of the therapist as simply a friend and a concerned helper is a valuable service that can be rendered.

5.8. Group Approaches

Group treatment approaches play a valuable role in the habilitation of mentally retarded citizens. These approaches may be used in inpatient or outpatient settings and are often employed in conjunction with individual psychotherapy. The remarks made earlier concerning desirable therapist and client variables in individual therapy apply to group approaches as well. Likewise, the techniques involved in building a therapeutic relationship in group therapy parallel those that were mentioned regarding individual therapy with the retarded. Mentally retarded persons are able to benefit from group approaches, and in particular, those individuals who are able to communicate with the therapist either verbally or nonverbally in an affective relationship[18] are appropriate candidates for group treatment.

5.9. Survey of the Literature

A brief review of the literature on group therapy reveals much experimentation in approaches and techniques across various treatment settings. An early pioneer in this endeavor was Cotzin,[19] who reported on the improvement in behavior and personality of retarded adolescent boys who were seen for group sessions in an institution. In the 1950s, many group leaders employed a passive leadership style and nondirective techniques, such as discussion or verbal communication. Astrachan[20] and Kaldeck[21] reported favorable results with such an approach, whereas Vail[22] found a permissive approach to be disastrous. Therapists in the 1960s initiated the use of novel techniques and often found that nonverbal activities were effective. Gorlow *et al.*[23] used a combination of procedures, including role play, films, parties, and psychodrama exercises in treating female residents in a state school setting. Sternlicht[24,25] included arm wrestling, pantomimes, and balloon breaking as techniques for establishing rapport and pointing out personality dynamics to adolescents.

Individuals with mild to moderate mental retardation were often the focus of group methods in the late 1960s and the early 1970s. Despite earlier experimentation, many authors during these years reverted to the use of nonthreatening, passive approaches. Miezio,[26] for example, placed an emphasis on group discussion of daily problems and the sharing of feelings and needs in a group of adolescent inpatients. Slivkin and Bernstin,[18] Baran,[27] and Richards and Lee[28] also employed verbal expression and communication as the primary therapeutic tool. These groups were generally open-ended in nature, with the discussion of topics chosen by the group members, such as family relationships or behavior problems. The therapist usually attempted to be supportive and encouraging but often had no set agenda or goals for group sessions. The evaluation of group effectiveness was characteristically based on the observations and feelings of the therapist, rather than on any objective measurement or criteria.

Since the mid-1970s, group leaders have made determined efforts to develop techniques that can be applied to the total spectrum of retarded citizens, especially those who are more severely handicapped. These efforts have led to the construction of social-skills-oriented approaches, which attempt to teach clients specific abilities that are needed in daily living. These behavioral strategies are usually highly structured, and the group leader functions as a teacher and a role model. Zisfein and Rosen[29] and Lee,[30] for example, designed social-adjustment group-training programs, complete with manuals and step-by-step instructions for group leaders. Instruction in areas such as assertiveness and the appropriate expression of feelings is carried out in these groups primarily via modeling and behavior rehearsal. Similar structured training was carried out by Perry and Cerreto,[31] Bates,[32] and Matson and Senatore.[33] These authors have claimed that their approach is effective, based on measurement tools such as ratings of videotapes by trained observers and the use of standardized tests.

5.10. Group Purpose

As in individual therapy, many problem issues in group treatment can be avoided by reaching a clear understanding with the group members about the group's purpose and goals. This process should begin with the group's first meeting. Szymanski and Rosefsky[34] have succinctly stated that the purpose of the group should be well defined in the mind of the leader, yet flexible enough to allow for change in necessary. This statement implies a willingness on the part of the leader and the group members to adapt to changing circumstances and conditions, depending on the unfolding progress of therapy. The adoption of a contract, either written or verbal, is once again a valuable tool in joint decision-making concerning group purpose. The contract can spell out the specific parameters of the group, including such important factors as group composition or the setting and duration of the group.

Groups of mildly retarded clients often work on global goals that are similar to typical goals in therapy groups with nonretarded individuals. For example, a group may develop a general goal of enhancing the growth and development of each participant, by helping the clients to learn to recognize and manage their feelings. Groups may also address problem solving in areas of daily living, such as in the family, at work, or at school. In such a group, the leader would often attempt to teach or model adaptive communication and peer interaction skills. In many groups, the clients develop goals related to self-assessment and self-image, in terms of honestly looking at personal strengths and gaining an understanding of their handicaps. As the clients begin to accept their personal or social deficits, they are able to develop and rehearse successful coping strategies in the group. These types of goals are generally appropriate for higher functioning retarded individuals who possess adequate verbal skills and comprehension.

In some instances, groups are initiated for specific, more narrowly defined purposes. One such example would be groups in institutional settings that are designed to teach clients the skills necessary for successful adjustment to community living. This type of group not only would be intended to produce better client adjustment within the institution but also would be purposefully directed toward preparing clients for adaptation to community environments. Other special groups may be developed for needs such as sex education, relaxation training, or assertiveness acquisition. Many retarded individuals exhibit deficits in various social skills, such as engaging in appropriate conversations, the expression of feelings, and social responsibility. These deficits can be specifically addressed in the small-group format.

The theme-centered model of groupwork, as proposed by Cohn,[35] provides a useful framework for group leaders in developing group objectives with retarded clients. This approach involves the selection of a distinct theme that is used as a focal point for group interaction and awareness. The group leader attempts to concentrate the attention of the members on the theme, discouraging distractions or nonrelevant verbalizations. Ground rules or procedures are used that are guidelines for the participants in structuring their dialogue. Examples of ground rules include responsibility for oneself and speaking one at a time. One advantage of such an approach with retarded persons is that it has wide applicability across a variety of treatment settings. It may be used to instruct severely handicapped clients in basic social-adaptive skills, or it would be useful in allowing higher functioning clients to explore areas of interpersonal relationships such as communication patterns and peer interactions.

5.11. Techniques of Intervention

Therapists who work with mentally retarded persons in group therapy should be careful to develop different types of interventions for clients of various intellectual and adaptive levels. Clients with mild retardation generally respond adequately to an open-ended, client-centered approach, yet they still require some direction and structure from the leader. Clients with moderate to profound retardation, on the other hand, need a highly directive approach, with clearly defined goals and expectations. In either case, the importance of establishing the therapeutic relationship at the outset of therapy is preeminent. This involves some of the same strategies as were mentioned earlier regarding individual therapy, namely, the warm human qualities of the therapist (use of self) and the deployment of active listening skills.

The techniques involved in working with groups of mildly retarded individuals are not greatly different from the methods that are commonly used in group therapy with other types of clients. Initially, the therapist must concentrate on establishing a relationship with the group characterized by mutual respect and trust, so that the clients will feel safe and comfortable within the group. This is accomplished by allowing the clients to have the freedom and the spontaneity to express their thoughts and feelings. The therapist must stimulate discussion and encourage self-disclosure; it is only in such an atmosphere that the clients will ventilate painful feelings. Once the clients are willing to risk self-disclosure, the therapist promotes feedback and acceptance from other group members. In addition, other techniques, such as clarification, interpretation, and support, are used to assist the clients in understanding their emotions and behaviors.

Frequently, clients will test group limits, deny their problems, or use various defense mechanisms to avoid facing reality. At these times, the therapist needs to challenge and confront the clients, inviting them to examine possible alternative behaviors. As the clients begin to gain insight into their actions, they are encouraged and supported in their efforts to learn and experiment with new adaptive behaviors. These new behaviors must be tried out in real-life situations and then discussed in the relative safety of the group. The therapist and the other group members reinforce the individual client's behavioral change through their praise and encouragement; new attitudes and behaviors are thus subject to continual refinement and clarification.

Groups of moderately to profoundly retarded clients derive the most benefit from techniques that are structured and directive. Therapeutic approaches with these groups are often based on behavior modification techniques and are directed toward teaching clients adaptive social skills. A theme-centered approach has been mentioned as a useful model for application to this population. Discussion and verbal instruction regarding the theme serve as a way of introducing the concept being taught. The therapist then models inappropriate and appropriate responses in order to present the clients with a visible picture of the desired behavior. The clients are then encouraged to take part in role-play exercises, rehearsing the behavior in front of their peers. Social feedback in the form of verbal praise and criticism from group members provides the clients with the correction and the redirection that they will require in order to further refine and master the behavior. Clients are also given "homework assignments" or tasks to perform in situations outside the group as a way of transferring their knowledge to other settings. This format is obviously much more specific and didactic than an open-ended traditional group approach, and it requires the leader to function as both a teacher and a role model.

Various types of interventions may be adapted for use with retarded adolescents in group therapy. With clients who are mildly handicapped, interaction may center on discussions or sharing of feelings concerning issues of importance to all adolescents, such as family interaction or problems in relationships with peers. Clients with severe retardation require a more structured group approach and the integration of planned activities into the group format. These activities might include social-recreational outings in the community or activities within group sessions such as games, films, educational projects, or role-play exercises.

It is common for group therapists to have clients of different intellectual-functional levels integrated into the same group. Often these individuals come from different backgrounds and possess divergent levels of verbal skills. In these groups, the therapist needs to be eclectic, selecting from various sources the techniques that work best with each particular group. This type of approach has been recommended by Laterza,[36] who noted that approaches such as modeling, behavior contracting, transactional analysis, and systems theory all have relevance to the retarded. Group leaders, therefore, need to be flexible and eclectic in approach, at the same time providing a moderate amount of structure and direction for the group.

Many of the strategies that are used in group (as well as individual) therapy with the retarded are directed toward the management of stress in the client. Retarded individuals are particularly vulnerable to the effects of stress because of their allied physical handicaps, their poorly developed defense mechanisms, and their failure to master key developmental tasks. The retarded person also may not understand the demands being placed on him or her, becomes easily frustrated, and then acts out in an impulsive manner. Group techniques should be modified and simplified in terms of educating clients about the sources of stress in their lives and pertinent management techniques. We have found that relaxation training can be integrated into group experiences as a means of teaching clients to facilitate relaxation on their own. This training may include breathing exercises, muscle relaxation, and visualization (use of imagination). The objective in using these techniques is to help clients to realize that stress is a necessary and normal part of daily living; although stress can not be eliminated entirely, clients can learn how to cope with it adaptively.

5.12. Leadership Style

The term *leadership style* in relation to group work with the retarded may initially seem to be an ambiguous concept. Admittedly, one's style of leadership is highly personal and is derived from the sum of the therapist's training and personal experiences. *Style* refers not only to the therapist's characteristic manner of expression in the group, but also to his or her design for group interaction and degree of control over group dynamics. We have found in several years of experience in group therapy with retarded individuals that, in general, an active, directive style of leadership is indicated, in which the therapist should clearly establish the structure and the limitations of group interaction.

The therapist's style and techniques should be geared toward encouraging interaction and expression among group members. Clients often need to learn how to verbalize their feelings, rather than acting them out irresponsibly or aggressively. The effective leader, therefore, allows freedom and spontaneity (within reasonable limits) of communication in the group. This communication must at the same time be clear and concrete, geared to the level of verbal ability of the members. Communication must also establish and reinforce reality for each client.

It is of crucial importance to group members that the therapist be a genuine, caring individual who is not afraid to bring up examples from his or her own experiences. Such examples demonstrate to the group that the therapist, too, continues to struggle with the vicissitudes of daily living. As the group progresses, the therapist should be perceived by the members as a warm, accepting individual who is able to respond in an uninhibited manner to others. The therapist ultimately adopts several different postures as part of his or her leadership style, including those of therapist, teacher, and role model.

5.13. Summary

Individual and group treatment approaches continue to be of fundamental importance in the evaluation and habilitation of mentally retarded individuals. This chapter has traced the historical roots of these approaches and the key therapist and client variables that are necessary for effective therapy. Other crucial elements in the helping process have also been explored, including the therapeutic relationship, the goals of therapy, techniques and approaches, common themes, and leadership style. Professionals from various disciplines may evaluate their own therapeutic work with the retarded in light of the framework and suggestions that have been presented here. By refining the techniques presented here for use with retarded persons in various settings, therapists will continue to enhance the growth and development of their clients and teach them the practical skills that are so necessary for successful community adjustment.

References

1. Rogers CR, Dymond RF: *Psychotherapy and Personality Change.* Chicago, University of Chicago Press, 1954.
2. Thorne FC: Psychotherapy in relation to mental deficiency. *Am J Ment Defic* 45;135–141, 1941.
3. Sternlicht M: Psychotherapeutic procedures with the retarded, in Ellis NR (ed): *International Review of Research in Mental Retardation,* vol. 2. New York, Academic Press, 1966.
4. Lott G: Psychotherapy of the mentally retarded: Values and cautions, in Menolascino FJ (ed): *Psychiatric Approaches to Mental Retardation.* New York, Basic Books, 1970.
5. Halpern AS, Berard WR: Counseling the mentally retarded: A review for practice, in Browning P (ed): *Mental Retardation Rehabilitation and Counseling.* Springfield, IL, C. C. Thomas, 1974.
6. Selan BH: Psychotherapy with the developmentally disabled. *Health Soc Work* 1;73–85, 1976.
7. Rosen M, Clark GR, Kivitz MS: *Habilitation of the Handicapped.* Baltimore, University Park Press, 1977.
8. Szymanski LS: Individual psychotherapy with retarded persons, in Szymanski LS, Tanguay PE (eds): *Emotional Disorders of Mentally Retarded Persons.* Baltimore, University Park Press, 1980.
9. Mackinnon MC, Frederick BS: A shift of emphasis for psychiatric social work in mental retardation, in Menolascino FJ (ed): *Psychiatric Approaches to Mental Retardation.* New York, Basic Books, 1970.
10. Perlman HH: *Relationship, the Heart of Helping People.* Chicago, University of Chicago Press, 1979.
11. LaVietes R: Mental retardation: Psychological treatment, in Wolman BB (ed): *Handbook of Treatment of Emotional Disorders in Childhood and Adolescence.* Englewood Cliffs, NJ, Prentice-Hall, 1978.
12. Wolberg LR: *The Technique of Psychotherapy,* part 2. New York, Grune and Stratton, 1977.
13. Bellak L, Small L: *Emergency Psychotherapy and Brief Psychotherapy.* New York, Grune and Stratton, 1978.
14. Gardner WI: *Behavior Modification in Mental Retardation.* Chicago, Aldine Atherton, 1971.
15. Prouty G: Pre-therapy—A method of treating pre-expressive psychotic and retarded patients. *Psychother Theor Res Prac* 13;290–294, 1976.
16. Skelton N, Greenland C: Social work and mental retardation, in Croft M (ed): *Tregold's Mental Retardation.* London, Bailliere Tindall, 1979.
17. Neugarten BL: Adult personality: Toward a psychology of the life cycle, in Sze WC (ed): *Human Life Cycle.* New York, Jason Aronson, 1975.
18. Slivkin SE, Bernstein NR: Group approaches to treating retarded adolescents, in Menolascino FJ (ed): *Psychiatric Approaches to Mental Retardation.* New York, Basic Books, 1970.
19. Cotzin M: Group psychotherapy with mentally defective problem boys. *Am J Ment Defic* 53;268–283, 1948.
20. Astrachan M: Group psychotherapy with mentally retarded female adolescents and adults. *Am J Ment Defic* 60;152–156, 1955.
21. Kaldeck R: Group psychotherapy with mentally defective adolescents and adults. *Int J Group Psychother* 8;185–192, 1958.
22. Vail DJ: An unsuccessful experiment in group therapy. *Am J Ment Defic* 60;144–151, 1955.
23. Gorlow L, Butter A, Einig K, *et al*: An appraisal of self-attitudes and behavior following group psychotherapy with retarded young adults. *Am J Ment Defic* 67;893–898, 1963.
24. Sternlicht M: Establishing an initial relationship in group psychotherapy with delinquent retarded male adolescents. *Am J Ment Defic* 69;39–41, 1964.
25. Sternlicht M: Treatment approaches to delinquent retardates. *Int J Group Psychother* 16;91–93, 1966.
26. Miezio S: Group therapy with mentally retarded adolescents in institutional settings. *Int J Group Psychother* 17;321–327, 1967.

27. Baron FN: Group therapy improves mental retardates' behavior. *Hosp Community Psychiatr* 23;7–11, 1972.
28. Richards LD, Lee KA: Group process in social habilitation of the retarded. *Social Casework* 53;30–37, 1972.
29. Zisfein L, Rosen M: Effects of a personal adjustment training group counseling program. *Ment Retard* 12;50–53, 1974.
30. Lee DY: Evaluation of a group counseling program designed to enhance social adjustment of mentally retarded adults. *J Couns Psychol* 24;318–323, 1977.
31. Perry MA, Cerreto MC: Structured learning training of social skills for the retarded. *Ment Retard* 15;31–34, 1977.
32. Bates P: The effectiveness of interpersonal skills training on the social skill acquisition of moderately and mildly retarded adults. *J Appl Behav Anal* 13;237–248, 1980.
33. Matson JL, Senatore V: A comparison of traditional psychotherapy and social skills training for improving interpersonal functioning of mentally retarded adults. *Behav Ther* 12;369–382, 1981.
34. Szymanski LS, Rosefsky QB: Group psychotherapy with retarded persons, in Szymansky LS, Tanguay PE (eds): *Emotional Disorders of Mentally Retarded Persons*. Baltimore, University Park Press, 1980.
35. Cohn RC: Style and spirit of the theme-centered interactional method, in Sager CJ, Kaplan HS (eds): *Progress in Group and Family Therapy*. New York, Brunner/Mazel, 1972.
36. Laterza P: An eclectic approach to group work with the mentally retarded. *Social Work with Groups* 2;235–245, 1979.

6

Specific Psychopharmacological Approaches and Rationale for Mentally Ill-Mentally Retarded Children

John Y. Donaldson

More than 20 years after their introduction, the use of psychotropic medications for psychotic children, particularly retarded children, remains somewhat controversial. Several factors appear to contribute to this controversy. These include a tendency toward unpredictability in response that is an especial problem in children with organic dysfunction; examples of abuses of these medications, particularly through excessive use; and the inherent, but often poorly understood, limitations of any pharmacological intervention.

Most experienced clinicians can think of specific case histories in which the use of psychotropic medication has been associated with dramatic improvement in a patient's overall ability to function. Usually, they can also think of examples where virtually every medication available has been tried on a certain psychotic child and none of these has been associated with significant improvement. They have also often seen cases where one set of symptoms was relieved only to be replaced by another, equally troublesome set of behavioral side effects.

Because of a variety of research efforts, especially in the past decade, it is now increasingly possible to understand why some of these patients are helped by medications and why others are not. Being familiar with this information can be of great help to the clinician in her or his efforts to predict which medication is most likely to help a given child and which children are unlikely to respond to medication, and to recognize and minimize problems with side effects. This chapter also identifies some frequent causes of medication failure and suggests alternative solutions if this should occur. Finally, it reviews the effectiveness of some frequently advocated nutritional adjuncts to treatment.

6.1. Factors Influencing Choice of Medication

The author has identified four principles that appear to be particularly helpful in deciding which, if any, medications are likely to be beneficial in the

John Y. Donaldson • Department of Psychiatry, Nebraska Psychiatric Institute, University of Nebraska Medical Center, Omaha, Nebraska 68105.

treatment of a given psychotic retarded child or adolescent. Briefly listed, these principles are (1) identifying as specifically as possible the abnormalities that can and cannot be remedied with medication; (2) understanding the pharmacological actions of the medications being used; (3) knowing the most commonly troublesome side effects of the medications; and (4) being aware of special problems that are somewhat more likely to occur when psychotropic medications are given to this particular group of patients.

6.1.1. Principle 1: Identifying Specific Abnormalities That Psychotropic Medications Can or Cannot Be Expected to Help

In many centers, it is still common to think in terms of using psychotropic medications to *control* abnormal or undesirable behaviors in mentally retarded psychiatric patients. This is a misperception that occurred for several reasons. When these medications were first introduced, they were used empirically without a clear understanding of their actions. Also, in acutely ill psychotic adult patients with normal intelligence, the response is often so rapid that it does appear that the medication controls the related behavioral problems. In addition, many experimental designs still focus on the control of unwanted behaviors simply because they are relatively easy to measure. Nevertheless, the whole concept of using these medications for behavioral control is really not very accurate. Unless one uses massive doses—medication as a chemical strait-jacket—the drugs do not control behavior. The medications are more appropriately used to correct certain abnormalities in neurochemical activity. This normalization of neurophysiology may directly reduce certain associated behavioral symptoms, but more important, it can facilitate a greater capacity for learned self-control on the part of the patient.

A related source of confusion about proper medication usage is the currently used psychiatric diagnostic nomenclature, which is based primarily on a description of patient behavior.[1] In several of these categories, including attention deficit disorders, schizophrenia, and autism, patient physiology may vary tremendously—from intense hyperarousal to profound hypoarousal to essentially normal. These differing physiologies imply differing biochemical etiologies for certain similar symptoms and suggest that differing types of medical interventions may be appropriate for patients having the same diagnosis.[2] Also, within the given diagnostic categories currently available, medications may still not be effective for significant subgroups.

A considerable amount of research in the past few years has shown that the psychiatric conditions that can easily be brought under control by psychotropic medications appear to resolve abnormalities of patient physiology and biochemistry at the neurotransmitter level.[3,4] The medications are of less help to patients whose problems are due to neurological deficit and are of very little help in learned psychosis.[5]

Because of these factors, the first principle—that of identifying the correctable abnormality—should shift from identifying a target behavior of a general diagnosis to identifying probable neurotransmitter defect or related physiological abnormality.

One may ask if it is currently a realistic goal for the average clinician to attempt to identify physiological or biochemical abnormalities. Admittedly, few programs or individuals have access to a polygraph, and fewer still have laboratories equipped to measure dopamine, norepinephrine, serotonin, the endorphins, acetylcholine, their metabolites, or their regulatory enzymes. Even without these important adjuncts, it is possible to begin to think in these terms and thereby to improve the quality of the assessment of the patient prior to the administration of neuroleptic drugs.

Certain patient behaviors, when correlated with clinically observable physiology, can give the clinician important clues to the presence or the absence of *probable* abnormalities of neurotransmitter activity. For the medications currently available, norepinephrine, dopamine, acetylcholine, serotonin, and the endorphins appear to be the most important neurotransmitters. It should also be stressed that, when apparent neurotransmitter abnormalities are described in this chapter, it is not always appropriate to think in terms of absolute levels of these substances. It is most accurate to think in terms of neurotransmitter *activity*. Neurotransmitter activity may be influenced by absolute levels, and also by the relative amount of substance compared to the total number of receptor sites or the sensitivity of these sites.[6,7] The following paragraphs contain summaries of behavioral symptoms and physiological signs that appear to be associated with certain abnormalities in neurotransmitter activity.

Decreased adrenergic (norepinephrine) activity appears to be associated with apathy and endogenous depression in older adults and with physiological hypoarousal and attention deficit disorders with hyperactivity in children who also have minimal brain damage or dysfunction.[8,9]

Increased adrenergic activity is associated with a sense of anxiety, increased alertness, peripheral vasoconstriction, and pressure of speech. In extreme cases, these may shift to the hyperalertness, irritability, hostility, and ideas of reference that characterize the paranoid state. Most acute schizophrenics, including some very young children, show this type of physiology early in their illness.[10]

Decreased dopaminergic activity is associated with a poverty of ideas, impaired spatial ability, learning disabilities in children, and, in extreme natural or medication-caused cases, symptoms of Parkinson's disease.[3]

Increased dopaminergic activity is associated with unusually good spatial ability, creativity, an ability to anticipate problems, and a tendency toward obsessive speech or compulsive behaviors. In extreme cases, the patient may have such an overwhelming level of mental activity that his associations become disorganized in a classical schizophrenic pattern. High levels of dopamine are also a cause of some stereotypical behaviors. This latter type of behavior and symptomatology seem to predominate in the middle portion of a schizophrenic illness.[3]

Decreased cholinergic activity may be associated with disinhibition, poor recent memory, and a lack of capacity for introspection. Both mania and schizophrenia can be precipitated by a marked decrease in cholinergic activity, but efforts to increase cholinergic activity are often not helpful because of their tendency to cause anxiety and depression.[10]

Increased cholinergic activity appears to contribute to introspection, hyperactivity, depression, inhibition, sweaty hands, and psychophysiological complaints.[11]

Decreased serotonergic activity has been associated with anxiety, depression, irritability, and diminished levels of other neurotransmitters.[12]

Increased serotonergic activity has been linked with drowsiness, a sensation of mental fogginess, and, when abnormal metabolites are produced, visual hallucinations.[13]

Decreased endorphin activity has been associated with hypersensitivity to pain and stress and an inability to experience pleasure.[14]

Increased endorphin activity has been associated with auditory hallucinations, catatonic posturing, insensitivity to pain, and midbrain seizures. In addition, some data suggest a link between increased endorphin production and catecholamine blockage.[15-18]

6.1.2. Principle 2: Knowing the Pharmacological Actions of Psychotropic Medications

With the information regarding principle 1 in mind, the second principle, regarding the pharmacological action of the various medications, becomes a relatively easy task. All medications commonly used in psychiatry work at least in part to counteract excesses or to overcome deficiencies of neurotransmitter activity. The table of commonly used medications (Table 1) summarizes the action of these drugs on neurotransmitter activity in its third column. In general, it can be said that the stimulants and the antidepressants all act to increase norepinephrine and/or dopamine activity, whereas the antipsychotic medications tend to block the action of these same substances. The more sedating major tranquilizers have a potent norepinephrine blocking action, whereas the more potently antischizophrenic medications tend to block dopamine more strongly. Most of the antidepressants act first by increasing serotonin and blocking acetylcholine and later by increasing adrenergic activity.

Several other medications in the table are technically not neuroleptics but are included because some retarded patients may come to you already on these drugs because of some other condition or because someone else thought they were required. Some of these may be essential for treating epilepsy, dystonias, or other problems. They are included mainly because they may facilitate (or complicate) the psychiatric treatment of a psychotic, hyperactive, retarded child. When behavioral problems are a primary concern, it is important to choose the medications having the fewest behavioral side effects whenever conditions permit. For example, we would generally recommend using phenytoin instead of phenobarbital if hyperactivity, aggression, and impulsiveness are serious problems for a patient with major motor or grand mal seizures. Carbamazepine is less likely to cause behavioral problems in patients with psychomotor seizures than is primidone, but it is more of a risk with regard to the patient's hematological status.

6.1.3. Principle 3: Knowing the Most Frequently Troublesome Side Effects

The most common side effects are summarized in the last column of Table 1. This is not meant to be an inclusive list of side effects, but it includes many of the problems that are most frequently encountered in clinical practice. Being aware of these can do much to prevent unnecessary discomfort in retarded patients.

Almost all medication appears to have a small potential to cause a variety of semiallergic idiosyncratic reactions. These adverse reactions are most likely to involve liver, bone marrow, or skin. The phenothiazines seem to be at somewhat higher than average risk to cause problems in any or all of those areas. In addition, the more sedative phenothiazines tend to accumulate in certain tissues when they are given in high doses for long periods of time. Although it is certainly important to be aware of the various idiosyncratic side effects of any medication—in the case of the psychotropic medications—it is particularly important also to be aware of side effects that are related to their *pharmacological action.*

The effect of the stimulants and the antidepressants is to increase the actual levels or the activity of catecholamines at billions of synaptic clefts. As a result, excessive amounts of these medications may create anxiety states, hyperarousal, and psychotic conditions almost identical to those that occur naturally when an endogenous excess of catecholamine activity is present. Similarly, the major tranquilizers block the activity of these same neurotransmitters, and it is very easy to create relative deficiencies of norepinephrine, dopamine, or acetylcholine. Excessive norepinephrine blockage can lead to sedation, depression, and apathy in some patients and to classical stimulus-bound hyperactivity in others. Excessive dopamine blockage is associated with Parkinson-like movement disorders, learning disabilities, and an impoverishment of thought. Excessive acetylcholine blockage is likely to impair recent memory, lead to poor impulse control, and potentiate dopamine and norepinephrine activity. In extreme cases, acetylcholine blockage can cause actual delirium. The development of any of these problems often does not mean that the patient cannot take a given medication. More accurately, it is an indication that the patient has been given an excessive amount of a specific medication. We would, in general, recommend using medication dosages that stop short of producing physiological states that are the opposite of those seen in the original condition. Patient responses to medication are often helpful in determining the severity of the physiological aspect of the overall problem. Often, the fact that high doses are tolerated supports the contention that a serious physiological cause exists for the emotional or behavioral problem. A great sensitivity to a specific medication would tend to indicate that an excess or a deficiency of the neurotransmitter activity that is blocked or enhanced by that medication is not a significant cause of the patient's problem.

Table 1. Specific Pharmacological Approaches and Rationale for Mentally Ill–Retarded Children

Representative types of psychotropic medications for retarded children and adolescents

Drug	Dose	Indication	Apparent action	Common problems
1. Dextroamphetamine (Dexedrine)	5–20 mgm/day	Classical or "stimulus-bound" hyperactivity with minimal brain dysfunction (MBD)	Mimics or releases norepinephrine	↓ Appetite ↓ Growth ↑ Anxiety ↑ Aggression when given to anxious children ↑ Stereotypical behaviors
2. Methylphenidate (Ritalin)	10–40 mgm/day	Classical or "stimulus-bound" hyperactivity with MBD; may be somewhat more helpful for learning disabilities	Releases norepinephrine and dopamine	↓ Appetite ↓ Growth ↑ Anxiety ↑ Aggression when given to anxious children ↑ Stereotypical behaviors
3. Pemoline (Cylert)	37.5–112.5 mgm/day	Classical or "stimulus-bound" hyperactivity with MBD; may be somewhat more helpful for learning disabilities	Thought to increase dopamine synthesis	↓ Appetite ↓ Growth ↑ Anxiety ↑ Aggression when given to anxious children ↑ Stereotypical behaviors ↑ Insomnia
4. Imipramine (Tofranil)	10–50 mgm/day	Familial enuresis, especially when associated with classical hyperactivity with MBD or in some cases of detachment	↑ Brain norepinephrine,[b] blocks acetylcholine,[a] ↑ brain serotonin[a]	Anticholinergic side effects ↑ Anxiety ↑ Aggression, may unmask latent schizophrenia
5. Chlorpromazine (Thorazine)	10–300 mgm/day	↑ Anxiety associated with aggression and/or psychosis, especially with intense peripheral vasospasm	Block norepinephrine[b] and dopamine[a]	Photosensitivity, leukopenia; occasional extrapyramidal side effects; tissue disposition with prolonged usage; tardive dyskinesia

6. Thioridazine (Mellaril)	10–300 mgm/day	Psychosis especially with aggression or epilepsy	Block norepinephrine,[b] dopamine,[a] and acetylcholine[a]	Headache, depression, weight gain, nasal stuffiness, retrograde ejaculation, tissue deposition, tardive dyskinesia; not antipsychotic in low doses
7. Trifluoperazine (Stelazine)	1–10 mgm/day	↑Anxiety with withdrawal and compulsive features and/or psychosis	Block norepinephrine[a] and dopamine[b]	Extrapyramidal side effects, leukopenia, ↑aggressiveness or hyperactivity in some patients with MBD, tardive dyskinesia
8. Fluphenazine (Prolixin)	1–10 mgm/day	Psychosis and ritualistic or stereotyped behavior or severe aggressive outbursts	Block norepinephrine[a] and dopamine[b]	Extrapyramidal side effects, leukopenia, ↑aggressiveness or hyperactivity in some patients with MBD, tardive dyskinesia
9. Haloperidol (Haldol)	0.5–15 mgm/day	↑Anxiety with withdrawal and compulsive features and/or psychosis	Block dopamine[c] and norepinephrine[a]	Severe extrapyramidal side effects, ↑hyperactivity in some patients with MBD, worsening of learning disabilities, tardive dyskinesia
10. Lithium carbonate (multiple trade names)	600–1800 mgm/day	Manic-depressive illness; may also be helpful in patients with severe obsessive speech patterns, auditory hallucinations, self-injurious behavior	Displaces sodium at neuronal cell membrane; appears to decrease adrenergic activity and decrease sensitivity to endorphins	Not approved for children under 12; therapeutic levels are close to toxic levels; nausea, vomiting, tremor, polyuria, diarrhea are usually dose-related; long-term effects on renal and thyroid functions are possible

Table 1. (*Continued*)

Representative types of psychotropic medications for retarded children and adolescents

Drug	Dose	Indication	Apparent action	Common problems
11. Benztropine mesylate (Cogentin)	1–4 mgm/day	Extrapyramidal side effects due to dopamine-blocking medications	Blocks acetyl choline[c]	Dry mouth, blurred near vision, constipation, reversible memory loss or confusion
12. Diphenhydramine (Benadryl)	25–300 mgm/day	Hyperactivity 2°, anxiety, allergies, restlessness 2° haloperidol	Antihistamine[b]; blocks acetylcholine[a]	Drowsiness, some anticholinergic effects; may worsen classical hyperkinesis
13. Diazepam (Valium)	4–15 mgm/day	Situational anxiety	This class of drugs appears to block purines at natural receptor sites; action is sedative	Possible impairment of recent memory, aggression in some children, some potential for dependence, loss of effectiveness after time
14. Chlordiazepoxide (Librium)	10–40 mgm/day	Situational anxiety	This class of drugs appears to block purines at natural receptor sites; action is sedative	Same as Valium except less problem with recent memory loss
15. Phenobarbital	30–240 mgm/day	For grand mal and petit mal epilepsy, situational anxiety	Sedative, anticonvulsant	↑ Aggressive behavior in some children, especially with MBD, impairment of recent memory, potential for dependence
16. Phenytoin sodium (Dilantin)	5 mg/kg/day up to 300 mgm/day	Grand mal seizures	Anticonvulsant	Leukopenia, gingival hypertrophy, skin rash, increased anxiety
17. Primidone (Mysoline)	250–750 mgm/day	Psychomotor (temporal lobe) seizures	Anticonvulsant	Metabolized to phenobarbital, ataxia, drowsiness, worsened hyperactivity or aggressiveness

18. Carbamazepine (Tegretol)	200–1200 mgm/day	Anticonvulsant	Psychomotor seizures, especially complex partial temporal-lobe seizures	Agranulocytosis, leukopenia, hepatic and renal dysfunction, drowsiness, dizziness, incoordination
19. Ethosuximide (Zarontin)	250–750 mgm/day	Anticonvulsant	Petit mal seizures	Blood dyscrasias, allergic reactions, drowsiness
20. Valproic acid (Depakene)	250–1250 mgm/day	Anticonvulsant (appears to increase GABA levels in brain)	Petit mal, simple and complex absence seizures; may be a useful alternative to phenobarbital	Hepatic dysfunction, nausea, blood dyscrasias, hyperactivity (less likely than with phenobarbital); sometimes is incompatible with phenytoin

[a] Pharmacological activity slight but significant.
[b] Pharmacological activity moderate.
[c] Pharmacological activity marked.

A side effect that is especially important to be aware of in long-term major tranquilizer use is tardive dyskinesia. This is an abnormal movement disorder that is now thought most often to be due to a reactive increase of dopaminergic activity in the basal ganglia of the brain. The condition appears most likely to occur when patients have had a prolonged, simultaneous blockage of dopamine and acetylcholine. It is probably part of an adaptive mechanism as the patient's physiology attempts to overcome the drug-induced neurotransmitter blockade. It can be prevented by avoiding excessive dopamine blockade, especially in combination with an acetylcholine blockade. One should, therefore, not follow the old adage of pushing the phenothiazines to the point of Parkinson-like effects and then adding anti-Parkinson medication on a chronic basis. Better long-term results are obtained by lowering the dose of dopamine blocker if Parkinsonism occurs or by using anti-Parkinson drugs only when needed, for as long as needed. In children and young adults, tardive dyskinesia is almost always reversible when it is diagnosed early and attempts are made to reduce or withdraw medication as soon as the problem is observed. This condition has been called rebound dyskinesia. In older patients who have had the symptom for a very long period of time, the condition is frequently not reversible and may be due to actual structural changes.[19]

Another condition has been recently described that can be a significant complication of long-term neuroleptic use. Supersensitivity psychosis may occur when the patient responds to long-term neurotransmitter blockade by developing more sensitive neurotransmitters or an absolute increase in neurotransmitters. If one suspects that a patient may no longer need a major tranquilizer, it is important to withdraw the medication slowly. A sudden withdrawal may cause transient behavior to appear within a day or two, which if not recognized as a rebound phenomenon could mean returning the patient to medication unnecessarily.[20]

It is relatively easy for the physician to see such obvious medication side effects as skin rash, pseudo-Parkinsonism, or tardive dyskinesia, but unpleasant symptoms can occur in patients who are not able to describe their discomfort. This is especially true of psychotic and retarded patients. This brings us to the final principle.

6.1.4. Principle 4: Special Problems of Psychotic Children Who Are Receiving Psychotropic Medications

In these patients, the clinician must be alert to certain uncomfortable side effects by looking for more subtle signs. These would include increased physiological signs of anxiety, restless behavior due to tension, loss of appetite, or crying spells—all of which are associated with excessive stimulant or antidepressant administration. If catecholamine-blocking drugs are used, drowsiness, classical hyperactivity, restlessness due to akathisia, apathy, and increased learning disabilities are all possible side effects.

Another problem with medicating psychotic children is that many of the abnormal behaviors they present are learned adaptations that are not directly related to abnormal physiology. A child with autistic features who makes strange noises and claps his hands may do this as part of a stereotypical schizophrenic pattern secondary to a relative excess of dopaminergic activity in one or both temporal lobes, whereas an almost identically appearing retarded child may have learned that hand clapping and the uttering of strange noises will allow him to achieve relief from the demands of concerned teachers and parents. The first child will commonly show a significant improvement with medication, whereas the second child may develop side effects at a low dosage and show no improvement. Often, one does not see a pure case of either type. It is more typical to see a situation where the stereotypical behavior improves only 50% with the medication. Too many clinicians are tempted to achieve 100% improvement with higher doses of medication and then give up altogether because of side effects. Ideally, the medication should be used only to normalize or optimize the patient's physiology. Once this is done, the clinician can shift his or her therapeutic efforts toward behavioral and psychotherapeutic interventions.

Another related problem is that many psychotic retarded children have not had a period of normal behavior. It is easy to treat the college student who presents in an acutely psychotic state, responds rapidly to medication, and soon returns to her or his usual activities with minimal disability. But a 17-year-old autistic patient who has been psychotic since age 2 can be helped only minimally by medication. If one is fortunate enough as to be able to correct such a patient's abnormal physiology, then years of additional work are required to overcome the developmental lags that are associated with a lifetime of psychotic behavior.

Closely related to this concept is a problem associated with the pharmacological action of most of the antipsychotic medications. They tend to interfere with conditioned learning. This appears to be especially true if the dosage of medication is high enough to cause significant sedation and the complete elimination of the physical signs of anxiety. Therefore, when dealing with a patient who requires a great deal of behavioral shaping, it is especially important to avoid overmedication. Occasionally, with older children, it may be necessary to use high dosages of medication to prevent repeated episodes of dangerously destructive behavior. If it is necessary to do this, one should not expect to see significant behavioral changes on a learned basis during the period of heavy medication. The optimal result in such a case is a return to a previous set of learned behaviors.

One type of child that is especially difficult to medicate combines high catecholamine levels with organic brain dysfunction. This category includes a considerable number of psychotic or prepsychotic children. These children are likely to become classically hyperactive or to function as having severe character disorders with the catecholamine blockade or sedation of the tranquilizers, and they are at very high risk of becoming psychotic if given stimulants. They seem to have a very narrow therapeutic window. Either type of medication alone is very likely to cause side effects. Fortunately, many of these children respond postively to a combination of medications. They react as though the stimulant or the antidepressant medication has reached the reticular activating system to improve impulse control while the major tranquilizers have decreased the excessive dopaminergic activity in the limbic area, thereby preventing or lessening psychosis. This is one of the few areas where polypharmacy seems to be indicated. It is important to note that a significant minority of this group of patients does not show a positive response to the combination but instead seem to show troublesome side effects from both types of medication. Some of them do better with very low doses of one or the other group of drugs, and some may be best without medication.

A subgroup of difficult-to-treat autistic patients is currently being described anecdotically at national meetings. Although no one has, to our knowledge, published a report of significant series of these patients, our own clinical observation would tend to confirm the existence of this subgroup. Some of the most refractory autistics appear to have signs of temporal lobe atrophy when evaluated by CAT scan. In our own experience, we have seen one mute autistic with bilateral temporal-lobe damage; two autistic adolescents with parrotlike speech and good musical ability, who lacked a capacity to synthesize useful speech, and in whom left-temporal-lobe damage alone was present; and one patient with right-temporal-lobe damage who can synthesize speech, but who is without spontaneity, totally anhedonic, and given to stereotypical behavior.

All of these patients have at some point shown serious behavioral outbursts. All were relatively sensitive to potent neuroleptics in that they developed extrapyramidal side effects at relatively low doses. The severity of their behavioral problems necessitated continuing efforts to find relief in medication. In all cases, partial relief was found in using a combination of high-dose potent neuroleptics and anti-Parkinson medications. In one case, dramatic relief was obtained with carbamazepine even though the patient's EEG was normal.

6.2. Neurotransmitter Mechanisms: Problems and Challenges

There is increasing consensus that schizophrenia is an extremely complex group of conditions and really no more a single disease than fever, pulmonary congestion, or cancer. The dopamine hypothesis holds some promise for one aspect of one subtype of condition, but when the number of factors that can affect dopamine activity alone is considered, it serves as an illustration of the extreme unlikelihood that one abnormality will be found that is always present in schizophrenia.

Dopamine production is regulated by the availability of its amino acid precursors and by tyrosine hydroxylase, a regulating enzyme in part triggered by stress. The reactivity of this enzyme is in part dependent on acetylcholine levels, in part on the related levels of the trace minerals—zinc and copper— and in part on the intactness of the sympathetic nervous system. Once dopamine is synthesized, its clearance from the synapse is controlled by cell reuptake and its metabolism by two more enzymes, monoamine oxidase (MAO) and dopamine beta hydroxylase (DBH). Although DBH can be temporarily

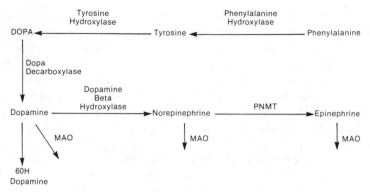

Figure 1. Biosynthesis and metabolism of dopamine.

increased by stress, the baseline levels of both enzymes appear to be genetically determined. They can also be altered by nutritional factors. Finally, the receiving cell can vary in its sensitivity to dopamine and its ability to send messages to the transmitter cell regarding the need for more or less dopamine.[2,5] Figure 1 illustrates a portion of the biochemical reactions in this complex system.

Dopamine-blocking neuroleptics appear to be most effective in acute psychotic reactions associated with intense physiological signs of anxiety. However, there is a need to develop a laboratory screening device that will help the clinician and document schizophrenic patients who have excessive dopaminergic activity. Such screening would increase the likelihood that dopamine-blocking medications would be given to patients who can be helped by them.

Hopefully, a time will come when all of the factors leading to abnormal neurotransmitter activity can be measured. Such a systems approach to diagnosis would allow us to choose psychotherapy for stress-related abnormalities, specific nutrients when indicated for correctable enzyme dysfunctions or substrate deficiencies, and psychotropic medications for the otherwise uncontrollable or genetically based abnormalities.

Another very important research frontier involves patients who are refractory to our present medications and other therapies. Many autistic children appear to be very much like chronic adult schizophrenics when viewed physiologically. It has been hypothesized that a schizophrenic who has excessive dopamine because of too little MAO and too little DBH has only one other metabolic option—to produce 6-hydroxy dopamine, a neurotoxic substance that destroys dopaminergic neurons. Over time, this would lead to decreased dopamine, decreased anxiety, loss of medication response, intellectual deterioration, and possible seizures. If correct, this hypothesis would imply an irreversible pattern; could explain that apparent fate of many psychotic children, especially those of the disintegrative type; and would correlate well with recent studies being carried out by many investigators, which indicate diffuse cortical atrophy in refractory schizophrenics.

The variability of symptoms in other refractory patients suggests a waxing and waning of a neurotransmitter. The endorphins give us another, perhaps more hopeful, hypothetical explanation for such patients. Endorphins are a group of recently discovered, morphinelike, naturally occurring polypeptides that have created considerable interest in adult psychiatry. When present in high levels, these substances decrease dopamine synthesis through an elaborate feedback mechanism. Endorphins are increased by an increase in catecholamine levels, pain, and a number of other factors, including diet. Normally, they appear to be a part of an adaptive physiological response; however, it has been shown that certain abnormal subtypes of endorphins or excessive amounts of normal types can cause sensory distortions, movement disorders, and midbrain seizure activity. Their presence could explain many autistic symptoms, as well as the decreased anxiety level seen in some of the more refractory of these patients. It could also explain the lack of effectiveness of the dopamine blockers in this group of patients.

At the present time, this entire area must be considered experimental. No oral endorphin blocker is available. The possibility of endorphin removal by dialysis has been explored in chronic adult schizophrenics, with very mixed results.

It is worth noting that some of the dietary changes that have been successfully used from time to time in refractory schizophrenics can now be more fully explained. Both wheat gluten and milk have the potential to produce abnormal endorphins in some patients.

6.3. Dietary and Nutritional Considerations

The long-standing observation that glutenfree and milkfree diets are help to a limited number of psychotic patients is well documented.[16] Many other dietary and nutritional factors seem to be helpful to some retarded patients with behavioral and emotional symptoms. The discussion in the previous section illustrates the extremely large number of factors that can influence neurotransmitter activity. Because of the complexity, most clinicians are aware of individual cases where a nutritional or dietary factor, apparently not known to be effective in most patients with that diagnosis, seemed to cause a marked improvement in the specific patient. Although nearly all authorities do not recommend across-the-board megadosages of vitamins for psychotic patients, it is worthwhile to have some understanding of why some of these approaches appear to work occasionally in some patients.

Supplemental vitamin B6 (pyridoxin) has the best documentation of its effectiveness in certain psychotic children. A review of its functions indicates that it increases DBH levels, thereby decreasing dopamine and increasing norepinephrine; it increases the natural inhibiting neurotransmitters serotonin and the natural anticonvulsant GABA.[21] Some autistic children seem to respond very positively to its administration.[22]

Other commonly used nutritional adjuncts that seem to have some rationale in their usage include niacin and vitamin C. Niacin has been hypothesized to act as a methyl group acceptance and in our experience has been helpful in patients who are troubled with vivid visual imagery or frank visual hallucinations. Similarly, vitamin C may help some schizophrenic patients by increasing DBH levels.[22,23] Massive doses of B complex cannot be recommended for most psychotic children. In general, these substances appear to increase acetylcholine, norepinephrine, and dopamine.

The Feingold diet and other similar efforts at dietary control of hyperactive impulse disorders have also been subjects of much controversy. Most of the early controlled studies using large samples of hyperactive children tended to discount this approach as not being associated with statistically significant positive changes in the group as a whole.[23,24] More recent studies have indicated that artificial food colors and preservatives are significant causes of impairment in a subgroup of children.[25,26] Animal experiments suggest that the disinhibition may be due to a sudden release of acetylcholine, followed by a refractory period in which little or no acetylcholine is released into the synaptic cleft.[27]

Our own observations tend to confirm that the elimination of artificial colors and preservatives is indeed helpful in some impulsive retarded children. One of the best means of determining the likelihood of a patient's responding to a diet is marked day-to-day variability in behavior. Often, children come to the physician already on a dietary program that their parents feel has been helpful. In some of these cases, the approach appears to be reasonable and to be consistent with known neurotransmitter mechanisms, whereas other approaches may seem irrational or unnecessary. Unless a diet or a dietary supplement is clearly dangerous, the clinician would do well to respect the findings of the parents, to work with them to systematically test the need for various parts of the program, and, above all, to try to understand why a certain approach is working with a given patient. To automatically reject these efforts risks alienating the patient's parents and also risks closing the door on approaches that could provide help to other patients. Also, although these adjuncts are often not adequate by themselves, they may aid in the regulation of other, more traditional medications.

6.4. Summary

Several points need to be stressed. It is no longer appropriate to think in terms of using psychotropic medications simply to control behavior. The function of these medications is more accurately that of correcting certain abnormalities of brain physiology and/or biochemistry that may lead to disturbed behavior. If through medications and other adjuncts these physiological abnormalities can be corrected, the patient then has a better opportunity to develop positive human relationships and to respond to traditional psychotherapy, relationship therapy, and behavior modification. If medications are not used when indicated, many patients remain too anxious or too psychotic, or too irritable to learn. In contrast, if excessive amounts of inappropriate types of medications are used, sedation, impaired learning, movement disorders, psychologically induced behavioral disorders, or even more severe psychosis can be side effects.

It is also essential to remember that, although neuroleptic medications can be very helpful in treating mentally disturbed retarded children, these patients are more likely than the general population to have unusual side effects, and that they are more likely to have only a partial improvement in symptoms associated with the use of medications.[28] Some may not improve because their illness has an unrelated etiology, and they should not be subjected to continual exposure to unnecessary medications. Retarded children receiving these medications require close attention—partly because of the complexity of their problems, partly because of their impaired ability to refuse the medication or to complain about any adverse effects, and partly because they will continue to require many other nonmedical approaches.

References

1. American Psychiatric Association: *Diagnostic and Statistical Manual of Mental Disorders*, ed 3. Washington, D.C., Author, 1980.
2. Satterfield, J, Cantwell D, Satterfield B: Pathophysiology of the hyperactive child syndrome. *Arch Gen Psychiatr* 31;838–844, 1974.
3. Snyder S, Banerjee S, Yamamura H, et al: Drugs, neurotransmitters, and schizophrenia. *Science* 184;1243–1253, 1974.
4. Cohen DJ, Young, JG: Neurochemistry and child psychiatry. *J Child Psychiatr* 16(3);353–411, 1977.
5. Donaldson JY, Menolascino FJ: Emotional disorders in the retarded. *Inter J Ment Health* 6(1);27–35, 1977.
6. Snyder S: The dopamine hypothesis of schizophrenia: Focus on the dopamine receptor. *Am J Psychiatr* 113(2);197–202, 1976.
7. Yepes L, Winsburg B: Vomiting during neuroleptic withdrawal in children. *Clin Res Rep* 134(5);574, 1977.
8. Schildkraut J, Kety S: Biogenic amines and emotion. Science 156;3771:21–30, 1967.
9. Skekim W, Dekirmenjian H: Urinary catecholamine metabolites in hyperkinetic boys treated with d-amphetamine. *Am J Psychiatr* 134(11);1276–1279, 1977.
10. Snyder S: Catecholamine in the brain as mediators of amphetamine psychosis. *Arch Gen Psychiatr* 27;169–179, 1972.
11. Ulus I, Wurtman R: Choline administration: Activation of tyrosine hydroxylase in dopaminergic neurons of rat brain. *Science* 194;1060–1061, 1977.
12. Greenberg AS, Coleman M: Depressed 5-hydroxyindole levels associated with hyperactive and aggressive behavior. *Arch Gen Psychiatr* 33;331–336, 1976.
13. Coleman M: Serotonin and central nervous system syndromes of childhood: A review. *J Autism Child Schizophr* 3(1);27–35, 1973.
14. Watson SJ, Akil H: Some observations on the opiate peptides and schizophrenia. *Arch Gen Psychiatr* 36;35–41, 1979.
15. Watson SJ, Berger PA, Akil H, *et al*: Effects of naloxone on schizophrenia: Reduction in hallucinations in a subpopulation of subjects. *Science* 201;73–75, 1978.
16. Bloom F, Segal D: Endorphins: Profound behavioral effects in rats suggest new etiological factors in mental illness. *Science* 194;630–632, 1976.
17. Urca G, Frenk H: Morphine and enkephalin: Analgesic and epileptic properties. *Science* 197;83–86, 1977.

18. Marx JL: Brain opiates in mental illness. Science 214;1013–1015, 1981.
19. Task Force on Late Neurological Effects of Antipsychotic Drugs. Tardive dyskinesia: Summary of a task force report of the American Psychiatric Association. *Am J Psychiatry* 137(10);1163–1173, 1980.
20. Chouinard, G, Jones BD: Neuroleptic-induced supersensitivity psychosis: Clinical and pharmacological characteristics. *Am J Psychiatr* 137(1);16–21, 1980.
21. Ebadi M: Vitamin B and biogenic amines in brain metabolism. *Nat Acad Sci* 8;129–161, 1978.
22. Rimland B, Callaway E: The effect of high doses of Vitamin B_6 on autistic children: A double-blind crossover study. *Am J Psychiatr* 135(4),472–475, 1978.
23. Pauling L: On the orthomolecular environment of the mind: Orthomolecular theory. *Am J Psychiatr* 131(11);1251–1257, 1977.
24. Wender E: Food additives and hyperkinesis. *Am J Dis Childhood* 131;1204–1206, 1977.
25. Swanson JM, Kinsbourne M: Food dyes impair performance of hyperactive children on a laboratory learning test. *Science* 207;1485–1487, 1980.
26. Weiss B, Williams J: Behavioral responses to artificial food colors. *Science* 207;1487–1488, 1980.
27. Augustine GJ, Levitan H: Neurotransmitter release from a vertebrate neuromuscular synapse affected by a food dye. *Science* 207;1489–1490, 1980.
28. Bruening SE, Poling AD: *Drugs and Mental Retardation.* Springfield, Il, C. C. Thomas, 1982.

Treatment Strategies in the Habilitation of Severely Mentally Retarded-Mentally Ill Adolescents and Adults

Jack A. Stark, John J. McGee, Frank J. Menolascino, Daniel H. Baker, and Paul E. Menousek

7.1. Introduction

The purpose of this chapter is to provide an analysis of habilitation (prevocational and vocational) intervention strategies for severely mentally retarded and mentally ill adolescents and adults. Educators, rehabilitation specialists, and community agencies are faced with a growing and critical problem in meeting the needs of this population. Because of recent legislative, judicial, and consumer advocacy pressure, these persons are beginning to be served in the mainstream of community life. However, even today, some professionals consider persons with these special needs as too severely handicapped to receive prevocational or vocational training. Because community agencies are faced with an increasing need to serve these individuals, new treatment strategies must be developed to meet their needs. Unless such strategies are developed, many of these persons will continue to be placed in nursing facilities or other long-term care institutions. In addition, it is the authors' intent that this chapter provide a framework for understanding the overall problems, needs, techniques, strategies, issues, and new findings in serving this challenging population.

7.2. Historical and Evolutionary Aspects of Habilitation for the Mentally Retarded-Mentally Ill

The history of the habilitation movement in this country has been described in great detail by Obermann[1] and by Cull and Hardy.[2] After a period of public

Jack A. Stark • Departments of Psychiatry and Pediatrics, Meyer Children's Rehabilitation Institute, University of Nebraska Medical Center, Omaha, Nebraska 68105.   *John J. McGee* • Department of Psychiatry, Nebraska Psychiatric Institute and Meyer Children's Rehabilitation Institute, University of Nebraska Medical Center, Omaha, Nebraska 68105.   *Frank J. Menolascino* • Departments of Psychiatry and Pediatrics, Nebraska Psychiatric Institute, University of Nebraska Medical Center, Omaha, Nebraska 68105.   *Daniel H. Baker and Paul E. Menousek* • Department of Psychiatry, Meyer Children's Rehabilitation Institute, University of Nebraska Medical Center, Omaha, Nebraska 68105.

apathy toward both the mentally retarded and the mentally ill, attitudes have changed to the recognition of an economic necessity and a social obligation to help the mentally retarded and the mentally ill move toward independence and vocational sufficiency.

The application of habilitation goals is a relatively recent phenomenon, first appearing in the mid-nineteenth century. This philosophy of rehabilitation regarding the mentally retarded has been described[3] as a shift from the *desire* to "make the deviant undeviant" (1850–1880), to a *concern* to "shelter the deviant from society" (1870–1890), to *alarm* over the "protection of society from the deviant" (1880–1890).

Historical records also show that the earliest institutions in this country for disabled people were designed for children and usually carried a vocational emphasis. Indeed, in 1885, the superintendent of the Utica New York State Lunatic Asylum wrote at some length on the subject of the conditions and the needs of mentally retarded people in that state:

> We are of the opinion that much may be done for their improvement and comfort, that many instead of being a burden and expense of the community may be so improved as to engage in useful employment and to support themselves; and also to participate in the enjoyments of society. (p. 124)[9]

The healers of the mid-nineteenth century gave way to the moral teachings of the early twentieth century. Some lived to see the pendulums swing back again and regretted their earlier words. In 1912, Fernald[9] generalized about the moral sensibilities of the mildly retarded and thought them all potentially to be criminals. The habilitation ideas of Itard and Seguin seemed all but forgotten in the early twentieth century, when there was little emphasis on preparing the mentally retarded for a return to society. The emphasis was on the elimination of these groups of human beings so as to prevent the contamination of the population. This eugenic scare seemed to peak in the 1920s and then to abate.[9]

The period between the late 1920s and 1960 was one of contradictory development. In general, the climate became more optimistic; there was a reawakening of the original habilitation and education principle, as well as a reaffirmation that retarded persons could be trained, some sufficiently to permit their functioning within a community setting. Yet, the large institutions during this period continued to be the dominant choice of treatment for mentally retarded individuals, and in many instances, conditions within institutions were directly antithetical to the idea of habilitation.

The passage of Public Law 236 by the Sixty-sixth Congress in June 1920 was a landmark in the history of rehabilitation in this country. The Civilian Vocational Rehabilitation Act, as it was called then, provided for the vocational rehabilitation of persons disabled in industry or in any legitimate occupation and for their return to civil employment. During the period between 1920 and 1943, vocational rehabilitation was a federal system serving only *physically* disabled persons. The Vocational Rehabilitation Amendments in 1943 (Public Law 113) extended the concept of vocational rehabilitation to "include any services necessary to render a disabled individual fit to engage in remunerative occupation." It meant for the first time that our mentally retarded and mentally

ill individuals, as well as the physically disabled, would be accepted as rehabilitation clients. However, little progress in serving these groups was made
until 1954 when rehabilitation services, training, and research were expanded.
The Office of Vocational Rehabilitation was established to prepare disabled
workers to engage in production essentially in industry and other peacetime
pursuits.

The 1965 amendments to the Vocational Rehabilitation Act further expanded research and demonstration projects, many of which developed new
methods and techniques for serving mentally disordered individuals. The 1968
amendments emphasized vocational evaluation and work adjustment services.
The Rehabilitation Act of 1973 included a strong mandate to state-federal vocational rehabilitation programs to serve the more severely disabled and to
actively involve clients in the planning and the delivery of vocational rehabilitation services.

The Rehabilitation Act of 1973 marked a major redefinition of the 53 years
of efforts of rehabilitation in this country. It no longer placed eligibility requirements solely on "substantial gainful activity." It also included comprehensive services for independent living, particularly designed for the severely
disabled. The purpose of this new eligibility requirement was to provide alternative living systems to help the individual to engage in employment or
simply to support his or her ability to function independently of a family or an
institution. The act, for the first time, also specified that such services could
include transportation and attendant care, recreational activities, health maintenance, services for children of preschool age, and appropriate attendant services to decrease the needs of the severely handicapped. These amendments
of 1973 were further strengthened by the 1978 amendments, in which Section
503 and 504 were enacted. These amendments created a great deal of controversy but strengthened the emphasis on reducing prejudices and on assisting
handicapped individuals particularly in the area of employment. They established a legal mandate in which a reasonable accommodation must be made
by each employer to hire a handicapped individual who has talents and skills
equal to those of a nonhandicapped person applying for the job. In short, every
piece of habilitation legislation since 1943 has contained references to the mentally disabled as a target population for vocational rehabilitation services.

Despite these tremendous advancements in the rehabilitation laws and a
new emphasis on the severely handicapped, we still see the *de facto* practice
in vocational rehabilitation programs across the country that most severely
handicapped individuals, who have been given priority by this new legislation,
have been declared too severely handicapped or medically unfeasible at this
time to receive vocational rehabilitation training. We had thought that the Rehabilitation Act of 1973 and its amendments of 1978 would put an end to hiding
behind the very restrictive "eligible but not feasible" criteria for providing
services. Legislation for other programs has also had an impact on the vocational rehabilitation program, particularly the legislation authorizing the development of community mental-health centers. The increasing awareness of
the necessity for vocational rehabilitation services to be an integral part of the

community mental-health-centers system culminated on June 1, 1978, with the signing of a joint agreement between the Rehabilitation Services Administration and the National Institute of Mental Health. This agreement sets out general guidelines for closer working relationships between the two agencies at the federal, state, and local levels.

7.3. Parameters of the Mentally Retarded-Mentally Ill Population

7.3.1. Definitional Issues

There is so much confusion about what constitutes mental illness in mentally retarded individuals that it has led to equivocation and inappropriate assumptions. Mental retardation implies both a symptom of an underlying developmental disorder and the assessment of an individual's potential to learn.[4] *Mental illness*, in this context, refers to abnormality of behavior, emotions, or relations sufficiently marked or prolonged for the handicapped individual in distress, as well as his family and community. In short, the etiological factors and functional conditions of mental retardation and mental illness in combination have a compounding effect in which strategies and techniques traditionally proven with each group will not automatically work.

The term *mental illness* is used in this chapter not according to the medical model, but to denote a severe and multiple condition that often requires the service of both mental health and mental retardation professionals. Other terms, such as *behaviorally impaired, emotional disturbance, learning handicap*, and *behavioral disorder* (all of which have an educational background and history), can be used synonymously with the term *mental illness* for the purposes of this chapter, only when these disorders meet the following criterion: the term *mental illness*, or other synonymously used terms, must refer to those categories that range from disturbances of high severity, encompassing psychosis and personality disorders, to minor disturbances and special symptoms such as hyperactivity, anxiety, and situational stress incidences.

Habilitation can be defined as an integration or reintegration, socially, educationally, vocationally, and psychologically, of the mentally retarded individual into the least restrictive environment possible. It is the authors' belief that this definition must be based on the conceptual premise that the developmental-learning-model approach is the *sine qua non* of the habilitation process. This process and model are dependent on several key premises: (1) habilitation may be viewed as a process of change that involves the development of behaviors compatible with the current and projected tasks affecting the individual; (2) all persons are continually developing and are capable of learning productive and socially acceptable behaviors; (3) all persons can develop skills suited to some level of productive functioning in an environment that fosters the maximum development of the potentials for independence; and (4) training processes and contingencies are more important in determining success than specific settings, although the goals are easier to accomplish in natural-environmental settings.

Traditional interpretations of habilitation have focused on its *vocational* aspects. However, habilitation should be interpreted more broadly as a habilitation of "life space." Greenblatt[5] viewed the habilitation of an individual's life space as consisting of a hexagon, with the six sides representing essential areas: psychological, educational, social, recreational, family, and community. Greenblatt's model refers especially to the habilitation of the life spaces of an individual with mental health needs. He described this hexagon as a symbol of the individual's adaptation to these six areas of living. He felt that deficiencies or imbalance in one given area could produce an asymmetrical hexagon and thereby lead to inadequate adaptation to one's environment.

7.3.2. Population Needs

There is an abundance of research studies highlighting the importance of the mental health needs of mentally retarded individuals and the roles that these needs play in determining whether a mentally retarded individual will adapt to the community. Emotional problems[6] have long been recognized as an important factor leading to the institutionalization of mentally retarded individuals. Even today, from a review of the various state developmental disability plans and the data analyses of those individuals entering the institutions, it is clear that the vast majority are being placed in such settings because of the community's inability to deal with their mental health needs.[7] There have been various hypotheses about the causes of these emotional-behavioral problems. Wortis[8] identified the causes as inadequate services and rejection by family, peers, and society. Menolascino[9] pointed out that the high frequency of sensory integration disorders associated with mental retardation hampers an individual's problem-solving ability and leads to a higher probability of his or her developing abnormal behavior. Menolascino[10] also noted that certain types of emotional disturbance are a function of responses partially gained as a result of institutionalization. Phillips[11] concluded that mentally retarded individuals are more vulnerable to defects in personality development because of their interpersonal experiences and their constitutional endowment. Cytryn and Lourie[12] also cited constitutional factors as leading to the mentally retarded individual's hypersensitivity to external and internal stimuli, hyposensitivity to sensory stimulation, aggressiveness related to irritability or inappropriate handling of situations, and inability to tolerate change. The consensus is that mentally retarded individuals do not necessarily develop mental illness; however, it is suggested that, because of the stresses that the mentally retarded individual encounters, he or she is vulnerable to developing mental illness. Regardless of the etiological reasons, mental illness and mental retardation often coexist.

The misunderstanding of the mental health needs of mentally retarded individuals has led to inappropriate service-delivery systems and complex unmet needs. These needs have not been met either by the community mental-health centers or by the vocational rehabilitation agencies because of inadequate training on the professional's part, lack of understanding of the mentally retarded's emotional needs, and referral breakdown between agencies.

7.3.3. Prevalence Studies

Determining the frequency and the types of emotional disturbance in the mentally retarded is beset by some major methodological problems. Studies before 1960 were conducted primarily in institutional settings. In these studies, the prevalence rate ranges from 16% to 40%. More recent studies on institutionalized retarded individuals report a similar range, but it is questionable whether they represent a cross section of this population. A series of reports on mentally retarded individuals who live with their primary families or in their primary community have consistently reported a 20%–35% frequency rate of emotional disturbance. Menolascino[10] stated that

> the frequency rates concerning the relationship between emotional disturbances and mental retardation reported in the literature should be placed in proper perspective as to the expected frequency rates of emotional disturbances in the non-retarded. A recent report of the Joint Commission on Mental Health in Children[13] suggests that emotional disturbances complicate the lives of 14 to 18 percent of the child population whereas scientific population studies on mental illness in adults suggest that the incidence of emotional disturbance in the general population approaches 20 to 40 percent. Viewed in these perspectives, the reported range of frequency of emotional disturbances in the mentally retarded suggest [sic] a moderately increased susceptibility to emotional disturbances for them as a group. (p. 23)

Epidemiological research indicates that there are approximately 6 million individuals in this country who have been identified as mentally retarded. Of this population, the U.S. Department of Labor has estimated that 87% have the potential to be employed in the competitive labor market (obviously, this percentage represents the moderate-to-mild population group). In addition, 10%, or approximately 600,000, are capable of working in a sheltered workshop setting, both with and without environmental and prosthetic support.[14] This chapter, however, focuses on the lower 3% of the entire population identified as severely and profoundly retarded. And it is this group—which represents some 200,000 people nationally, of which those with severe behavioral impairments comprise some 50,000–80,000 individuals—whose needs we have not adequately addressed. Once again, however, it is this small, but very difficult-to-serve, population, averaging 1,000 plus per state, that has proved the most controversial of any group in the state institutions. It is argued that because this particular population is virtually all that is left in the state institutions around the country, and because we have not adequately developed techniques for training them to leave these facilities, it is therefore best that we continue to maintain them there. Hopefully, the contents of this chapter will dispel this myth.[15]

7.4. Research

Research into the interrelationship between mental retardation and mental illness had been approached by researchers in their respective fields without much collaboration or interdisciplinary effort until the late 1970s. Psychiatrists, most notably Menolascino[16] and Chess,[17] delineated the psychiatric approaches to mental retardation, and educators have begun to develop educational programs for the classroom instruction of this population.[18] Likewise, habilitation and vocational rehabilitation programs have focused on this population.[19–24]

There is a need to bring together the most recent advances of the various disciplines involved in the diagnosis of, the treatment of, and the research on those individuals with severe mental retardation and mental illness. Over the years, researchers and practitioners have developed a variety of valid treatment approaches for the population. Now there is a need to bring these approaches together in order to develop comprehensive service-delivery systems and to provide a continuum of care from birth to death for these most challenging individuals.

7.5. Client Profiles: Who Are the Mentally Ill-Mentally Retarded?

Mentally retarded adolescents and adults with psychiatric disorders encompass the entire range of psychiatric diagnoses. Wing and Gould[24] have described these individuals as having severe abnormalities of interaction and communication, as well as a behavioral repertoire consisting of repetitive, stereotyped activities. Menolascino[10] portrayed them as demonstrating primitive, atypical, or abnormal behavior. They represent a complex developmental and psychiatric challenge regardless of their level of retardation or psychiatric involvement.

The following client profiles are a sample of five adolescent and adult clients who have participated in a prevocational-vocational program sponsored by the Meyer Children's Rehabilitation Institute (MCRI) and the Nebraska Psychiatric Institute (NPI) located at the University of Nebraska Medical Center (Omaha). These five individuals symbolize the practical challenges that the mentally retarded–emotionally disturbed present to professionals and family members. In spite of multiple and complex needs, these five cases also symbolize the fact that this population can be served in the least restrictive environment and that personnel can be prepared to provide such services. Typically, the clients in these profiles demonstrated a combination of developmental and behavioral problems that resulted in extreme difficulties relative to their treatment, whether at home, in school, or in a vocational training program. Their ages ranged from 17 to 27 years. All demonstrated, on entrance into the MCRI/NPI program, severe social impairments, moderate to severe communication deficits, and a repertoire of primitive or atypical behaviors. These profiles provide a complete picture of the individuals served by the MCRI/NPI program and the challenges that the mentally retarded–behaviorally impaired present to the mental retardation and mental health professionals:

Steve (born September 24, 1954) was a 26-year-old young man who had been rejected from his local school system when he was 10. (See Table 1.)

Table 1. Client Profile—Steve

Diagnoses	Behavioral descriptors	Placements	
A. Organic brain syndrome with psychotic reactions	—Primitive behaviors	1954–80	Home
	—Ingests anything	1959–64	Attended school from
B. Severe mental retardation	—Yells for attention		ages 5–10 with "no
—Organic autism	—Self-abusive		success"
—No expressive language	—Eats with hands	1980	Nebraska Psychiatric
—Minimal receptive language	—Refuses to wear clothes or		Institute
	wears extra layers	1980–	Home and
	—Multiple scars on face and	present	prevocational program
	forearms		

According to his school records, he had learned all that he could learn, and his behaviors were so disruptive that he could no longer remain in school. Steve spent the next 14 years of his life isolated at home. His parents cared for him as best as they could, but in reality, Steve dominated and controlled his home. His mother had responsibility for him 24 hours a day, seven days a week. Steve would roam his house, squat in the corner, strip his clothing off, cover himself with blankets, scream, batter himself, and so on. The parents report that nobody would serve Steve. They did not want to institutionalize him; yet there were no community resources available. Their only option was to do their best in maintaining him at home. Finally, the parents admitted him to the Nebraska Psychiatric Institute and the MCRI/NPI prevocational program in order to stabilize his behaviors and to prepare him for possible placement in a community-based program. The parents had been so convinced by this time that nobody could handle Steve that it had taken them a year to make this temporary placement decision.

Upon entering NPI, Steve displayed a wide range of primitive behaviors. He screamed incessantly and squatted on the floor with a blanket wrapped around his head. His cheeks were bloody from his hitting himself. He had no functional expressive or receptive language. As he entered the MCRI/NPI prevocational program, he spent 30 minutes a day in a one-to-one teacher-to-client setting learning to assemble an 18-step flashlight and a 39-step bicycle brake. His first reaction to such a structured learning situation was to continuously leap out of his chair and attempt to wander around the room, hitting his cheeks with his hands and screaming. Within the first week, he began to acquire the assembly skill and therefore became more manageable. The trainer began to introduce various management techniques to control the environment so that maximum attention could be given to the acquisition of skills rather than focusing on the "inappropriate" behaviors. Staff positioned Steve at a work table in such a way as to prevent him from sliding his chair away from the table. A layout board was designed so that he could select only the correct responses in his work tasks. He was taught basic manual communications so that he could express some of his basic needs. As he began to acquire the assembly skills, his behaviors began to deteriorate and more appropriate relationships began to build.

Table 2. Client Profile—Leeann

Diagnoses	Behavioral descriptors	Placements	
A. Chronic undifferentiated schizophrenia	—Biting	1961–68	Home
	—Striking out	1968–73	Institution
B. Moderate to severe mental retardation	—Twirling	1973–74	Group home and school
	—Jumping up and down		
—Marked mood swings	—Banging head	1978–80	Nebraska Psychiatric Institute
—Echolalia	—Feces smearing		
—Minimal expressive language		1980– present	Residential and vocational program
—Moderate receptive language			

After three months in the MCRI/NPI program, Steve was placed in a community-based mental retardation program in his home community. He now spends six hours per day in a prevocational setting. Steve lives at home, and follow-up reports from his mother indicate that he is doing well. He is acquiring a number of daily living skills and no longer dominates the household.

Leeann (born March 27, 1961) was a 19-year-old woman who had spent the last 12 years of her life in a series of institutional settings, continuously being moved from one institution to another because of her "violent" behaviors. (See Table 2.) She had been generally considered unmanageable. When confronted with any structured, demanding learning situation, Leeann would typically begin to wave her arms, hit anyone near her, bite, scratch, and lie down on the floor kicking and screaming. Staff were literally afraid to work with her.

Leeann spent approximately 12 weeks in the MCRI/NPI prevocational program. Initially, her primary negative response was to pinch the trainer's forearms when manual guidance was used. Leeann would also shake her head, laugh inappropriately, sing out irrelevant phrases, and flap her arms in the air. In the first 10 days, there were four major temper tantrums. After several experimental sessions to help her become accustomed to a structured learning environment, she spent 12 weeks in daily 90-minute training sessions. Leeann learned to assemble an 18-step flashlight. The trainer sat across the table from Leeann in order to prevent her hitting and pinching behaviors. When she started to flap her arms in the air, the trainer would instruct her to "sit on your hands" and redirect her to the task. In a short time, Leeann learned to return to her task. By the third month, Leeann's behaviors were reduced to a manageable level. She was then able to be placed in a small, structured residential day-program, where she still resides.

Phillip (born October 17, 1953) was a 27-year-old man who had spent the last 17 years of his life in a series of institutions because of extremely violent behavior. On admission to the MCRI/NPI program, he was virtually unmanageable. During the first week, when asked to perform basic daily

Table 3. Client Profile—Phillip

Diagnoses	Behavioral descriptors	Placements	
A. Organic brain syndrome with psychotic reactions	—Self-abusive	1953–63	Home
	—Refuses to cooperate	1963–69	Private institution
B. Mild mental retardation	—Obstinate	1969–76	State institution
—Moderate expressive language	—Numerous scars from self-inflicted wounds	1976–80	State institution
—Moderate receptive language		1980	Nebraska Psychiatric Institute
		1981–present	Group home and community-based retardation system

tasks, he responded by ramming his head through two windows and breaking a toe by kicking a wall. His expressive and receptive language were adequate, although extremely institutionalized.

During the first day in the MCRI/NPI prevocational program he frequently refused to participate in the instructional process. When asked to attend, he would begin to tremble, jump up and down, and threaten violence to himself and others. His staff person did not threaten him but gave him the option of either participating in work tasks or remaining in his residence. Because Phillip liked mechanical work, he eventually agreed to participate in the program.

Through a delicate balance of psychotropic medications and behavioral intervention, Phillip soon became receptive to learning vocational tasks. He currently resides in a community-based group home and participates in a sheltered workshop.

Jim (born October 15, 1962) was an 18-year-old young man who had been placed in the MCRI/NPI prevocational program because of a number of unmanageable behaviors in his local school program, including walking through a plate-glass window. He had lived at home all of his life and had no obvious expressive language other than grunts.

When confronted with a structured learning situation, Jim would slide out of his chair and lie down on the floor. He was over six feet tall and

Table 4. Client Profile—Jim

Diagnoses	Behavioral descriptors	Placements	
A. Organic brain syndrome with psychotic reactions	—Poor attention span	1963–80	Home
	—Wanders	1980	Nebraska Psychiatric Institute
B. Severe mental retardation	—One- or two-word vocabulary		
C. Behavior disorder of adolescence	—Uncooperative	1981–present	Home and public school
—No expressive language	—Lies on floor		
—Moderate receptive language	—Runs away		

Table 5. Client Profile—David

Diagnoses	Behavioral descriptors	Placements	
A. Organic brain syndrome with psychotic reactions	—Aggressive and violent behavior	1963–77	Home
B. Low moderate mental retardation	—Destructive behavior	1969–71	Home and school
	—Marked mood swings	1971–77	Home and halfday school
C. Grand mal seizures	—Hitting and striking out	1977–79	Institution
—Minimal expressive language	—Scratching	1979–80	Nebraska Psychiatric Institute
—Moderate receptive language		1981– present	Residential facility for the retarded; sheltered workshop

weighed over 230 pounds. It was impossible for his teacher to get him back in his seat, either physically or by verbal coaxing.

Jim spent five days in the MCRI/NPI prevocational program for one hour per day, learning to assemble a complex 36-step stopvalve. When he had difficulty with the task, he would invariably drop the materials and either stand up and walk away or slide to the floor and lie there. Jim would use his stature and weight to control the situation and to avoid the training when he did not understand the task presented to him. It quickly became obvious that Jim could not be physically coaxed back into his seat without escalating his out-of-seat behaviors. Jim's staff person discovered that placing that task in his hands and demonstrating what had to be done would result in Jim's returning to his seat and to the task. Initially, this meant giving the task to Jim while he was lying on the floor or while he was standing. Jim is now back in his classroom and living with his mother.

David (born July 25, 1963) was a 17-year-old young man who had been institutionalized since age 14 because of violent and unmanageable behavior. He would hit himself and others with tremendous force. While in the institution, he spent most of his time tied "spread eagle" on his bed. He had no expressive language on admission to the MCRI/NPI program, and it was felt that much of his "violent" behavior was due to his inability to communicate his needs. During his first month in the MCRI/NPI prevocational program, David was extremely prone to striking out. It became obvious that he needed an extremely structured and consistent training environment with minimal external distractions. David spent approximately six months in the prevocational program. A careful analysis of his hitting behaviors indicated that they were closely related to either changes in routine or errors in work performance. When these situations were minimized and controlled by the trainer, his hitting decreased. His aggressive behaviors decreased to a manageable level within two months. He currently participates in a residential-vocational program near his home community.

Regardless of diagnostic classifications, these five persons indicate an array of significant behavioral problems and functioning levels. Functionally, parents and professionals working with mentally retarded and emotionally disturbed adolescents and adults are confronted with

1. Behavior problems such as
   a. Self-abusive behavior—hitting, scratching, and head-banging.
   b. Abusive behavior toward others—hitting, biting, and scratching.
   c. Abuse of property—breaking windows and throwing objects.
   d. Bizarre, repetitive behaviors such as spinning and twirling.
2. Communication disorders ranging from
   a. No or minimal expressive and/or receptive language to
   b. Moderate expressive and/or receptive language.
3. Cognitive deficits ranging from
   a. Severe and profound mental retardation to
   b. Moderate mental retardation.

All of the families appeared to be able to cope fairly well with their children from infancy to early childhood. Two out of the five families still maintain their son or daughter at home, although with occasional difficulty and a deep concern about the future. Three of these persons had been in and out of mental health and mental retardation institutions since childhood because of their extreme behavior problems.

More often than not, programs and services for this population are caretaking at best and physically and psychologically abusive at worst. For those who had been institutionalized, the use of physical restraint, chemical restraint, and physical seclusion appeared to have been the rule rather than the exception. Case records gave abundant evidence of prolonged seclusion, two-point restraint (being "hogtied"), and four-point restraint (being "tied spread eagle"), as well as other forms of punishment.

Perhaps the key variable that characterizes this entire population is adverse reactions to developmental demands. When presented with appropriate developmental demands (e.g., the performance of a work task), these individuals typically become emotionally disorganized. This disorganization expresses itself in the form of self-abusive, aggressive, or avoidant behaviors, such as hitting, biting, scratching, or running away. The introduction of structure into the person's life—without appropriate strategies and techniques—invariably results in self-abusive or aggressive behaviors. There is an apparent resistance to the introduction of an appropriate set of expectations and demands. Without adequate programs, services, staff, and technology, it is clear that this resistance could easily become insurmountable and frustrating. However, with adequate programs and services, each of these persons rapidly began to acquire appropriate behaviors and meaningful interpersonal relationships. Their post-treatment placements indicate that all can clearly live, work, and play in the mainstream of community life if adequate support systems and trained help are available.

7.6. Alternatives to Traditional Approaches

The array of services that professionals working with this population provide can be organized into a number of approaches. Although the more traditional approaches have been found to be ineffective with the mentally retarded–behaviorally disordered population, effective service alternatives do exist. Professionals working in this area need to be aware of the existence of these alternatives, as well as of the ineffectiveness of more traditional postures. We have identified seven approaches to serving this population. Six of these can best be described as dichotomies of effective alternatives versus traditional approaches; the seventh is best conceptualized as two traditional extremes, with the most effective alternative consisting of a balance between the two. In this section, we examine the implications of these traditional approaches and offer progressive alternatives to each. The alternate approaches and their traditional counterparts are

1. Comprehensive community-based programs versus institutionalization.
2. Functional, individualized approaches versus preconceived approaches.
3. Training versus testing.
4. Unconditional positive regard versus professional inflexibility.
5. Behavioral communication versus volitional aggression.
6. Ecological behaviorism versus behavioral myopia.
7. Medical or behavioral extremes versus a balanced approach.

7.6.1. Comprehensive Community Programs versus Institutionalization

A basic characteristic of all learning is that it should occur within a real-life context. Traditionally, we have accepted the "institutional mentality" that suggests that we can teach a number of general skills in all real-life contexts. In comprehensive community programs, training takes place in ever-increasing approximations to real-life situations. All learning should place the individual within the context in which he or she will actually function.

Community-based systems offer a wide variety, both qualitatively and quantitatively, of learning opportunities and experiences. Qualitatively, a community program offers exposures to a variety of social, cultural, leisure-time, vocational, and educational experiences. Quantitatively, a community-based system can provide exposure to a greater variety of each of these experiences. This exposure increases the probability of the generalization of skills because, although adaptive skills may be difficult to generalize beyond a specific situation, the opportunity to perform these skills in a wider variety of situations increases the probability that such generalization will occur.

Traditional approaches have accepted the premise that the retarded person with severe behavioral disorders requires institutional placement. However, when reviewed from a historical perspective, it is apparent that this population, when institutionalized, does not develop the skills that a few progressive programs have clearly demonstrated as possible in community settings.[25] The primary reason is that the institutional model lacks individualized and adaptive programming. Too often, this population, because of the complexity of its needs, is institutionalized and forgotten. The people with the greatest needs receive the fewest services.

Although almost every institution in the country writes individual program plans, these in fact are frequently mechanical, irrelevant programs that exist on paper merely to satisfy the Intermediate Care Facility-Mental Retardation/Developmental Disabilities (ICF-MR/DD) standards. When they are examined and scrutinized thoroughly, there is little carryover to the real world and little benefit to the individual. In addition, there is very little opportunity for individualized programming in an institutional setting, as there is very little opportunity for individualized activities. In the institutional model, residents must get up and dress with the group, are often given little or no choice in the clothes they will wear, practice certain hygiene activities in a group, walk together to the cafeteria or the classroom, and so on. Modern treatment approaches must thus emphasize the integration of this population into community life as much as possible. Institutionalization and mere custodial care must be forsaken for the development of comprehensive educational, vocational, and residential alternatives in the community.

7.6.2. The Functional, Individualized Approaches versus Preconceived Approaches

The functional approach is based on individualization. It focuses on the individual's needs and strengthens and develops individualized training programs and teaching techniques based on them. The functional approach looks at the individual in relationship to his or her environment and asks what training or learning experience can be provided so that this person can develop more adaptive skills within the environment.

The content of each individual's program curriculum should be drawn from real-life settings. That is, the curriculum must come from the daily routines and activities to which the individual must adapt. Therefore, programmatic content can be derived from any requirement that the environment places on the individual from the time he or she wakes up in the morning until bedtime. To develop this *curriculum* content, one simply asks what type of training is needed to enable the individual to get out of bed unassisted (or with minimal assistance), toilet, dress himself or herself, or prepare a morning meal. In order to determine these training needs, it is necessary to observe the individual over several days or weeks to see whether she or he can, in fact, get out of bed, toilet, and dress appropriately. It is this real-life "evaluation" that provides information on an individual's strengths and deficits and thus pinpoints target behaviors for program content.

The end result of this functional approach is that it allows the client to more appropriately control his or her environment rather than the reverse being true. Hence, the client can now interact more successfully with the environment, which becomes a more reinforcing set of circumstances. This self-reinforcement provides a built-in maintenance of the behavior, minimizing the need for staff supervision and maximizing the independent potential of the client—our goal in education and human services.

Traditionally, one of the major reasons for the use of "canned" systems was to provide readymade curriculum content for a human service agency. This content is often a composite drawn from a wide range of environments and the demands that they place on an individual. The skills needed to meet these demands become the training objectives of the "canned system." For example, in developing a vocational curriculum, the demands and skills required in a wide variety of jobs are determined. Based on this list, a composite of skills required for "work in general" is transformed into curriculum objectives. The problem that this approach presents is that these objectives are frequently taught in the absence of any real-life context and that they disregard the emotional needs of the person. The assumption is that the basic "skill" can be taught and utilized in any environment. However, the generalization that such a transfer requires frequently does not occur with the mentally retarded-mentally ill individual.

Each mentally retarded–mentally ill person must receive highly individualized programs and intervention strategies. There is no easy answer. The acquisition of skills and the deceleration of inappropriate behaviors require functional and individualized programs. It is our experience that the teaching of a vocational task is secondary to the formulation of a strong, dynamic relationship with the person. No "canned" training system can create such a relationship.

7.6.3. Training versus Testing

Training offers the opportunity to observe the learner interacting with her or his environment, whereas testing simply describes the problem. The reactions and accommodations made by the individual are studied when we manipulate variables in the environment and provide information on how she or he learns.[26–29] This approach begins to demonstrate what the individual is capable of doing and identifies her or his skills and deficits. This is vital in the training process. It is urged by some that if we did not take the more traditional testing approach, we would not know where to begin. It seems that this is a very myopic approach to understanding an individual, who must constantly interact to some degree with the environment. It is the observation of this interaction that gives clues to where to begin in the training process. Many of the individuals in the MCRI/NPI prevocational program have never seen the tools or the work samples that we ask them to work with. We simply bring them in, ask them to sit down, and begin teaching them to assemble some of the work samples. This interaction, then, not a percentile score or a position on a normative curve, provides us clues to how to go about training.

The traditional response when one is presented with a profoundly retarded, combative individual is to test. However, from a psychometric perspective, there is very little that is appropriate in the way of validated assessment for these individuals. The tests available have been developed for people who have more skills than many severely retarded people.[30] Many of the tests rely on language, or on the ability to reason abstractly, such as recognizing symbolic representation. The majority of this population possesses very little ability in these areas, and most test scores adequately reflect this fact. The test data merely provide a measure of the individual in his or her present situation and offer little help in developing intervention and teaching strategies, short-term objectives, or long-range goals.[31] It is a descriptive rather than a prescriptive approach.

The same can be said of another type of instrument frequently used with the severely retarded individual: the behavioral checklist. The information provided is also descriptive in nature and provides little in the way of viable recommendations or treatment strategies. A second undesirable characteristic of checklists is their increased emphasis on the negative behaviors of the individual. Although it can be argued that the data represent an accurate picture of the person, such information not only provides little help in developing meaningful recommendations, but also helps develop a negative bias toward the individual for all those who come in contact with the test results. Data from these instruments represent responses to a particular environment at a particular time and cannot be used to predict response patterns in new environments and new circumstances. Unfortunately, admission to or rejection by a variety of training programs is often based on negative checklist data.

It cannot be denied that testing is an established part of many vocational systems and, as a result, is often a necessity at times (e.g., to establish eligibility, to meet accreditation standards, or to meet legal requirements). Under these conditions, the best alternative is to limit the amount of testing to the bare essentials and to accept the results for what they are: descriptive rather than prescriptive information. The real test of the success of any program is not the number of test scores, but the integration of the client into community life.

7.6.4. Unconditional Positive Regard versus Professional Inflexibility

Although we do not propose a Rogerian-like reflective method of interacting with this population, we do mean to suggest that there are some significant and necessary characteristics that staff must possess before they train and interact with them. These characteristics are very difficult to measure but are readily observable in most cases. The first and foremost characteristic that is necessary in working with the mentally retarded–mentally ill is respect for the client as a *human being* who happens to lack a variety of developmental experiences. This means that the individual is given all the courtesy, attention, interest, concern, and affection that any other person is afforded. It also means that it is understood that the individual has certain needs and responses that are for the most part the results of past history and environment—factors that are out of the client's control and, therefore, for which he or she should not be blamed.

Parents and professionals need to cultivate the attitude that learning can and will occur, given the right set of conditions. This means that the trainer must accept total responsibility for whether or not learning occurs, given an opportunity to explore and discover those variables that seem to be salient in the learning process for the client. If learning does not occur, the problem lies in the strategies used by the trainer—not in the learner. In addition, we have a growing body of research findings that demonstrate the severely retarded individual's ability to learn.[32-37]

It is important that parents and professionals nurture the development of a sharing relationship. Activity is shared in the training process, with the degree of responsibility gradually shifting predominantly from the trainer to the learner. During the initial trials in any learning situation, the trainer provides a great deal of assistance to the learner—his or her hands may manipulate the learner's hands, or he or she may perform some difficult aspects of the task. The trainer must be willing to be part of such a cooperative relationship, in spite of the knowledge of the client's past or present aggressive or inappropriate behavior. This willingness requires a patience and a perseverance that often result in a very close and lasting relationship.

Traditionally, it is not uncommon for professionals in the field, especially paraprofessionals, to have the expectations—oftentimes shared with and fostered by professionals—of being responsible for the *control* of the client or of the total programmatic situation. There may also develop a considerable degree of professional pride, ego involvement, job satisfaction, and performance evaluation in the maintenance of this control. Often, aggressive or combative clients can gain control of the situation from the trainer by engaging in aggressive, avoidant, or otherwise inappropriate behavior. This loss of control by the staff is often taken as a personal affront, and a strong, emotional, retaliatory response is the result. A variety of punitive responses thus occur through which the staff attempts to reestablish control and thereby regain professional pride. Some of the most common examples of such responding are "That is not allowed in my building" (my room, on my shift, etc.); "Because you did that, you will pay the following price"; "You're going to do it my way"; or "You have to apologize before you can."

Such inflexible approaches typically result in more inappropriate behaviors. It may seem paradoxical, but a patient, persevering, and sharing relationship is essential in meeting the needs of this population.

7.6.5. Behavioral Communication versus Volitional Aggression

One of the descriptors of mentally retarded and mentally ill persons seen earlier in our client profiles was that of communication disorders ranging from total absence to moderate development of verbal (expressive) language abilities. However, it becomes apparent in working with those individuals who do not have at least a modest control of expressive language that they develop alternate means for expressing themselves (i.e., nonverbal communication). When aggressive behavior occurs, staff are quick to interpret it in many ways other than as a form of communication. However, it is often simply a form of communication and should be seen as such. It should not be taken personally, nor should an individual staff person become too emotionally involved, as such involvement may inhibit the ability of reading nonverbal behavior, which has tremendous communicative potential. Aggressive behaviors have often been observed when clients are introduced to new tasks or new training, or when something that was not planned occurs in their environment. As a consequence, the first reaction is confusion, which leads to frustration and ultimately to some form of *self-defense*, either aggressive or avoidant.

In most cases, there appear to be a number of physiological precursors to aggressive behavior. For example, we may see increased stereotypical behaviors such a rocking, biting, or self-slapping. We may see muscle tightening (e.g., a clenched masseter muscle protruding at the jaw) or changes in complexion, activity level, and alertness. These precursors indicate that some appropriate action should be taken to deescalate the impending outburst. This may include providing additional cues, removing ambiguous stimuli, or performing a difficult segment of the task for the client. One of the most important factors to consider is avoidance of the escalation of behaviors that may ultimately end in confrontation and/or aggression. One technique that is extremely beneficial in preventing inappropriate behaviors is errorless learning. As stated above, aggressive or avoidant behaviors often occur when an error or a confusing situation is encountered. By restructuring the environment to allow only the correct response to occur, all incorrect responses are prevented. This prevention frequently leads to a deceleration of aggressive and avoidant behaviors and to an increase in the acquisition of skills.

Traditionally, one of the primary errors in providing services for this population is that staff frequently view aggressive acts as volitional and as being exhibited solely to inflict injury or cause damage. Because there is often no obvious, rational cause for the behavior, the cause is assumed to be internal and pathological, and generally, the person is viewed as deliberately acting out or avoiding required tasks. When this type of behavior is viewed as premeditated or volitional, the obvious response by staff is to "treat" the client on a cognitive or mediational level, punishing the individual each time the behaviors occur. The punishment most often takes the form of restriction of privileges, restitution for damage, restraint, or time-out. The underlying intent is to make the client "understand" the connection between his or her inappropriate behavior and the negative consequences in the hope of making him or her more "responsible" for his or her actions. However, a common result of such an approach is the escalation of inappropriate client behaviors (and the escalation of "negative" staff interventions) and the development of a negative relationship between staff and client.

7.6.6. Ecological Behaviorism versus Behavioral Myopia

Although it is a given fact that behavior is a function of antecedents and consequences, it must also be recognized that behaviors occurring in a natural environment are much more than a composite of simple stimulus–response units. In providing services on a day-to-day basis, a perspective that is both behavioral and ecological is essential to effective positive service delivery. This combined perspective views behavior not as a combination of individual, dissectable units, but as a complex unit of interrelationships and interdependencies with a delicate organism–behavior–environment system.[38,39] There are two aspects of this ecobehavioral perspective that impact on the delivery of services to this population: one relates to viewing an individual's behavior as a complex interrelated system, and the other is related to the influence of the environmental setting on an individual's behavior.

The notion of behavior as part of a complex, interrelated and interdependent system has several implications for the provision of services to this severely handicapped population. The first is awareness of and attention to the fact that a change in one aspect of this system can have multiple effects, both positive and negative, on all other aspects of the system. As trainers and modifiers of the individual's behavior, we must not only be aware of potential negative "side effects"[39] but must also *plan*, to the best of our abilities, for such interactive effects of our intervention strategies. In essence, our whole approach of focusing on the positive acquisition of skills as replacements for inappropriate behaviors is based on this notion. We assume that by providing learners with functional skills, we also give them a positive impact on their own environment, and thus a number of things will "fall into place." Learners will acquire more "acceptable" methods of interacting with their environment. As this happens, more unacceptable methods will decrease. As the learner's behaviors become more acceptable, interactions with him or her become less aversive to others, and the probability of more positive relationships is increased. As they do, the probability of the client's engaging in additional learning situations is greatly increased. Thus, by focusing on only one small aspect of an individual's "system" (i.e., the acquisition of a functional skill), a "snowballing" of positive results can be accomplished.

It becomes clear then that this ecobehavioral perspective can have a definite effect on the goal-setting procedure. Thus, rather than designing specific programs to decelerate targeted inappropriate behaviors, an intervention strategy that focuses on the acquisition of functional skills has an overall positive effect on this deceleration.

An important aspect of this ecobehavioral perspective is its attention to the effects of the environment on an individual's behavior. This perspective gives a great deal of credence to the notion of antecedent control. If an analysis of an individual's behaviors indicates that inappropriate behaviors are more likely to occur under certain stimulus conditions, modifying the environment to eliminate or greatly reduce these stimuli can result in a considerable reduction or elimination of these inappropriate behaviors. When training an individual who is likely to pinch, scratch, kick, or bite the trainer, it is more practical to arrange the training environment so that the probability of the inappropriate behaviors occurring is reduced. For example, if a particular client is likely to hit the trainer while learning a skill, it is logical that the trainer should sit across the table from the learner. The trainer sits at arms length from the learner and is able to react much more quickly and pull back from any attempted hits, scratches, or bites, thus preventing the inappropriate behavior from occurring, and allowing the trainer and the learner to focus on the acquisition of skills.[40,41]

Unfortunately, there is considerable evidence of a more traditional and narrow-minded behaviorism in a great many service-delivery systems today. This simplified version of behaviorism is evidenced in a number of ways. First, behaviors are dissected from the environment and the system in which they occur and are targeted for acceleration or deceleration. These behaviors are singled out as either problem behaviors, which must be eliminated before effective functioning can occur, or as in some way important to effective functioning, in which case they are "programmed" regardless of the context in which they occur or are expected to occur. Examples of this traditional approach include such things as attention to task, remaining seated, and punctuality, regardless of the work environment or the work task involved. The result of this approach is an attempt to shape the "perfect worker" in an imperfect environment.

In addition, many professionals assume that all negative, inappropriate behaviors must first be eliminated before any positive functional skills can be taught. It is frequently felt that it is inappropriate to begin training on improving self-feeding skills before self-abusive or self-stimulatory hand movements or head banging is decelerated. It is also not uncommon to find the absence of self-stimulatory or aggressive behaviors as a prerequisite for entry into various training programs. If the focus is on the elimination of negative behaviors— rather than on the acquisition of skills—the learner will never learn appropriate behaviors.

Another counterproductive, traditional posture is a complete reliance on the manipulation of consequences as the primary intervention strategy. In attempting to modify undesirable behavior in this manner, the only intervention choices are negative: aversive therapy, time-out, restraint, chemical intervention (overdosing), positive practice, or "forced" realization. Such intervention strategies have their own negative side effects, such as continued escalation of inappropriate behaviors to the point of danger to the client or others, ethical and legal considerations, and the difficulty in maintaining positive relations with the client, which are essential to teaching positive skills.

Thus, there needs to be a much broader interpretation of the principles of behavior management. Consequences are important. But even more important are the conditions that lead up to the inappropriate behaviors and the replacement of those behaviors with appropriate skills.

7.6.7. Medical or Behavioral Extremes versus a Balanced Approach

There has long been a dichotomy between advocates of the medical model and advocates of the behavioral model relative to the management of persons with mental retardation and behavioral disorders. The one side has argued that drugs are the "cure," and the other side has presented the same argument in favor of behavioral management. Frequently, the client has been left in the middle, pulled apart by an extreme of one treatment procedure or the other.

It is our position that there needs to exist a delicate balance between the use of psychotropic medications and behavioral programming, and that each is a valid tool for assisting a person to grow and develop toward independence. Both of these positions are all too frequently subjected to abuse because neither has a broad enough vision of the individual's needs and thus narrowly addresses retarded citizens' right to receive and participate in programs that meet their *total* needs in the most individualized and sensitive manner possible. Neither approach gives the definitive answer to the clients' basic human needs. Both are simply tools in a large arsenal of approaches. Each has a legitimate place in treatment and management.

Perhaps the most reasoned way to reach this balance is to first examine the precipitating causes for the use of psychotropic medications. There are three: (1) the client displays motoric overactivity; (2) the client displays motoric underactivity; and (3) there is evidence of slowly or rapidly escalating behaviors. All three of these symptoms produce serious interference with the person's ability to learn or to interact appropriately in the mainstream of community life. Putting aside the extensive list of psychiatric syndromes, it is important to analyze the behaviors that are interfering with the person's ability to learn and to live in normalizing environments. This process involves (1) pinpointing these interfering behaviors; (2) measuring their extent and frequency; and (3) arriving at an objective conclusion about whether the behaviors are sufficiently disruptive to learning or to the maintenance of the person in the normalizing social-recreational routines of life.

It is clear that this treatment-delineating process involves a close working relationship between parents, behavioral-analysis-oriented programmatic staff, and psychiatric professionals. If not, the needed balance is lost.

Practically speaking, a teacher, a parent, or a workshop trainer is confronted with a person who presents motoric underactivity, overactivity, or escalating behaviors. The client is referred to a cooperating mental-health specialist. The interfering behaviors are described; their frequency and extent are measured. If the behaviors are deemed to be of low frequency and can be rather easily redirected by program or personnel intervention tactics, then the use of psychotropic medications is not warranted. However, if these and similar first-level extrinsic modification tactics are unsuccessful, a psychoactive agent may be warranted. A mutually arrived at decision is reached based primarily on what psychotropic medication would best allow programmatic staff to most effectively, developmentally, and behaviorally work with the person. The basic question becomes what medication, dosage, and schedule would enable programmatic staff to assist the person in initially becoming tractable so that he or she can begin to acquire appropriate and normalizing behaviors.

For example, an adolescent may be hitting others 30 times per day, running away 2 times per day, and biting his wrists 10 times daily. This behavior obviously presents many barriers to the teaching and training process. The dosage of the medication, if necessary, should reduce those behaviors enough so that programmatic staff can work on the acquisition of appropriate skills and behaviors. Thus, in this example, the medication might serve the purpose of reducing the inappropriate, disruptive behaviors by one third—just enough to enable the teaching process to take place.

The initiation of the use of psychotropic medications requires close monitoring by the psychiatrist, with frequent descriptive input by the programmatic staff. Adjustment relative to the type of medications, the dosage, and the schedule is made based on this and other relevant input. All concerned persons should understand the basic process involved in balancing the use of medications with intensive ongoing developmental programming. This typically can be described as

1. Initiation phase. There is a gradual growth of the drug's effect in reducing the inappropriate behaviors to the point where programming "takes hold." This effect needs to be closely and sensitively monitored so as to avoid sedative effects.
2. Catching-on phase. As the effect of the medication joins forces with the intensive developmental programming, the acquisition of appropriate behaviors and skills begins to accelerate, multiplying by its own power, and the inappropriate behaviors begin to decelerate, often in direct proportion to the accelerating appropriate learning.
3. Reduction phase. Once the second phase begins to stabilize, it is time to focus on the reduction and/or the elimination of medication. Concomitantly, intensive developmental programming must continue and extend into extrinsic interpersonal transactions that permit the recently acquired behavioral improvement to stabilize.

If there are problems in the initiation or the catching-on phase, three questions should be asked relative to the drug management: 1) Is it the correct drug? 2) Is it the right dosage: too little, too much, side effects? 3) Is the correct administration schedule being utilized? These questions clearly indicate the need for constant and rapid feedback between the cooperating professionals and the parents.

A careful review with the physician or the pharmacologist of dosage levels and a gradual reduction or titration can be accomplished. Flexibility should be built into the use of medications. The reduction of medication enables staff to observe and describe behaviors without the drug variable. Typically, 48–72 hours without drugs gives those concerned a clear picture regarding the need for the drug. Adjustments can and should be made accordingly. The scheduling of the drugs should be flexible enough to coincide with the times when the impact of the medication is most needed; that is, the half-life of the drug and how quickly it is absorbed into the bloodstream should be taken into account. The impact should occur when behavioral tractability and "cooperative" behaviors are most needed by the client in order to truly profit from ongoing programmatic efforts.

As previously noted, the balance between the use of psychotropic medications and developmental and behavioral programming is delicate. The primary purpose of the medication should be to help the person arrive at a threshold state of readiness for learning and thus to make the person maximally accessible to the ongoing teaching and training process. Both behavior management and drugs are tools: behavioral management can be viewed as an external behavioral prosthesis; drugs can be viewed as internal prostheses. Both can be abused, just as a knife can be used to hurt a person or to create a sculpture. Both can be food for thought or poisons that destroy thinking, memory, and thus learning.

In using either tool, the right balance must be struck. Just as behavioral techniques are gradually faded in and out, the use of medications must be faded in the same way. There is a minimum and maximum therapeutic use for each psychoactive drug. It is the professional team, including the client's parents, who must decide when to increase and decrease each so that the mentally retarded person with severe behavioral disorders can grow and develop as independently as possible in the mainstreams of community life.

7.7. Intervention Strategies

In the previous section, we attempted to clarify the progressive postures that parents and professionals must take if mentally retarded persons with severe behavioral disorders are to grow and develop. These progressive postures require a rethinking of past stances. Because the needs of persons who are mentally retarded and mentally ill are so individualized, it is impossible to give "recipes" for appropriate intervention strategies. The current state of research clearly indicates that this population is able to learn, to acquire skills, and to reduce inappropriate behaviors. There are two thematic areas that relate to pragmatic intervention strategies: specific teaching strategies and programmatic issues/staff–management concerns. Based on our experiences, we briefly review these two areas.

7.7.1. Teaching Strategies

Various strategies that are effective in teaching individuals who find it difficult to learn complex tasks have been identified in the last two decades. However, the literature does not mention techniques that are effective with those individuals who not only find it difficult to learn but also display aggressive or disruptive behaviors or are less than compliant in a learning situation (i.e., the behaviorally impaired–mentally retarded). Although the strategies developed by Zeaman and House,[42] Gold,[43] Crosson,[44] and Bellamy[41] serve as the basis for training this population, we have found that additional techniques and strategies or modifications of existing methods are required for replacing aggressive behaviors with functional skills.

7.7.1.1. Errorless Learning

In providing one-to-one, multiple-step assembly training with emotionally disturbed–mentally retarded persons, observations indicate an increase in the frequency of avoidant or aggressive behaviors (e.g., hitting, leaving their chair, lying on the floor, hand biting, and self-stimulation). Further observation reveals a close relationship between these behaviors and errors in performance or confusion about the next correct response. Whereas previously developed technology would seem to indicate a strategy of allowing an incorrect response to occur with a correction following (e.g., "Try another way"), we have found that this strategy often results in inappropriate behavior in the form of aggression and/or violence. The strategy that has been found to be more effective in both increasing correct performance and preventing inappropriate responses has been an "errorless learning" approach. This involves structuring the learning environment so that the correct response is possible and all incorrect responses are minimized or impossible. Specific examples of this approach would include covering all parts on a layout board except the trough that holds the correct part, performing a difficult portion of the assembly for the learner, or increasing the frequency and the intensity of the prompts provided during training.

In using this approach, successful completion of the total task, regardless of the amount of assistance provided by the trainer, appears to be the key variable. Once acquisition is apparent, the fading of this highly structured situation can be initiated. Overall, this approach seems to build a strong, positive reinforcement history and provides a positive base for continued training.

7.7.1.2. Redirection

As stated above, the emphasis of our program is on the positive rather than the negative aspects of behavior. The resultant course of action when negative behaviors occur is to redirect the behavior back to the positive: the acquisition of skills. Several things are accomplished with this strategy. First, negative behaviors are not attended to. Second, attention becomes contingent on positive, appropriate work behavior. Third, a message is communicated to the learner that the behavior that is expected and the only behavior that is acceptable is participation in a learning activity. One example of this strategy involved a client's raising a wrench over his head as if to strike the trainer. The trainer simply said, "No, Jim, try this one," replaced the wrench with the appropriate tool, and redirected the client's hand back to the task. A second example is attempted hits that are caught in midair. Once their physical precursors are recognized, the learner's hands can be caught before striking the trainer and can be physically directed back to the task. A third example involved a young man sliding out of his chair. Instead of attempting to pull him back into the chair, he was simply given parts of the task while lying on the floor. He quickly returned to his chair and continued working. A key aspect of this strategy, which is exemplified by this third situation, is the importance of successful experience in maintaining participation in the task. It was not simply the placing of parts in this young man's hand that reestablished his participation in the task, but the manipulation of the task to a point where this young man could again achieve the success that appeared to result from his "reentry" into the training process.

7.7.1.3. Environment Engineering

Although a wide variety of strategies that employ some aspects of stimulus control are used in training all individuals who find it difficult to learn, there are certain aspects of this strategy that are particularly effective with individuals with aggressive behaviors. The observation and analysis of aggressive behaviors and their precursors often lead to the identification of certain stimuli that are more likely to cue specific inappropriate behaviors. For example, there was a high probability of one particular client's striking or swinging at a person's glasses when upset. The frequency of these behaviors decreased considerably when the trainer simply removed his glasses when working with this individual. This same individual would also throw objects on the floor when upset. The result of this act (i.e., various parts of an assembly task strewn across the floor) increased the likelihood of a further escalation of these behaviors. By removing all nonessential training materials from the table when working with this individual, the frequency of these inappropriate episodes was greatly decreased.

7.7.1.4. Fading Assistance

Although this aspect of the total training procedure has again been identified and employed with individuals who need it, feedback—auditory, visual, tactile, or a combination thereof—is utilized. However, with this population, we have found that the use of the inappropriate modality often results in inappropriate behaviors. For example, one client responded most effectively when provided with verbal input: "Pick up the nut"; Thread it on"; and so on. However, training procedures based on the tactile modality (i.e., a high frequency of physical prompts) were most likely to result in slapping or pinching the trainer's hand. Another client appeared to become greatly frustrated by a high degree of verbal input and would engage in self-abusive behaviors when this technique was utilized. By reducing the verbal input and utilizing primarily visual and physical input, the self-abusive behaviors decreased and effective learning occurred. Other individuals were consistently limited in their verbal language abilities, which, in essence, precluded the use of any verbal input. With these individuals, training input that was completely visual in nature was necessary for successful learning to occur. Thus, with all individuals, the choice of the appropriate input–feedback modality is necessary not only for learning to occur, but also for avoidant and/or aggressive behaviors to be decelerated.

There is no magic answer to the question of how to work with behaviorally disturbed retarded persons. However, the teaching and training strategies cited above have proved to be effective tools in the acquisition of skills and the deceleration of inappropriate behaviors. Professionals have to be competent in such strategies and apply them with sensitivity case by case.

7.7.2. Programmatic Issues

Even with the acceptance of the progressive postures and the specific teaching and training strategies that we have reviewed, there remain a number of programmatic issues that must be resolved. These issues deal with general practices and procedures in providing programmatic services for this population. They are not specifically applied in one-to-one individual program training; rather, they are applicable to the general approach and expectations of staff.

7.7.2.1. Programmatic Consistency and Scheduling

The daily activities of the learner should be prearranged in a schedule of activities that is followed as consistently as possible. The specific activities may include the acquisition of skill training, performance or the maintenance of skills already acquired, or "free time" that is structured but nondemanding. A consistent schedule of this nature provides an established structure of activities for the learner and avoids the increased probability of negative behaviors during unstructured "downtime." The consistency of this structure also provides more predictability in the environment for the learner and appears to reduce the probability of the inappropriate behaviors that frequently occur in a more unpredictable environment. This emphasis on consistency should not be construed as support for a static or unchangeable schedule. Changes in schedule or programmatic activities are not only acceptable but essential to continuous learning. They do, however, need to be introduced in a gradual, consistent, and planned manner. Thus, changes in the number of work units produced or in the nature of the task taught may be made as long as they are introduced gradually and consistently.

7.7.2.2. Individualization

We have previously stated that program goals should be based on the individual's environment and/or anticipated environmental demands and the skills needed to function effectively. We have also stated that the trainer must be attentive to the learning modalities that are most effective with each individual learner. In addition to these two areas, individualization must be a goal for the total programmatic activities for the behaviorally impaired–mentally retarded individual. Such factors as the length of training time, the complexity (demands) of the training tasks, the physical arrangements of the training environment, and the particular style of verbal and social interactions with a learner must all be individualized (i.e., they must all be developed programmatically, based on experimentation with a variety of approaches, and refined, based on the learner's response to each). This type of individualization requires several weeks of one-to-one staffing, until the learner reaches the point where a lower staff-to-client ratio is feasible.

7.7.2.3. Flexibility with the Learner and Staff

Although the two points above are based on maintaining as consistent an approach as possible, it is essential in dealing with this population to allow flexibility in activities, interventions, and teaching strategies. The majority of these individuals have well-developed response tendencies to overly demanding or aversive situations. These response tendencies generally have negative consequences for the trainer and others in the environment. A trainer who respects the learner as a human being should avoid backing the learner into a corner where her or his only option is to respond aggressively. In these situations, a program that is sufficiently flexible to allow the learner a number of options is a necessity. Providing the learner options not only allows him or her to avoid an aversive situation but also teaches appropriate responses to such situations. This is not to suggest that the trainer should back down completely and allow the learner to obtain control of the situation by threatening aggressive acts. However, if the situation is moving toward confrontation, it is best to find an alternative that will terminate this trend. Options that are based on some form of compromise are usually preferable. Staff should, however, be willing to, in some way, "lose the battle" in an overall effort to "win the war," backing off on client demands on that particular day, but ready to "try another day" and ready to introduce new training strategies for improving the situation.

7.7.2.4. Staff Feedback

In working with mentally retarded–mentally ill persons, it is essential to provide adequate feedback to staff regarding their work behaviors. In dealing with the complex behaviors that this population presents, it is essential that staff be able to periodically analyze their interactions with clients, both in specific acquisition training and overall interactions with the learner. Videotape has been found to be particularly useful for the analysis of staff and client interactions. Trainers can review the effectiveness of their teaching techniques, supervisors can review the same techniques with trainers, and the entire staff can review problem behaviors in an effort to brainstorm effective solutions.

An additional source of feedback for the entire staff of the program is periodic external feedback. Professionals involved with this population on an ongoing basis frequently get "stuck in a rut" with a limited number of solutions to problem behaviors and situations. Professionals from outside the agency who are not involved in day-to-day contact with the particular clients and programming often bring a new perspective to problem situations. New ideas in relation not only to specific problem behaviors but also to the total programming approach are often the result of periodic feedback from "visiting" professionals.

7.7.2.5. Positive Staff Relationships

Providing services to this population typically involves concentration on and attention to individual learning situations, calm but rapid responding to problem situations, and perseverance in the face of numerous frustrations and, at times, physical abuse. Although it is necessary to control "gut-level" emotional responses to these situations while working with the client, staff must realize that these responses will occur. Being able to openly discuss and at times joke about interactions with these clients is often an effective and useful means of venting emotional responses. Positive relationships among staff that are conducive to open discussions of one's feelings about one's interactions with clients are thus very helpful in maintaining an effective program. Such open discussions frequently lead to a more objective viewing of one's own responses to client behaviors and to creative problem-solving in terms of more effective means of dealing with such problems.

7.8. Conclusions

There has been a clear demonstration that all levels of mentally retarded persons, including mentally retarded persons with severe behavioral problems, can grow and develop, gain functional skills, and be integrated into community life. However, severely mentally retarded persons with behavioral disorders are often the last population to receive systematic, individualized, informed technology in community-based settings. An extension of the same techniques that are being used with all levels of mentally retarded citizens is being shown to be effective with persons with severe behavioral disorders. Nevertheless, it is obvious that this population requires a special sensitivity and even intensity in terms of programming.

References

1. Obermann CE: *A History of Vocational Rehabilitation in America.* Minneapolis, T. S. Dennison, 1965.
2. Cull JG, Hardy RE: *Vocational Rehabilitation Profession and Process.* Springfield, IL, C. C. Thomas, 1972.
3. White WD, Wolfensberger W: The evolution of dehumanization in our institutions. *Ment Retard,* 7;5–9, 1969.
4. Menolascino FJ, Egger ML: *Medical Dimensions of Mental Retardation.* Lincoln, University of Nebraska Press, 1978.
5. Greenblatt M: The rehabilitation spectrum, in Greenblatt M, Simon B (eds): *Rehabilitation of the Mentally Ill.* Washington, D.C., American Association for the Advancement of Science, 1959.
6. Penrose LS: *The Biology of Mental Defect.* New York, Grune and Stratton, 1963.
7. Stark JA: A systems approach to barrier analysis, in Schalock R (ed): *A Model Comprehensive Delivery Service System for Persons with Developmental Disabilities.* Springfield, IL, Illinois Developmental Disabilities Council, 1979.
8. Wortis J: The role of psychiatry and mental retardation service, in Mittler P (ed): *Research to Practice in Mental Retardation,* vol 1: *Care and Intervention.* (Proceedings of the Fourth Congress of the International Association of Scientific Study of Mental Retardation.) Baltimore, University Park Press, 1977.
9. Menolascino FJ: *Challenges of Mental Retardation: Progressive Ideology and Services.* New York, Human Sciences Press, 1977.

10. Menolascino FJ: Emotional disturbances and institutionalized retardates: Primitive, atypical and abnormal behavior. *Ment Retard* 10(6);38, 1972.
11. Phillips I: Psychopathology of mental retardation, in Menolascino F (ed): *Psychiatric Aspects of the Diagnosis and Treatment of Mental Retardation*. Seattle, Special Child Publications, 1971.
12. Cytryn L, Lourie RS: Mental retardation, in Freedman AM, Kaplan HI (eds): *Comprehensive Textbook of Psychiatry*. Baltimore, Williams and Wilkins, 1967.
13. Joint Commission on Mental Health in Children. *Annual Report*. Washington, D.C., Bureau of Maternal and Child Health, U.S. Department of Health and Human Services, 1980.
14. President's Committee on Mental Retardation. *Report of the Liaison Task Panel on Mental Retardation*, vol. 4. Washington, D.C., Government Printing Office, 1978.
15. Stark JA, Baker DH, Menousek PE, *et al*: Behavioral programming for severely mentally retarded/behaviorally impaired youth, in Lynch KP, Kiernan WE, Stark JA (eds): *Prevocational and Vocational Education for Special Needs Youth: A Blueprint for the 1980s*. Baltimore, Paul H. Brookes, 1982.
16. Menolascino FJ: *Psychiatric Approaches to Mental Retardation*. New York, Basic Books, 1970.
17. Chess S: Emotional problems in mentally retarded children, in Menolascino FJ (ed): *Psychiatric Approaches to Mental Retardation*. New York, Basic Books, 1970.
18. Blatt B: *Souls in Extremis: An Anthology on Victims and Victimizers*. Boston, Allyn and Bacon, 1973.
19. Bellamy GT, Inman DP, Horner RH: *Design of Vocational Habilitation Services for the Severely Retarded: The Specialized Training Model*. Ninth Banff Conference Proceedings, Banff, Alberta, 1977.
20. Bellamy GT, Irvin L: Habilitation of the severely and profoundly retarded: An applied research perspective, in Cleland J, *et al* (eds): *Research with the Profoundly Retarded*. Second Annual Conference Proceedings, Austin, Texas, Western Research Conference and Hogg Foundation, June 1976.
21. Bellamy GT, Sheehan M, Horner RH, *et al*: *Community Programs for Severely Handicapped Adults: An Analysis of Vocational Opportunities*. Position Paper, Center on Human Development, Eugene, OR, 1980.
22. Karan O, Wehaman P, Renzaglia A, *et al*: *Habilitation Practices with the Severely Developmentally Disabled*. Madison, University of Wisconsin, Waisman Center on Mental Retardation and Human Development, 1976.
23. Karan O: *Project Deinstitutionalization: Using Extended Evaluations to Enable Institutionalized Severely Developmentally Disabled Persons to Demonstrate Their Vocational Rehabilitation Potential*. Progress Report. Madison, University of Wisconsin, Waisman Center on Mental Retardation and Human Development, 1980.
24. Wing L, Gould J: Severe impairments of social interaction and associated abnormalities in children: Epidemiology and classification. *J Autism Devel Dis* 9;1, 1979.
25. Karan O: From the classroom into the community, in Lynch KP, Kiernan WE, Stark JA (eds): *Prevocational and Vocational Education for Special Needs Youth: A Blueprint for the 1980s*. Baltimore, Paul H. Brookes, 1982.
26. Fisher M, Zeaman D: An attention-retention theory of retardate discrimination learning, in Ellis N (ed): *The International Review of Research in Mental Retardation*, vol. 6. New York, Academic Press, 1973.
27. Gold MW: Stimulus factors in skill training of the retarded on a complex assembly task: Acquisition, transfer, and retention. *J Ment Defic*, 76;517–526, 1972.
28. Horner RH, Bellamy GT: A conceptual analysis of vocational training with the severely retarded, in Snell M (ed): *Systematic Instruction of the Moderately, Severely, and Profoundly Handicapped*. Columbus, Charles E. Merrill, 1978.
29. Irvin L, Bellamy GT: Manipulation of stimulus featured in vocational skill training of the severely retarded: Relative efficacy. *Am J Ment Defic* 81;486–491, 1977.
30. Botterbusch K: *A Comparison of Commercial Vocational Evaluation Systems*. Menomonie, Materials Development Center, Stout Vocational Rehabilitation Institute, University of Wisconsin-Stout, 1980.

31. Gold MW: Research in the vocational habilitation of the retarded: The present, the future, in Ellis N (ed): *International Review of Research in Mental Retardation*, vol. 6. New York, Academic Press, 1973.

32. Bateman S: Application of Premack's generalization on reinforcement to modify occupational behavior in two severely retarded individuals. *Am J Ment Defic*, 79(5);604–610, 1975.

33. Bellamy GT, Inman DP, Yeates J: Workshop supervision evaluation of a procedure for production management with the severely retarded. *Ment Retard*, 17(1);37–41, 1978.

34. Boroff GS, Tate, PR: Training the mentally retarded in complex production: A demonstration of work potential. *Excep Child*, 33;405–408, 1967.

35. Crosson JE: *The Experimental Analysis of Vocational Behavior in the Severely Retarded Males*. Final report (Grant No. OEG32-47-0230-6024). Washington, D.C., U.S. Department of Health, Education, and Welfare, 1967.

36. Crosson JE: The functional analysis of behavior. A technology for special education practices. *Ment Retard*, 7(4);15–19, 1969.

37. Gold MW, Barclay CR: The learning of difficult visual discrimination by the moderately and severely retarded. *Ment Retard*, 11;9–11, 1973.

38. Rogers-Warren A, Warren SF: *Ecological Perspectives in Behavioral Analysis*. Baltimore, University Park Press, 1977.

39. Williams EP: Behavioral technology and behavioral ecology. *J Appl Behav Anal* 7;151–165, 1974.

40. Bijou SW: Behavior modification in teaching the retarded child, in Thoresen CE (ed): *Behavior Modification and Education*. Chicago, The National Society for the Study of Education, 1973.

41. Bellamy GT, Horner RH, Inman DP: *Vocational Habilitation of Severely Retarded Adults*. Baltimore, University Park Press, 1979.

42. Zeaman D, House B: The role of attention in retardate discrimination learning, in Ellis N (ed): *Handbook of Mental Deficiency*. New York, McGraw-Hill, 1963.

43. Gold MW: Vocational training, in Wortis J (ed): *Mental Retardation in Developmental Disabilities*, vol. 2. New York, Brunner/Mazel, 1975.

44. Crosson JE: *Experimental Analysis of Vocational Behavior in Severely Retarded Males*. Doctoral dissertation, University of Oregon, 1966. Dissertation Abstracts International, 27;3304.

Multimodal Treatment of Mental Illness in Institutionalized Mentally Retarded Persons

William J. Bates

8.1. Introduction

The recognition that mental illness can strike mentally retarded persons, as well as those of normal intelligence, is not new. During the nineteenth century many psychiatrists were actively involved in the field of mental retardation. They provided enlightened clinical care, pursued research, filled important administrative posts, and were effective advocates for the mentally retarded. However, during the period referred to by Menolascino[1] as the *tragic interlude* (1900–1920), psychiatric interest in mental retardation waned. In fact, it was replaced largely by an attitude of despair and helplessness—a change that led to the relative withdrawal of psychiatry from the field. During the last two decades (since the early 1960s), psychiatrists have begun to return to the treatment of mentally retarded persons—especially those with allied symptoms of mental illness—with modern treatment tools and techniques that promise to improve the lives of these individuals.

8.2. Scope of the Problem

The psychiatrist providing services to the mentally retarded is working at the forefront of an important and expanding movement within psychiatry. Although the true prevalence of psychiatric disorders in the mentally retarded is uncertain, it is clear from many studies that retarded individuals are highly susceptible to the development of mental illness, and therefore that they require and deserve appropriate psychiatric services.

As Wortis[2] stated, mentally retarded individuals "are subject, probably to an enhanced degree, to all the psychiatric disease and disorders that can befall a normal population" (p. 412). Rutter,[3] in his well-known Isle of Wight study, found that the mentally retarded persons he studied had more than three times the frequency of psychiatric impairment found in a control population. The 1976 annual report of the President's Committee on Mental Retardation[4] indicated that over 40% of mentally retarded persons suffered an emotional or

William J. Bates • Department of Psychiatry, Ohio State University, Columbus, Ohio 43210.

behavioral disorder of sufficient magnitude to be considered a partial or severe handicap. Further data to support the high rate of psychiatric disorders in the retarded have been supplied by Menolascino[5-7] in studies that reveal a prevalence of 33%. An extensive review of the data on the incidence and the prevalence of emotional disturbance in retarded persons, both institutionalized and noninstitutionalized, has been provided by Balthazar and Stevens.[8]

8.3. Treatability of the Mentally Retarded

In the field of mental retardation, the psychiatrist may function in a variety of roles, ranging from the provision of direct care to institutional administration. Between these extremes lie many other important functions, including the role of this author: the challenging role of a psychiatric consultant to a large state institution for the mentally retarded. Mentally retarded persons who live in such "total institutions" frequently have problems (e.g., psychological, social, or physical) that are so extreme that they necessitate residential placement outside their primary home. Often, these individuals have needs for services in excess of those retarded persons who can remain in their natural homes, or who can live independently. The magnitude of these needs makes the role and the involvement of the psychiatric consultant in institutional care of critical importance to the retarded. The psychiatrist who accepts this challenge must initially resolve some persistent diagnostic and treatment myths. One such myth is the oft-repeated statement of the nontreatability of mentally retarded persons with mental illness. As noted by other colleague-contributors to this book, mental illness in the retarded tends to respond to modern treatment interventions in the same fashion as mental illness in the nonretarded. Unfortunately, the medical records of mentally retarded persons in state institutions indicate that many community-based psychiatrists still need to be persuaded of this fact. Repeatedly, respected community-based psychiatrists continue to write brief referral–admission reports such as "Mentally retarded, hyperactive, uncontrollable young child. Recommend institutionalization as soon as possible."

In the retarded, treatable mental illness should be sought for, diagnosed when found, and treated appropriately. Unfortunately, there are still colleagues who believe that it is normal for the retarded to talk to themselves and to act "psychotic." This professional belief is a myth, as the clinical syndrome of mental retardation does not include hallucinations, delusions, or incapacitating depression. These later phenomena are symptoms of severe mental illness—not mental retardation—and demand treatment just as they would if found in the nonretarded.

8.4. Role of the Psychiatric Consultant in Institutional Care

In the large public institutions for the mentally retarded, the psychiatrist usually serves as a consultant rather than as a direct care provider. General medical care is usually provided by the nonpsychiatrist physician, who may be so overworked that he or she has the medical responsibility for serving 300–600 or more patients. Under these circumstances, it is quite difficult to maintain a focus on the larger picture of individual patients who have special social, educational, vocational, or other "nonmedical" needs.

Psychiatrists are in a unique position to help their colleagues by putting the treatment focus back on the broader goal of total adjustment of the patient, rather than just medical treatment. It is important, however, that the psychiatrist not simply make recommendations and then offer no further input in a given case. He or she must return frequently to supervise the recommended treatment, or to take over treatment responsibilities temporarily until the patient's situation is stabilized.

In the institution where I provide consultation services, it has been my policy that if the patient's best interests are not served by a regular consultative visit, I have the privilege of assuming responsibility for the case and providing direct care until the situation becomes stable. When I began assuming this role and its allied responsibilities, I was concerned that the other physicians would feel threatened and reject my intervention. Instead, I have found my colleagues grateful for these interventions in cases where they lack the time or the expertise to provide optimal care. In the consultative role, I have also found opportunities to educate the medical staff through the use of in-service training on the use of psychopharmacological therapy. But again, just as with a consultation on a patient, a simple presentation on a subject like drug interventions does not alter the quality of care appreciably. Just as in prescribing medication, these presentations must be individualized and must include provisions for follow-up and direct or indirect supervision of one's audience. Many physicians pick up good ideas from in-service presentations, but they either do not apply them because of feelings of insecurity or misinterpret and misapply the information. Helping one's nonpsychiatric colleagues use psychopharmacological treatments more effectively and helping them become more aware of the adjunctive role of such medications are contributions to the treatment of emotionally disturbed mentally retarded patients that require commitment and follow-up.

8.5. Psychopharmacological Treatment

The goals of psychopharmacological treatments may be many and should not be geared solely to the treatment of clear-cut mental disorders. We must additionally recognize that the retarded patient, even more than the nonretarded patient, has many treatment needs. In the general adult psychiatric population, we may occasionally encounter patients for whom the prescription of medication, accompanied by routine outpatient follow-up, is all the treatment that is needed. However, such individuals must be sufficiently in control of their lives so that once the acute symptoms of mental illness are alleviated by psychopharmacological treatment, they can return to their previous, reasonably balanced life situation.

Retarded patients usually lack a background of sufficient stability to allow us to treat only their mental illness and literally to ignore the rest of their life situation. Frequently, they have been institutionalized, are socially isolated, are financially fragile, have severe or troublesome physical handicaps, and have limited psychological resources. Many of these patients are involved in community- or institution-based programs aimed at alleviating their developmental and adaptational problems. Consequently, one must not only treat the mental illness but also be careful not to interfere unduly with the patient's other treatment programs. As the medications treat basic disturbances, we hope to improve the effectiveness of other ongoing programs for the retarded. This treatment approach involves considering carefully the positive benefits of the psychopharmacological agents that we prescribe—and being highly sensitive to their potentially adverse or negative aspects. Retarded patients are already handicapped, and we do them a great disservice if, in our effort to treat their allied psychiatric problems, we handicap them in other areas by causing undue sedation or other troublesome side effects.

8.6. Psychopharmacological Treatment of Diagnosable Mental Illness

There are two basic ways in which psychopharmacology can contribute to the overall programmatic goals of many retarded individuals. The first is the treatment of diagnosable mental illness, and the second is treatment of symptoms. The treatment of clearly diagnosed psychiatric illness includes the treatment of such disorders as schizophrenia, bipolar affective disorder, major depression, psychotic organic brain syndromes, other psychoses, and occasionally neuroses. In many patients, drug therapy is not sufficient alone and should be buttressed by psychotherapy. In the more severely retarded, however, psychotherapy may be less valuable, and drug therapy may be even more important.

In many cases of psychiatric disorders in the retarded, the presentation of a mental illness such as depression is straightforward and obvious. For instance, a previously well-adjusted individual may become withdrawn rather acutely, lose his or her appetite (with an accompanying loss of weight), develop anhedonia and crying episodes, lose interest in previously enjoyable activities, and experience early-morning awakening. This person is most likely experiencing an episode of diagnosable and treatable depression. In our institution, we have observed a number of such patients, as in the following case illustration.

A 53-year-old moderately retarded woman, previously married and living in the community, was totally independent in function. When psychiatrically ill, she became dependent, and her activities were severely constricted. She also became socially withdrawn and isolated, reluctant to communicate with anyone, apathetic, and anhedonic. She spoke of the future in bleak terms. No programmatic activities or reinforcers were effective in changing her behavior. She refused to participate in the unit token-economy program, neglected her personal appearance, and stopped attending the many programmatic activities available to her. She needed prompting to eat, and eventually, she refused to walk to the cafeteria; her food was then brought to her. This patient showed severe impairment in many spheres of her life because of an underlying psychiatric illness.

The psychiatric consultant diagnosed major unipolar depression and instituted treatment with a tricyclic antidepressant agent. Because of side effects and a suboptimal response, the patient was later given a course of eight electroconvulsive treatments. Her response was quick and dramatic.

On follow-up review two years later, she was alert and cheerful, ready to engage in conversation, active and helpful in her living unit, conscientious in her personal habits, and productively engaged in a vocational rehabilitation program. The ward staff continued to make comments such as "She is her old self again."

This example illustrates the pervasive benefits of the somatic psychiatric treatment of mental disorders in the retarded. Her severe mental illness was identified and treated, and more important, she became effectively engaged in programming efforts that may eventually allow her to resume a life outside the institution. Without effective psychiatric treatment, the other treatments could not proceed.

Psychosis in any form can interfere greatly with efforts to help the retarded move toward more independent and satisfying lives. Delusions and hallucinations always render the most well-designed behavioral programs ineffective. Psychosis interferes with independence and may make community placement difficult or impossible. Consider paranoid patients who hate everyone and feel "they" are all out to "get" them. These are patients who often respond minimally and in peculiar ways to behavioral programs. They may do a few things for reinforcers, but they always participate grudgingly. They never quite trust "the system," which they feel is exploiting them, and they often display a great deal of psychological discomfort even as they participate for reinforcers.

In other words, the behavioral approach may alter some surface behaviors but ignore the underlying mental illness. Psychopharmacological agents prescribed to treat the paranoid disorder can eliminate the suspiciousness, the hostility, and the delusions. Once this is accomplished, the patient can participate in programming and benefit from the experience.

A moderately retarded 35-year-old male patient living in the highest level unit in the institution was a clear example of paranoid schizophrenia. He had never been properly diagnosed or treated. His hostility, which was expressed through surly behavior and verbalizations, and his social isolation led the staff to avoid contact with him. They did plan and make available a full program of activities for him, but he never participated. He would get up early every morning, dress, swear at anyone around, and proceed to walk downtown. No one was quite sure where he went or what he did, and no one bothered to find out.

The staff were able to justify their lack of interest in this gentleman by assuming either that he could not profit from the planned activities or that he would not participate anyway. Efforts had been made in the past to reduce his hostility, his suspiciousness, and his delusions of persecution by prescribing psychopharmacological agents. One or two efforts with the sedating phenothiazines had proved useless, and the patient had been left on a small but ineffective dose for the past few years: the often-noted "traditional" 25 mg of thioridazine three times daily. At most, he took two doses a day, and usually only one.

As the consulting psychiatrist, I did a careful psychiatric examination. The patient was obviously suffering a clear-cut psychiatric disorder with target symptoms that normally respond to major psychopharmacological agents. Because of the patient's failure to respond to previous treatment efforts, I initially concluded that he may have been a nonresponder to oral medications, and I chose the depot neuroleptic fluphenazine decanoate for a treatment trial. A test dose of 0.1 ml was given intramuscularly. When reexamined two days later, the patient approached me, called me by name, and proceeded to talk about his present interests. He did not mention his delusions or his preoccupations with imagined or real past injustices. Because of these encouraging results, a second injection, of 0.5 ml, was ordered. This dose rendered the patient immobile and Parkinsonian and caused profuse drooling. Though toxic, the patient did not display any of the signs or symptoms of the paranoid psychosis that had been the target of the treatment. The ultimate goal of psychopharmacological treatment was to get this client actively and profitably involved in social, educational, and vocational activities. Thus far, the goal had not been reached and, because of the medication's side effects, could not be met. As a result, further adjustments were made in the dosage of the fluphenazine decanoate. Eventually, the patient was stabilized on 0.3 ml injected intramuscularly every three weeks. At that dose, the target symptoms continued to be absent, and the patient was free of any toxic drug effects. Moreover, he began to involve himself actively in programs he had previously rejected. Finally, we decided that, because this patient displayed a tendency toward lethargy on the day or two following his injection, he should be given his injections on Fridays in order to reduce any possible interference with the scheduled programming, which was mostly available on weekdays.

Intramuscularly injected, long-acting psychopharmacological agents such as fluphenazine decanoate have a particularly useful role in institutionalized mentally retarded–mentally ill patients who are unresponsive to orally administered neuroleptics. However, these drugs tend to be misunderstood and hence rather underutilized in institutions for the mentally retarded. A carefully individualized trial of such agents is indicated for patients who have target symptoms such as hallucinations, delusions, and unprovoked aggression, and who do not respond to ongoing programming or to adequate doses of oral psychopharmacological agents. However, their utilization must be highly individualized and closely monitored because these agents are difficult to regulate prop-

Table 1. Single Symptoms or Behaviors That Respond to Psychotropic Medications

Persistent uncooperativeness	Agitation
Destructiveness	Hallucinations
Irregular sleeping habits	Delusions
Explosive behavior	Hostility
Social withdrawal	Chronic anxiety
Apathy	Repeated self-injury
Hyperkinesis	Assaultiveness

erly. The patient must be carefully followed as one titrates the dose to the quantity and the interval that provide maximal benefit with minimal side effects. In contrast, the inflexible and routinized prescription of 1 ml every two weeks generally leads to poor results and troublesome side effects. Accordingly, what could have been a useful treatment fails, and this is one of the major reasons that such highly specific—and helpful—treatments often fall into disrepute.

8.7. Treatment of Nonspecific Symptoms

The second important approach to psychopharmacological intervention with the retarded is the less clear-cut area of treating specific symptoms (as opposed to diagnosable diseases or syndromes). Many specific symptoms, which may or may not be part of a more definite psychiatric illness, are known to be responsive to psychotropic medications. Table 1 lists the *single* symptoms or behaviors that may respond to psychotropic medications.

Although these symptoms and behaviors are not clearly definable mental illnesses or even necessary elements of identifiable mental illness, their control can benefit the patient greatly. Careful titration of dose, as well as a highly individualized approach to the patient, can result in the elimination or reduction of these undesirable behaviors and experiences, while allowing the patient to benefit maximally from involvement in his or her ongoing treatment program.

One must recognize, however, that psychopharmacological interventions should not be invoked to treat trivial instances of such symptoms. Only when symptoms are refractory to available social, behavioral, or other treatment interventions should drug therapy be initiated in these clinical instances.

An example is a moderately retarded 22-year-old man who never really displayed any definite evidence of psychosis, such as hallucinations or delusions, but might have been regarded as having a "psychotic" disruption of his personality that kept him from integrating his thoughts, feelings, experiences, and actions effectively. Behaviorally, he possessed all self-help skills, had a good vocabulary for his developmental status, was capable of interpersonal skills, but generally seemed to have a chip on his shoulder. He was passive-aggressive and obstructionistic when asked to do anything. His quick temper and argumentative approach to people led him into daily fights with staff and other clients. Frequently, if he could not promptly have his demands met, he destroyed property.

This young man had various target symptoms that are ordinarily responsive to psychopharmacological medications: aggression, uncooperativeness, destructiveness, poor disposition, explosive behavior, agitation, assaultiveness, and so on. Whether these medications were specifically justifiable at the time was problematic. The patient was questionably mentally ill, although clearly emotionally disturbed. The staff who dealt with this patient were able and well trained and had the personnel and the professional training resources to work one-to-one with him in a highly behavioral setting. When the patient first came to the unit, the staff asked the psychiatrist to discontinue the psychopharmacological agent that had been previously prescribed. Because it was an ineffective small dose of thioridazine, it was discontinued. After a few months, during which the patient showed no improvement, some members of the staff now asked if there were some psychopharmacological medication that would be helpful. Still other staff members remained opposed to the use of medications. Because of the lack of consensus, as well as the absence of a prescriptive diagnosis, psychopharmacological therapy was not instituted. After four months, however, the primary-care staff as well as the support staff unanimously agreed that their behavioral, social, and psychological interventions were not producing positive changes. At this time, there was general agreement that a psychopharmacological medication should be tried.

For a number of reasons, depot fluphenazine was chosen: absorption and compliance are guaranteed; the patient had previously resisted taking medications and frequently missed oral doses; and the patient had tried other medications without success.

Within two days, his spontaneous and unprovoked aggression largely disappeared. The patient still became angry if confronted by peers, but he retaliated with words rather than actions. He remained somewhat passive-aggressive, but he was considerably more cooperative. These clinical changes were noted not only on the unit, but in the classroom, in off-ground activities, and in his prevocational training program. Adjusting the depot fluphenazine to the optimal dose took about three months, during which time the staff were extremely helpful in reporting on behavior and side effects that interfered with other ongoing treatments. Eventually, the dose was stabilized at 0.7 ml intramuscularly every three weeks.

One year later, this patient was placed in a community group home. After successfully completing his six-week trial placement, he was discharged from the institution where he had lived for the previous 15 years to take up permanent community residence. He continues to receive his medication and supportive psychotherapy from a local community mental-health center.

Here, then, was a patient who had behavioral symptoms that were responsive to psychopharmacological intervention, but not the specific mental-illness diagnostic configuration noted in the first case illustration. Empirically, many such patients profit from the use of the major psychoactive agents. These patients deserve treatment despite our inability to arrive at a specific pretreatment or prescriptive diagnosis.

Often, in clinical psychiatry, it is the patient's response to a clinical trial of medication that helps to make the diagnosis. When persistent and consistent modern programming efforts fail to elicit positive changes in a behaviorally disturbed retarded individual, and the patient has symptoms that are known (empirically) to respond to psychopharmacological agents, the patient should be considered for an adequate clinical trial of psychopharmacological treatment. A definite diagnosis makes it easier to choose any appropriate treatment, but the absence of a definite diagnosis should not preclude a clinical trial of these medications.

8.8. Benefits of Psychopharmacological Medications

Quite often, specific psychopharmacological therapy opens doors to effective schooling, vocational training, normalized social environments, community placement, and independent living. When properly administered, these medications may produce one of the following benefits: (1) make the patient more alert, communicative, and interested in school and living area; (2) reduce restlessness, irritability, and aggression; (3) improve personal effectiveness; (4) improve interpersonal interactions; (5) improve intellectual performance; (6) possibly prevent institutionalization; (7) permit function in a less restrictive environment; (8) control explosive behavior; (9) minimize social withdrawal and apathy; (10) reduce hyperkinesis and excitability; (11) provide an altered climate within which other interventions are more effective in benefiting overall adjustment; and (12) reduce hallucinations, delusions, anxiety, and tension.

Such improvements are of vital importance for the continuation of effective community living, and they help to enhance the possibility of the return of institutionalized retarded citizens to group homes or their own families.

8.9. Role of Psychotherapy

Mentally retarded individuals, just like nonretarded persons, are vulnerable to emotional conflict, the pain of loss, blows to self-esteem, and, within institutions, a sense of isolation and alienation. Like everyone else, they desire acceptance. Rejection, failure, the frustration of difficult competition, and the impact of being labeled "retarded" all present difficulties for the retarded— difficulties that can be appropriately addressed by interpersonal psychotherapy. Although individual therapy is frequently indicated, family therapy and especially group approaches can also be effective and should be available when needed.

Interestingly, some professionals have argued in general against the applicability of psychotherapy to the retarded. Countering these arguments, Szymanski[9] has concluded that the opposition to psychotherapy for retarded persons is most often based on ignorance. A strong advocate of psychotherapy for the retarded, Szymanski provided the following criteria for its applicability:

(1) the presence of mental disturbance in which psychological factors play an etiological and/or an aggravating role; (2) the patient's potential to form a sufficient relationship with the therapist and to communicate to some degree verbally or nonverbally; and (3) an expectation that amelioration of the psychological symptoms will improve a patient's ability to utilize her or his cognitive potential.

These observations and the contributions of other colleagues to this book clearly show that psychotherapy is an appropriate and a potentially helpful therapeutic tool that can be incorporated into the overall treatment program for the mentally ill–mentally retarded person. Unfortunately, it remains overlooked in many institutions, perhaps as a result of limited access to trained personnel, a misplaced emphasis on a undimensional "behavioral" orientation, or, as Szymanski suggested, "ignorance." However, with the increasing number of institutionalized residents now receiving social security, Medicaid, or other forms of financial assistance, they can make greater use of community resources such as community mental-health centers, private practitioners, and other mental-health treatment resources.

Special problems confront the therapist dealing with institutionalized patients. Foremost among these is the difficulty inherent in eliciting and coordinating the efforts of many colleagues in the team approach to psychiatric care. If the therapist works in the community, it is especially important to maintain close contact with the various institutional staff involved in the patient's case, and thereby to achieve effective goal-setting, feedback, and interpersonal-environmental modification. The therapist working within an institution may adopt a "family" approach, recognizing the staff as the patient's surrogate family. This particular approach presents a challenge in terms of building a specific treatment prescription for each patient via the multidisciplinary team. However, when met successfully, such challenges enhance the value of therapy and also underscore the need for a flexible approach to psychiatric care that is carefully attuned to the specific realities of each patient's life.

8.10. Relaxation and Biofeedback

The effectiveness of muscle relaxation as a therapeutic treatment for various psychological and physical disorders has been demonstrated by Wolpe[10] and Jacobson.[11] Budzynski and Stoyva[12] have shown that biofeedback is a useful technique for eliciting deep-muscle relaxation. Although these newer approaches are gaining acceptance as treatment modalities in their own right, there is little research available to assess their effectiveness with mentally retarded patients.

In a unique project, Frankenberger[13] studied the individual and differential effectiveness of biofeedback and progressive relaxation with adult residents of a large state facility for the mentally retarded. His subjects ranged from severely to mildly retarded individuals. They were selected for the study on the basis of being the most aggressive clients in the institution. Frankenberger encountered some initial difficulties in that the subject often did not understand what "relaxation" meant. However, when using biofeedback, he was able to induce muscle relaxation by instructing the subjects to reduce the frequency of the click-feedback sounds. He also noted that aggressive retarded persons had higher baseline electromyograms (EMGs) than nonaggressive control retarded persons. Both during progressive relaxation exercises and with EMG-assisted biofeedback, all of the subjects but one were able to reduce muscle tension levels significantly. The effect of these treatments on the frequency of aggression suggests that this type of treatment can be of great potential benefit to mentally retarded persons. For example, within an institutional setting, biofeedback could be offered through a centralized service, and with the automated equipment now available, a small number of clients could be monitored at the same time by a single technician. Thus, a small biofeedback service in an institutional setting could serve a large population of aggressive clients, with the focus on teaching them enhanced self-control of their ongoing behavior.

General-relaxation and deep-breathing exercises are perhaps simpler to implement than biofeedback and can be quickly learned by institution staff members. I have found that the professional recommendation of such treatment interventions is quite effective for aggressive mentally retarded individuals. Generally, there is good staff acceptance of these interventions because staff members can readily implement them as part of a regular treatment plan.

8.11. Conclusion

The psychiatric evaluation and treatment of mentally retarded patients who are also mentally ill represent a relatively recent and growing area of psychiatric services. Increasingly, psychiatrists are recognizing that mental illness is not a natural concomitant of mental retardation, and that, when it occurs, it can be diagnosed and treated effectively. Certainly, the challenges that these patients pose are greater because of their multiple life problems and the complexity of the resources required for their care. However, our experiences have shown that successful psychiatric treatment endeavors are possible in institutions for the mentally retarded, especially if the consulting psychiatrist is attuned to the challenges presented by the dually diagnosed and takes an active role in coordinating the complex treatment efforts of the staff.

Assisting the physicians and the other health professionals who work in these institutional settings in the effective use of psychopharmacological treatment is one of the major goals of the consulting psychiatrist. The proper use of psychopharmacological treatment for mentally retarded persons who have a concomitant emotional disturbance, whether it be a diagnosable mental illness or a set of severely disruptive symptoms and/or behaviors, must strive to maximize the patient's overall well-being and not just his or her medical status. In evaluating treatment, the psychiatrist and other physicians must rely on feedback from all treatment team personnel who have an active part to play in the total treatment of the patient: nurses, teachers, case manager, ward personnel, peers of the patient, the family, and so on.

Psychotherapy is an additional, effective therapeutic modality that is too often ignored in the institutional setting. Additionally, one should not overlook the potential benefits of newer interventions such as biofeedback and relaxation techniques. Armed with these tools, and working within the scope of an interdisciplinary team, we can help mentally retarded patients to regain their mental health and to lead fuller, more productive lives.

References

1. Menolascino FJ: Psychiatry's past, current, and future role in mental retardation, in Menolascino FJ (ed): *Psychiatric Approaches to Mental Retardation*. New York, Basic Books, 1970.
2. Wortis J: The role of psychiatry in mental retardation services, in Mittler P (ed): Research to Practice in Mental Retardation, vol 1. Baltimore, University Park Press, 1977.
3. Rutter M: Psychiatry, in Wortis J (ed): *Mental Retardation: An Annual Review*, vol 3. New York, Grune and Stratton, 1971.
4. President's Committee on Mental Retardation: *Mental Retardation: The Known and the Unknown*, DHEW Publication No. (OHD) 76-21008. Washington, D.C., Government Printing Office, 1976.
5. Menolascino FJ: Emotional disturbance and mental retardation. *Am J Ment Defic* 70(2);248–256, 1965.
6. Menolascino FJ: The facade of mental retardation: Its challenge to child psychiatry. *Am J Psychiatry* 122(11);1227–1235, 1966.
7. Menolascino FJ: *Challenges in Mental Retardation*. New York, Basic Books, 1977.
8. Balthazar E, Stevens H: *The Emotionally Disturbed, Mentally Retarded: A Historical and Contemporary Perspective*. Englewood Cliffs, NJ, Prentice-Hall, 1975.
9. Szymanski L: Individual psychotherapy with retarded persons, in Szymanski L, Tanguay P (eds): *Emotional Disorders of Mentally Retarded Persons*. Baltimore, University Park Press, 1980.
10. Wolpe J: *Psychotherapy by Reciprocal Inhibition*. Stanford, CA, Stanford University Press, 1958.
11. Jacobson E: *Progressive Relaxation*. Chicago, University of Chicago Press, 1938.
12. Budzynski T, Stoyva J: An instrument for producing deep muscle relaxation by means of analogue information feedback. *J Appl Behav Anal* 2;231–237, 1969.
13. Frankenberger W: *Effects of Progressive Muscle Relaxation and Electromyographic Feedback Training on Aggressive Institutionalized Mentally Retarded Adults*. Unpublished doctoral dissertation, Ohio State University, 1979.

III

Special Systems of Services

Introduction

Hopefully, the reader has acquired by now a thorough overview and understanding of what individuals with mental illness and mental retardation are, as well as of what treatment, intervention strategies, and techniques can best be used in improving their behavior. In building on this understanding, we now focus in this section on the delivery service systems in which various models and programs are evaluated and presented for replication.

Chapter 9 presents a nationally acclaimed day-program model by the Rock Creek Foundation developed in 1973 for emotionally disturbed-mentally retarded persons in community-based settings. This model of habilitation draws on technology and assumptions from both the mental retardation and the mental health fields. These authors present the principles and the components in developing and operating a psychiatric day-treatment and outpatient program for this population. Successful techniques are analyzed, and specific habilitation skills are presented that are essential in developing independence in a community setting.

Independent living and residential programs are also reviewed in such a way that the more recent cycle of the community placement–decompensation–reinstitutionalization process is broken and a rationale is presented for maintaining a complete community-based system.

In early 1983, the Division of Hospital and Community Psychiatry of the American Hospital Association presented an award to the Nebraska Psychiatric Association for its outstanding inpatient program for the mentally retarded-mentally ill. This award came as no surprise to those familiar with model programs in the United States, for in the early 1960s, it was the Nebraska Psychiatric Institute that became the first psychiatric facility in the country to provide services to mentally retarded individuals who had psychiatric disorders. Over 20 years ago, this facility received federal funds to provide services, to conduct research, and to train medical and allied health personnel in working with this dually diagnosed population.

In Chapter 10, the authors explain this award-winning inpatient psychiatric program, demonstrating a continuum of services from the inpatient program to a community-based service system. The specific focus is on an analysis of 305 mentally retarded-mentally ill individuals for whom services were provided and on whom extensive data were collected. Eight diagnostic categories are presented and reviewed, ranging from schizophrenia, organic brain syndrome, and personality disorders to affective and neurotic disorders. Specific problems and concerns associated with each level of mental retardation, particularly medical problems, are also discussed. Most impressive in this chapter, however, is a model for a continuum of care ranging from long-term institutionalization to acute inpatient psychiatric care to an array of services in community-based settings. Specific strategies and techniques are presented at each step of the continuum. In addition, 81 dually diagnosed clients within the community-based Eastern Nebraska Community Office of Retardation (ENCOR) are presented, and evidence supports the viability of providing services to this population in a comprehensive community-based model system. Treatment issues are presented that the authors feel are essential in developing a comprehensive model that contains ingredients that others may want to replicate. Seldom will the reader find a more comprehensive model for the deinstitutionalization of the dually diagnosed, particularly based on the long history of successfully treating so many mentally retarded-mentally ill individuals.

Chapter 11 should prove to be both enjoyable and informative to the reader as its style and content are considerably different from those of any of the other chapters in this manuscript. It contains a detailed account of how one can set up services step-by-step to serve mentally retarded-mentally ill individuals. The author provides insight into the process of setting up a treatment unit in New York State and presents a convincing rationale of why such a program is needed for this population.

The goals for setting up such a unit, the actual early steps necessary to establish the unit, the resistance that one might meet, and then the actual maintenance and development of the unit are all clearly presented to the reader. Dr. Houston delineates the controversial and frequent roadblocks that one must overcome in order to achieve a smoothly operating program that can truly handle this population. Dr. Houston presents a blueprint for planning, developing, and establishing such a treatment unit.

Chapter 12 presents a model day-treatment service program for the dually diagnosed population that builds on and specifically addresses some of the programs more generically described in earlier chapters. The author specifically presents the Beacon House Program, which is a psychosocial rehabilitation center serving mentally retarded-mentally disabled adults. This model program follows a psychosocial club model, in which the patients become members and are encouraged to take on active roles in a therapeutic community atmosphere. Mr. Fletcher goes on to point out the specific therapeutic approaches and techniques and strategies used in treating the members. Sensory integration therapy, horticultural therapy, dance–movement therapy, music therapy, and art therapy are analyzed and presented for reader analysis as subcomponents of the overall model. A theme also reported by Mr. Fletcher, which exists throughout this book, is that there tends to be a great deal of emphasis on process (how to train or teach) rather than on content (what to teach or curriculum) because active involvement in the process is indeed frequently the treatment curriculum content.

Finally, in Chapter 13, the authors present a valuable alternative that is gaining popularity via a home intervention program for this population involving their families and the community. This home intervention program is intended to fill the gap in services offered to individuals with a dual diagnosis. The advantage of providing services in the natural environment, utilizing a variety of approaches to treatment, is also reviewed. In this chapter, the authors present a very specific blueprint that one can follow in providing a home-based treatment and intervention program supportive of the dually diagnosed individual and her or his family in the community setting.

Case studies are presented in the context of comprehensive service-delivery-system objectives, for evaluation, monitoring, and maintenance. The reader should find it particularly helpful to observe a listing of the major problems identified by both the clients and the parents and families of children who have this particular combination of impairments.

Rarely does one see any data presented on the impact on the family and how one actually goes about working with family members in the natural environment, as well as on the importance and effectiveness of such efforts. Utilizing the team approach via an *in vivo* strategy has long been recognized but seldom used in a model demonstration program such as the one described in this particular chapter.

In short, this section provides us with both general and specific service-delivery-system models, at each step of the continuum, which should demonstrate a need for the successful development of community-based services for the dually diagnosed population.

9

Value-Based Programming for the Dually Diagnosed
The Rock Creek Model

Michael W. Smull, Ellen S. Fabian, and Frederic B. Chanteau

9.1. Introduction

Over the past decade (1973–1983) the Rock Creek Foundation (RCF) has developed a comprehensive community support system to meet the needs of mentally retarded persons with severe mental-health problems. The array and content of the components of the service system reflect both the needs of dual diagnosis persons and the resources in the Washington Metropolitan environment. Although it is neither feasible nor appropriate for other regions to develop programs that replicate Rock Creek's programs, what can be replicated are the components of the programs.

This chapter details the general principles and the basic components of the Rock Creek Foundation's service system. The actual programs are reviewed to illustrate one way in which components can be put together to ensure the needed service continuum.

Our service system demonstrates that mentally retarded persons with severe mental-health problems can be served in a community-based setting. While representing a full continuum of services, the configuration of the service system reflects the resources available to it as well as the needs of the consumers. The services began with a program that borrowed freely from both existing mental-retardation and existing mental-health technology. This process of melding technology from a variety of disciplines has become basic to the evolution of programs of the Rock Creek Foundation.

Model program activities were supported, in part, by a Project of National Significance Grant (No. 54-P-71338) from the United States Department of Health and Human Services, Administration on Developmental Disabilities.

Michael W. Smull • Deputy Director, Mental Retardation Program, University of Maryland School of Medicine, Baltimore, Maryland 21201. He held the post of Director of the Rock Creek Foundation for 8 years.   *Ellen S. Fabian* • Director of Research and Training, the Rock Creek Foundation, Silver Spring, Maryland 20910.   *Frederic B. Chanteau* • Executive Director, the Rock Creek Foundation, Silver Spring, Maryland 20910.

The professional practices and techniques developed are rooted in value-based assumptions that are reviewed, discussed, and, where appropriate, adopted. Equally important is the simultaneous endorsement of the developmental model, with its programming dictates and its perception of mental health problems as conditions separate and distinct from mental retardation. With the recognition that both mental retardation and mental illness may require lifelong supportive services, the result is a synergistic mix of habilitation and treatment representing a multidisciplinary blend of technological modalities. All program values and assumptions (person, staff, environmental, and program) have at their core an acknowledgment of fundamental human worth and dignity regardless of handicapping conditions.

9.1.1. Person Assumptions

The core value of the Rock Creek Foundation is recognition of basic human worth and dignity.

It is here that normalization is endorsed proactively by stating that mentally retarded persons have a right to treatment and habilitation in community settings that use "culturally valued means, in order to enable people to lead culturally valued lives"(p. 8)[1]. It is also here that emphasis is placed on the separate and distinct nature of mental retardation and mental illness and on the recognition that most mentally retarded persons do not experience mental illness.

The assumption is balanced, though, by the recognition of the detrimental effects that the cultural stigma of mental retardation can have on development and function, especially the consequences of growing up as a devalued and stigmatized person.

For the persons who come to the attention of the Rock Creek Foundation, the stigmatizing effects have often been devastating. They have been denied the supportive opportunities to make choices (with the inherent risks) that are prerequisites to learning. In addition to the mental retardation and the mental health diagnosis, the person often experiences a developmental arrest, learned helplessness, or a failure–avoidance syndrome that cannot be attributed to mental retardation. The impaired ability to reason abstractly is seen as the loss of a coping mechanism that would otherwise help compensate for a culturally based stigma.

These assumptions also include the family, especially the parents, as valued members of the habilitation and treatment team. Their frequent mistrust of professionals has been painfully learned. Their feelings of hopelessness must be seen in a context of repeated efforts that have failed and the absence of effective treatment or support.

9.1.2. Staff Assumptions

The most fundamental of the staff assumptions is that staff must accept the person assumptions listed in Section 9.1.1. This is not an endorsement of a particular type of therapeutic modality or approach, but the fundamental acceptance of our clients as people more similar to ourselves than different from us.

Beyond acceptance of the handicapped individual as a person, staff need to share other characteristics to work effectively with this population. These characteristics may not sound special or unusual, but when looking for staff, we find that only a minority of professionals meet these criteria. Because the handicapping conditions transcend disciplinary boundaries, so must the professional. This relatively simple statement is, in fact, a challenge to the "lone-ranger" approach that most mental-health professionals have appropriately adopted in their view of their professional role. Traditionally, psychotherapy has been offered in a relatively isolated context, the assumption being that clients or patients will work out their problems in therapy and carry those solutions into their environments of work, family, social life, and so on. Because mentally retarded persons frequently have limited control over the environments in which they live and work, and as one effect of mental retardation can be a diminished ability to generalize, the concept of a holistic approach to treatment has to be endorsed and operationalized. Thus, the professional staff must actively seek out cooperative solutions to client problems by continually framing emotional, behavioral, vocational, or social treatment solutions in a holistic approach. In addition, the pervasive and complex nature of the disabilities often requires a problem-solving approach that emphasizes flexibility and creativity. Although previously developed techniques will work, they must be adapted to the circumstances and identified as worthy of a therapeutic trial that may require extensive efforts and multiple attempts at intervention. At times, it is the lack of resources present in our service systems that accounts for clinical failures. Where it exists, this lack must be identified, and the failure must be analyzed without affixing blame.

In general, the staff at the Rock Creek Foundation are not highly identified with their individual professional disciplines; they endorse the team concept, where professional turf is not as important as individual talents and competencies.

9.1.3. Environmental Assumptions

All persons admitted to Rock Creek's programs and services are admitted with the expectation that they will have the potential for community living. It is also recognized that the literature reports that the single greatest reason for reinstitutionalization is maladaptive behaviors.[2] Because these behaviors occur in an environment, a holistic approach to habilitation and treatment requires that the environment be assessed, as well as the individual and that individual's interaction with the environment.

Environmental norms and expectations demand conformity to certain standards and reflect tolerance of other behaviors. Therefore, it is essential to assess the "macro" environment, as well as the "micro" environment. For example, the Rock Creek Foundation is located in the Washington, D.C. metropolitan area, a mix of suburban and urban environments. Clients have complete access to the community and this access to public transportation, stores, shops, and other places of business demands certain behavioral conformities of the client. Our programming needs to account for these community expectations and integrate them within the program planning process. The environment itself becomes part of the "treatment" process. Often, the surrounding community works with the treatment team in the development of strategies to effectively facilitate community integration. When accounted for and actively made use of in the development of programs and programming, environmental constraints are not seen as barriers to movement as much as very real, behavioral goals which our clients can attain.

9.1.4. Program Assumptions

Programming brings together the previous three sets of assumptions and puts them into practice. Above all, the programming is client-centered. There is an active and ongoing effort to adapt programming to the needs of the client, rather than trying to adapt the client to the programming available. It is this orientation that has driven the evolution of Rock Creek's service system from a single day program serving a handful of individuals to a multiplicity of day and residential and support services assisting over 200 persons. Meeting client needs also demands flexibility and creativity in finding and using funding resources to develop appropriate programming.

All of the programming begins in a treatment–habilitation and planning process, where the client is seen within the context of the environment and the service system. Programming assists the staff and the individual to function with the greatest personal autonomy, the highest degree of "social potency," and the greatest self-satisfaction. Where the individual has not met the demands of the environment programming can be designed to compensate for those functional deficits. This requirement of community integration is rooted in the concept that a positive view of oneself is enhanced by taking part in valued activities which are valued by society as well as the individual or the staff. For example, to perform what our society labels as "make work" is not seen as a goal of independent vocational development. And, mastering public transportation is not only viewed as a skill building exercise, but is the vehicle for clients to get to Rock Creek. Because local public transportation is available, transporting adults in labeled vans is an unnecessarily stigmatizing activity whereas mastering public transportation enhances esteem and reinforces the client's perception of himself or herself as a capable person.

9.2. Program Development

The systemic components that underlie comprehensive community support systems designed to meet the multiple needs of the mentally retarded persons with severe emotional problems require:

1. Assessment of individuals in the context of environmental functioning and movement across less restrictive environments.[3]
2. The assessment of habilitation needs and the development of an individual plan in which the client has meaningful input and, to the degree feasible, control.[3]
3. Interdisciplinary staffing leading to the diagnosis of an emotional problem and a recommendation for treatment.[3]
4. A treatment team that acts on the recommendations.[3]
5. Flexibility in the development of program techniques, which are combined to meet individual needs.
6. A multidisciplinary blend of professional techniques that meet individual needs.
7. Variable and creative funding resources and patterns that enable program development to respond to needs.

These conditions describe the development and implementation of the client-based service system at Rock Creek.

Operationalizing the assumptions articulated earlier led to the development of a community support system that maximized resources through careful methods of program development mediated by an assessment of client needs. The Rock Creek Foundation has found that a client-based service system is one that evolves through the continuous process of evaluating needs and negotiating and/or developing systems to meet those needs within the context of environmental constraints. Pragmatic decisions are made about those compensatory mechanisms required to assist the individual in functioning in the current therapeutic environment, about the programming and services that will enable the person to live in the next environment, and about whether those programs and services are available or adaptable. With modification that reflects licensing and accreditation requirements, this treatment-planning process runs throughout all agency services. It operationalizes all the assumptions previously stated.

The treatment planning is designed to reflect the major technologies that it borrows from: mental health, mental retardation, psychoeducational, or vocational. For example, the mildly retarded person who is severely emotionally disturbed needs some technology drawn from mental retardation but is in primary need of technology developed for the mentally ill. Conversely, the person who is severely retarded and mildly disturbed is in primary need of technology from mental retardation but still requires some mental-health technology, particularly the nonverbal and behavioral modalities developed for work with severely regressed disabled persons.

At the core of this client-based service system is the criterion of ultimate functioning[4] and the corollary of client movement across less restrictive treatment environments. The clients are assessed according to their service system needs; their functional levels are defined; and program components are provided that address the needs identified. The process of treatment planning is viewed from both an individual and a systemic perspective. The results of this process are the driving force behind the continued and careful development of programs and services. Ultimate environmental functioning is evaluated on an individual basis. Program components as well as treatment strategies are then designed to address the barriers to movement across the treatment environments. This continued process of evaluating client needs and of matching needs to the available services is the operationalizing of the concept of a client-based service system and becomes the rationale behind program evaluation and quality assurance activities.

Treatment planning is based on four underlying conditions:

- Assessment takes into account not only the functional levels but also the developmental patterns of the individual. It allows for prescriptive programming that is targeted at critical skill deficits and that is presented within the developmental context of the individual.
- Clients have different needs in different areas of functioning. Thus, a client may be assessed at a vocational level requiring prevocational skill development and at a social level requiring only supportive networks to encourage activities. Assessment is not only a multidisciplinary but a multileveled process.
- Whenever possible, the service needs or the remediating programs necessary for movement are provided through generic service networks, or if not available, they are developed and implemented. Thus, for the client with a dual diagnosis, services may need to be developed that will meet special needs not provided for in other community settings.
- Modification of current technologies in vocational, social, rehabilitative, psychiatric, and educational systems is necessary in order to provide for appropriate client growth and development.

9.3. Description of Services

Currently, our service system spans environments by offering a continuum of care across less restrictive environments with ongoing client support and maintenance activities built into the clients' movement.

The program components described, represent not an exhaustive list of potential services, but the result of specific modifications and development utilizing existing technologies and adapting techniques from the mental retardation and the mental health disciplines to promote comprehensive client-based system development. Described are psychotherapeutic services, social survival services, vocational services, and residential services.

9.3.1. Psychotherapeutic Services

Psychiatric services are an integral part of the programs available at the Rock Creek Foundation and form the core of the day treatment program. The services offered include medication evaluation and chemotherapy; individual, group, family, and behavior therapy; psychiatric and psychological evaluations;

and expressive arts therapies. The services needed and the intensity and frequency of the service to be provided are a part of the treatment-planning process that identifies the barriers to movement across treatment environments and designs specific strategies to remediate these barriers. Consequently, individual therapy might initially be provided on a daily basis and later on a weekly basis after specific objectives have been attained. Or conversely, clinical therapies might be inappropriate for clients whose maladaptive behaviors prohibit the internalization of psychotherapeutic gains. In these cases, behavioral management programs may be initiated first, and once behaviors are modified, individual or group therapy may be initiated to facilitate the internalization of the new behaviors.

The goal of all psychotherapeutic intervention services is to enable clients to recognize their feelings, to assign labels to those feelings, to rehearse them, and to finally enhance or elaborate them. The holistic framework for this process is designed to teach problem-solving stategies that will enable the clients to transfer learning across environments and situations. In order for this transfer of learning to take place, the therapeutic services are offered within an interlocking system of all other services. A holistic framework emphasizes the acquisition of new behaviors and new coping skills in each different environment; the therapist is actually present in that new environment if necessary.

Other modifications and adaptations of existing mental-health technology are made in order to meet the needs of a population whose cognitive limitations dictate an eclectic, directive therapeutic modality. For example, because many of the clients have never had the opportunity to be involved in ongoing therapy, many experience initial difficulties in making active use of the forum. Additionally, the lack of previous experience in therapeutic intervention, combined with organic handicapping conditions, requires an adjustment to be made in the frequency and the length of therapeutic sessions. Therapy sessions are generally limited in length (20–30 minutes) in order to compensate for the clients' ability to concentrate and assimilate learning, and the frequency of sessions is increased to reinforce appropriate behaviors and thought processes.

9.3.1.1. Day Treatment Programs

The day treatment program functions as a highly integrated service and a careful blending of mental health and mental retardation technology. The program can be broken down into three major components: (1) formal psychotherapy (assessment, individual therapy, group therapy, and dance and movement therapy); (2) social survival/activity programming (assessment, task-oriented groups, community meetings, community-oriented activities, guided experience, travel training, and individual instruction); and (3) vocational services (assessment, individual counseling, group counseling, transitional employment placements, and job development, placement, and follow-along).

Currently, the day treatment program includes two separate components: psychiatric and behavioral programming. This separation arose from the effort to meet the needs of those recently deinstitutionalized clients coming to Rock

Creek and requiring intensive day programming in order to facilitate community maintenance. Many of these recently deinstitutionalized clients manifested severe maladaptive behaviors that were determined to be more amenable to behavioral programming than to a therapeutic milieu with intensive psychiatric services. These two programs are equal in cost and are organizationally defined as clinical day programs. Daily activities are differentiated between the two groups, but community meetings and some activities are done jointly.

The individual therapist, overseeing a multidisciplinary team, is charged with the coordination and the implementation of the client's treatment plan. Because of the interdisciplinary structure of the day treatment program and the use of these highly integrated treatment teams, professional boundaries are easily crossed and blurred. Thus, there is less territoriality programmatically, as professionals become cross-trained to the point where a psychiatric social worker or a psychiatric nurse will train a client employing behavior chaining, and a vocational counselor will substitute as a mental health worker. For the therapeutic process to be successful, the clients must have the opportunity to build on their existing strengths as well as to develop new ones. It is here that the availability of social survival and vocational programming becomes critical.

As the client displays increasing emotional stability and incorporates life skills development (such as being travel-trained), vocational activities are slowly integrated into the treatment plan. This process, during which all clients receive a minimum wage, may start with a highly supervised in-house job (e.g., maintaining the juice or coffee machine or acting as janitor) that evolves into transitional employment (4–10 hours per week) and hopefully to competitive employment. Or an individual may move into the psychosocial rehabilitation program, where support (both therapeutic and vocational) can be maintained, but within a less intensive and consequently a less costly program.

9.3.1.2. Outpatient Psychotherapeutic Services

Apart from the intensive psychiatric services offered in day treatment, a wide variety of outpatient services is available. These include group and family therapy, as well as psychiatric and psychological assessment. The outpatient program grew out of our experience that as clients moved into the community, an ongoing support system was needed in order to preclude regression and potential decompensation. Beyond the structured outpatient therapy, a 24-hour crisis service was developed and made available to all clients within the Rock Creek Foundation service system. Often the opportunity simply to talk to a staff member suffices to see the client through a troubling evening or weekend. Any necessary psychiatric intervention or hospitalization can also be accomplished via the on-call system.

9.3.2. Social Survival Services

Social survival/life skills training was developed by Ron Ward to meet the needs of specific clients. A critical role of social survival programming is to define treatment goals in terms of observable behaviors. Success is determined by the client's meeting the change criteria defined by the treatment team. Because the desired changes may be subtle, the approaches must be constantly appraised and adjusted.

The goal of providing social survival services is to assist persons in the acquisition of those adaptive skills and behaviors necessary for integration into community life. The programming is rooted in the behaviorally oriented psychoeducational technology developed over the last 20 years. Central to the success of the programming is assessment that takes into account not only skill levels, but the developmental pattern of the individual.

The developmental typology is derived from the work of Hewitt and Erickson.[7] Once the developmental level is identified, a specific intervention strategy follows. Programming is developed that will also address a consistently negative history as a learner, which many of the dually diagnosed persons in our program have experienced. Many have developed a failure avoidance syndrome and no longer try so that they will not experience other failures. Assessment begins with the independent living curriculum. This taxonomy of living skills does not produce a quantified score but clearly indicates the areas of competency and deficit. Observation and discussion with mental health personnel then determine the individual's development level. Further observations within the "classroom" assess the learning style of the client. All of these assessments are then combined to produce prescriptive programming and intervention strategies.

The areas of concentration are activities involving money, time, communication, and public transportation.

As a result of years of responding to client needs, social survival/life skills instructors have developed a repertoire of response alternatives. These sets of responses have been formalized as a set of programming alternatives that may be implemented by persons with varying amounts of training. Instruction in the use of these strategies is specific to the needs of the client. Of necessity, the approaches differ greatly, ranging from behavior serialization and environmental manipulation (which may be used with clients who are not subject to verbal mediation of behavior) to self-directed activities (for individuals who may be operating at the achievement level academically but who may have other behaviors that interfere with optimal social functioning, such as compulsive behaviors or conditioned inhibitons).

9.3.3. Vocational Services

Vocational (re)habilitation services were developed by Gary Donaldson. They represent an essential element of the service system at Rock Creek. In a work-oriented society such as ours, vocational success reflects on our self-esteem, our attitudes toward the community, and even our assessment of our growth and achievement. Therefore, prevocational and vocational development is a common thread that runs through our continuum of services, reflecting the importance of work to our clients, the difficulties that their multihandicapping conditions present, and the lack of previous successful work experiences.

The program goals cover four concept areas with a central theme of person–environment factors related to adaptation: (1) awareness of developing values, abilities, interests, limitations, identity, and motivations as they relate to occupational experience; (2) the development of decision-making skills to aid the individual in maintaining self-regulation; (3) the development of an awareness of the occupational and social environment in terms of work and social roles, related lifestyles, potential satisfactions, and potential dissatisfactions; and (4) the development of the interpersonal and work behavior skills necessary to maintain employment and adequate social adaptation.

These goals are presented within three major program divisions: day treatment, outpatient treatment, and psychosocial treatment.

All the programs share the primary goals of providing structured and guided work-adjustment training experiences within community-based employment situations accomplished through group and individual placements. Selective job placement is provided on completion of the training. A comprehensive follow-up program is also involved to assist in the maintenance of employment. Individuals in all three programs receive career guidance and skill development in decision making and problem solving around work-related issues.

The following section describes specific Rock Creek Foundation programs, including the residential and day programs and the outpatient services.

9.3.3.1. Psychosocial Rehabilitation

The psychosocial rehabilitation program began as an outpatient vocational service provided to people in all of our programs as well as to those community people requesting services. When it became clear that those persons who no longer needed intensive behavioral or psychiatric services still required a structured day program as part of a continuum of services, a vocationally based psychosocial rehabilitation program was developed.

This day program is based on a traditional psychosocial rehabilitation model with certain modifications made to meet the needs of developmentally disabled clients. The rationale behind the selection of the psychosocial model was the recognition of the psychosocial aspects of the rehabilitative process as it applies to the dually diagnosed population, as well as the continued blend of mental health and mental retardation technologies necessary to address the multiple disabling conditions present.

The original psychosocial clubhouse model of clients as members with responsibility for maintenance of and programming for the clubhouse was endorsed. As the Rock Creek service system evolved toward meeting the needs of recently deinstitutionalized persons, the emphasis in the program shifted toward increasingly structured life-skills management groups, prevocational and presocialization skills group, and active psychiatric and/or behavioral programs. Although adaptations in the program structure were required, it became even more important for the staff to view the psychosocial rehabilitation program as a critical step in the continuum of services. Staff in this program had to actively avoid viewing it as a maintenance or catchall for those clients whom we began to despair of. Therefore, a deliberate decision was made to provide vocational development and work adjustment training at community sites, rather than purchasing contracts for use within the treatment facility.

These transitional employment-placement sites are built on a framework of increasing vocational autonomy along with increasing responsibility and hours at work as one moves toward vocational independence. The ultimate goal for all clients is competitive placement in the community. Competitive employment is always attained through selective employment procedures and is defined as any employment for any number of hours that a client engages in in the community for at least the minimum wage. This broad definition allows those clients who can work only one hour per week to define their jobs as competitive employment and to see these jobs as valued by themselves, by the staff, and by society. Simultaneously, by avoiding placement criteria based on production standards, the clients are not maintained for indefinite lengths of time in workshop settings, as staff seek to increase their production ratio to over 50% of competitive employment. Focusing on developing appropriate work attitudes and behaviors both increases the chance of success in the community and allows the client to develop vocational skills and productivity rates within a normal, nonstigmatized environment.

The negative aspect of this active vocational-development model is the increased effort that the staff must maintain around work adjustment training and competitive placement. The staff work alongside the clients at all transitional employment placement sites and often for the first one to two weeks after competitive placement. We have found that this step increases the chances of successful community employment and is thus worth the investment of staff time and effort.

9.3.4. Residential Services

Residential programming was begun by the Rock Creek Foundation in 1979, following a lengthy debate over whether it was appropriate for the day program provider to become the provider of residential services as well. The services were begun with some reluctance, and those concerned with replication should consider the issues carefully. The advantages of maintaining both day and residential programs are:

- Consistency of treatment and habilitation.
- An assurance that the needed psychotherapeutic or behavioral support services will be provided.
- Enhanced communication between program elements.

The disadvantages are rooted in the negative effects of having one agency with 24-hour control over the lives of the consumers. This pervasiveness is inherently nonnormalizing. For most Americans, the day environment is quite separate from the residential environment, and the person occupies different roles and exercises different behavioral patterns. Excessive consistency between the environments may impede this normal aspect of development.

On balance, however, the lack of sufficient numbers of viable community residential alternatives has resulted in the establishment and the continued growth of the Rock Creek Foundation residential program services, ranging from apartments rented by consumers with drop-in supervision to a 24-hour-a-day, seven-day-a-week intensive behavioral unit. The number of hours of supervision provided in each unit fluctuates with the needs of the residents. Movement toward less restrictive (less supervised) settings is encouraged and expected.

With the exception of the intensive behavioral unit, the residential programming content is similar to that of other mental retardation providers. Adaptive behavior is assessed, and a mix of programming is provided that compensates for skill deficits while remediating those deficits. Goals and objectives are established and reviewed quarterly. For those persons in drop-in supervision settings, the majority of the goals relate to skill maintenance; the monitoring of emotional and behavioral status is a significant function as well.

The single major difference between the Rock Creek Foundation's programming and that of most mental retardation providers is the ability to program for maladaptive behaviors within the residential setting. This is accomplished by drawing on the psychotherapeutic service of the agency. All residences with live-in staff have group counseling sessions weekly. The individual therapists are expected to assist the residential counselors in coping with maladaptive behavior. Where warranted, specific behavioral programs are developed by a consulting psychologist with the active participation of the residential staff and the individual in question. Weekly problem-solving sessions are held by the staff, with a psychotherapist in attendance to give advice and to facilitate understanding of the meaning of the behavior.

The Intensive Behavioral Unit (IBU) was begun as a pilot deinstitutionalization project. The experience of the Rock Creek Foundation has been that behaviorally disturbed persons are placed from institutions with inadequate preparation. Their maladaptive behavior precludes community acceptance but is very difficult to mediate in the institution. What was hypothesized was that a transitional community-based environment that offered controlled community integration was required.

The program serves five mentally retarded persons from either the mental retardation or the mental health institution serving the District of Columbia. Referral is made by the responsible government agency, and admission is controlled by the agency, based on the assessed prognosis given the available resources. Maladaptive behaviors are assessed, programming is developed, and transitional support is provided to ensure successful placement in a less restrictive setting.

The innovative nature of the program does not lie in its theory base or its broad program content. It simply operationalizes good behavior theory in a community-based home. Although this process is often more easily stated than practiced, the key elements to success lie in the execution of well-conceived treatment plans compiled with effective linkage to the rest of the service system.

It is this linkage and its implications that are too often absent. The targeted behaviors must relate to the next less restrictive level of programming available. As the person begins to meet the necessary criteria, transitional programming is developed and a support system is designed. The aggressive and disruptive behaviors present at admission are eliminated or significantly decreased; the transitions have begun, but as of this writing the long-term success is unknown. It does hold out the promise of a rational approach to the deinstitutionalization of this population.

9.4. Summary

The overall service system that the Rock Creek Foundation has developed is conceptualized from a matrix based on the balanced service system.[5]

The matrix divides the continuum into crisis stabilization, growth, and sustenance. *Crisis stabilization* is a descriptive label for the protective services that an individual needs because of an emotional crisis. The *growth* dimension refers to the services that we all like to provide—those that lead to skill acquisition, maturity, and general developmental progress. *Sustenance* is a recognition that we are dealing with people for whom cure is not an appropriate term. Services on the sustenance continuum consist of compensatory mechanisms to help the clients cope with long-term organic and emotional deficits.

Living environments that are sufficiently supportive are not always available and not always sufficient. In such instances, we have made effective use of mental health and mental retardation institutions, but our preference is the psychiatric ward of the general hospital. General hospitals are more a part of the community and are generally responsive to the idea of early, brief intervention—typically 3–4 days—which assists us in breaking the cycle of community placement, subsequent decompensation, loss of community placement, reinstitutionalization, and reinitiation of the cycle. As the individual progresses, services from the growth and the sustenance continuum are utilized. Many persons with whom we have worked successfully continue to be seen in weekly counseling groups or maintain their social network through the social program.

The service system developed by the Rock Creek Foundation is complex, diverse, integrated, and modular. We have attempted to help this multiply handicapped population by addressing the needs presented by each handicapping condition. This approach has required simultaneous perception of the individual served as a whole person (with diverse capabilities, desires, and handicaps) and as a discrete set of problems. Few single handicapping conditions present overwhelming difficulty in treatment. In almost all cases, we have found that the necessary technology has already been developed and tested. Some of the techniques are quite complex, and most require specialized training, yet professionals with an in-depth grasp of the requisite specialties are available.

What is difficult to find are professionals who will transcend the narrowly defined boundaries of their own disciplines. We seek professionals who will recognize that they have only part of the answer for this population and that providing the services needed requires not just cooperation between disciplines but the integration of disciplines.

The programming developed not only must reflect the handicapping conditions and the local resource base but must respond to the changing needs of the population. The structure must be sufficiently complex to contain the services needed, yet fluid enough to allow for the client's growth. The content of the programming must seek not only to impact on those conditions that are disabling but to provide mechanisms to enhance self-concept as well. Travel training may be as important to a client as psychotherapeutic intervention.

Intensity, range, and complexity are required of the service system. Too often, there appears to be roughly an inverse relationship between degree of impairment and appropriateness of deinstitutionalization program plans.[6] The difficulty of developing the service system is a reflection not only of "turf" issues among the various professionals but of the value that society ascribes to this neglected and doubly stigmatized population. It has been only through a demonstration of the efficacy of the service system that the Rock Creek Foundation has been able to impact on the attitudes of professionals, advocacy groups, parents, and concerned citizens.

ACKNOWLEDGMENT. The authors would like to acknowledge the assistance of Ron Ward, Jayne Englert-Burns, Gary Donaldson, and Nading Giani in the preparation of this chapter.

References

1. Wolfensberger W: A brief overview of the principal of normalization, in Flynn RJ, Nigsch KE (eds), *Normalization, Social Integration, and Community Services*. Baltimore, University Park Press, 1980.
2. Holzer A: *Summary of Articles Pertaining to the Placement of Institutionalized Retarded Persons into Community Settings*. Office of Policy Analysis Program Evaluation, Department of Health and Mental Hygiene, Washington, D.C., 1983. (Unpublished manuscript.)
3. Reiss S, Levitan G, McNally R: Emotionally Disturbed Mentally Retarded People: An Underserved Population. *American Psychologist*, 1982, *37*(4),361–367.
4. Brown L, Nietupski J, Hure S: The criterion of ultimate functioning in public school services for the severely handicapped, in Thomas A: *Hey, Don't Forget about Me: Education's Investment in Severely, Profoundly, and Multiply Handicapped Children*. Reston, Va, Council for Exceptional Children, 1976.
5. Melville C (ed): *The Balanced Service System*. Georgia, Mental Health Institute, February 1977.
6. Bachrach L: The conceptual approach to deinstitutionalization of the mentally retarded: A perspective from the experience of the mentally ill, in Bruininks RH, Meyers CE, Sigford BB, Lakin KC: *Deinstitutionalization and Community Adjustment of Mentally Retarded People*. Washington, D.C., American Association on Mental Deficiency, Monog. 4, 1981.
7. Hewett F: *The Emotionally Disturbed Child in the Classroom*. Boston, Allyn & Bacon, 1970.

A Model Inpatient Psychiatric Program

Its Relationship to a Continuum of Care for the Mentally Retarded-Mentally Ill

John J. McGee, Larry Folk, Donald A. Swanson, and
Frank J. Menolascino

10.1. Introduction

The purpose of this chapter is to review the needs of the mentally retarded-mentally ill and to outline the range of programs and services that persons with these needs require. The mentally retarded-mentally ill represent the last group of retarded persons in the United States to move into the mainstreams of family and community life. They present multiple programmatic and environmental challenges. Their needs are often poorly identified. Services to meet their needs are few, and professionals often refer them from agency to agency because they fall between the cracks of most current human-service systems.

In this chapter, we first identify the psychiatric dimensions of mental retardation through an analysis of the needs of 305 mentally retarded-mentally ill individuals and outline the range of programs and services that this population requires. Recent studies confirm the fact that 25%–35% of the mentally retarded have associated signs and symptoms of mental illness.[1–6] The dual diagnosis of mental retardation and mental illness presents unique clinical and programmatic challenges to professionals in the fields of mental retardation and mental health. These challenges are further heightened by the escalating integration of mentally retarded children and adults into the mainstreams of family and community life.[7] As retarded persons are served in public schools, group homes and sheltered workshops, and other community-based programs, professionals are confronted with the challenge of serving persons who are not only mentally retarded but also mentally ill.

John J. McGee • Department of Psychiatry, Nebraska Psychiatric Institute and Meyer Children's Rehabilitation Institute, University of Nebraska Medical Center, Omaha, Nebraska 68105.   *Larry Folk* • Mental Health Coordinator, Dual Diagnosis Service, Nebraska Psychiatric Institute, University of Nebraska Medical Center, Omaha, Nebraska 68105.   *Donald A. Swanson* • Department of Psychiatry, Nebraska Psychiatric Institute, University of Nebraska Medical Center, Omaha, Nebraska 68105.   *Frank J. Menolascino* • Departments of Psychiatry and Pediatrics, Nebraska Psychiatric Institute, University of Nebraska Medical Center, Omaha, Nebraska 68105.

10.2. The Psychiatric Dimensions of Mental Retardation

When the lives of mentally retarded persons are further compounded by allied psychiatric disorders, their integration into community life becomes a dual challenge. In order to determine the range of programs and services necessary to meet the needs of the mentally retarded-mentally ill, it is first important to review the types and frequency of psychiatric disorders found in the mentally retarded. Therefore, in the initial part of this chapter, we report the findings of a recent study of 305 mentally retarded persons with coexisting mental illness. This study was conducted in an acute-care psychiatric unit at the Nebraska Psychiatric Institute. This unit provides backup support to Nebraska's community-based mental retardation programs and institutions for the mentally retarded.

From June 1979 through December 1981, 305 persons with a dual diagnosis were seen. Each was individually evaluated by an interdisciplinary team. The study group ranged in age from 3 to 76 years. Those aged 5 and under represented 1.6% of the study group; age 6–10 years comprised 2.6%; age 11–15, 8.8%; age 16–20, 23.2%; age 21–25, 20.6%; age 26–30, 10.8%; age 31–35, 9%; and over 36, 22.9%. The group was 66% male because of a disproportionately large number of adolescent males. For all other age groups, males and females were found in approximately equal numbers. Diagnoses in this sample were based primarily on DSM-III criteria. The types of psychiatric disorders and their frequency are seen in Table 1. The psychiatric disorders in their order of frequency were (1) schizophrenic disorders, 29%; (2) organic brain disorders, 19.6%; (3) adjustment disorders, 16.3%; (4) nonspecific mental disorders, 13.1%; (5) personality disorders, 10.8%; (6) affective disorders, 6.5%; (7) neurotic disorders, 2.2%; and (8) special symptoms, 1.3%.

10.2.1. Schizophrenia

The 88 patients in the study group with schizophrenia included 39 with undifferentiated schizophrenia; 7 displayed schizoaffective schizophrenia; 13 patients displayed paranoid schizophrenia; 6 patients displayed catatonic schizophrenia; and 23 patients displayed residual schizophrenia. Schizophrenia remains the most frequently reported type of major mental illness in mentally retarded individuals.[8]

Psychotic reactions of childhood have presented a major challenge to the clinician since their early recognition as distinct entities by DeSanctis in 1906. Delineation of types of etiologies has been delayed, in part, by the fact that psychotic children frequently function at a mentally retarded level, and early observers believed that all psychotic children "deteriorated." In 1943, "early infantile autism" was described by Kanner.[9] Yet, to label a child *autistic* introduces some formidable problems with regard to diagnosis and treatment. A number of follow-up studies,[10,11] coupled with the rediscovery of the wide variety of primitive behavioral repertoires in the retarded, have tended to mute

Table 1. Mental Illness in the Mentally Retarded ($N = 305$)[a]

Psychiatric Diagnoses	1–5	6–10	11–15	16–20	21–25	26–30	31–35	Over 36	Totals
Organic brain disorders									
Organic brain syndrome									
Psychotic reaction	1			1	7	4		2	15
Behavioral reaction		3	11	1	11		7	3	36
Presenile dementia							3	7	10
									61
Schizophrenic disorders									
Catatonic	1			3		1		1	6
Chronic paranoid				9				4	13
Schizoaffective				1	5		1		7
Chronic undiff.				12	4	8	3	12	39
Residual					5			18	23
									88
Affective disorders									
Unipolar manic disorder				3	2				5
Bipolar affective								2	2
Depressive disorder					1	1		1	3
Unspecified			3	1		2		4	10
									20
Neurotic disorders									
Anxiety				1					1
Depression				1	1		2	2	6
									7
Personality disorders									
Schizoid				1	3				4
Explosive						1	1		2
Passive-dependent				1		2		2	4
Narcissistic						2	3	1	6
Avoidant				1	1			1	3
Passive-aggressive				3	3		5	2	13
Unspecified				1					1
									33
Special symptoms									
Anorexia nervosa		1	3						4
									4
Adjustment reactions									
Childhood and adol.	3	2	6	23					34
Adulthood					6	3	3	4	16
									50
Nonspecific mental disorders									
Pervasive developmental			1	4	1				6
Disturbance of conduct		1	2	4	9	8	2	2	28
Undersoc.-aggressive			1		4	1		2	8
									42

[a] A review of retarded patients at NPI: June, 1979 through December, 1981

the earlier clinical enthusiasm concerning the functional psychoses and their interrelationships with mental retardation.

In this study, it was noted that 25 adolescent patients displayed indices of both mental retardation and schizophrenia—the latter having been noted since very early in life. For example, there was a striking presence of bizarre behavior, persistent withdrawal, echolalic speech, and affective unavailability in early adolescents who had clearly experienced regressive symptomatology from an earlier higher level of functioning. Three of these adolescents illustrated the superimposition of childhood schizophrenia (i.e., by past history, the schizophrenic illness in all three had begun between ages 4 and 6) on etiologically clear instances of mental retardation (e.g., one had Down's syndrome, one was postrubella, and the third had a major cranial malformation as the cause of his mental retardation). Because the treatment guidelines are markedly different for youngsters with "autistic" reactions to extremely bewildering extrinsic circumstances, and the combined mental retardation–childhood schizophrenia syndrome noted herein, this differential diagnosis is therapeutically significant beyond academic interests.

Although some clinicians seriously question whether the markedly primitive behaviors noted at certain levels of mental retardation (e.g., severe level with associated poor language evolution) can be separated from schizophrenia, this was not our experience. Significantly, the instances of paranoid schizophrenia were noted in both verbal and nonverbal patients. Included in our sample of the latter were three adults who drew out on paper their "attackers," replete with nonverbal gestures. One such young man would label his separate fingers as the "source" of his common delusions, which he would portray symbolically in crude drawings. Paranoid and catatonic features were the hallmarks of the acute/chronic undifferentiated schizophrenic groups. In the entire group of combined diagnoses of mental retardation and schizophrenia, it was noted that the altered affect responses, hallucinatory phenomena, bizarre rituals, and utilization of interpersonal distancing devices clearly marked the observed behaviors as being in the schizophrenic repertoire.

10.2.2. Organic Brain Syndrome

The diagnosis of organic brain syndrome (OBS) with a behavioral or psychotic disorder has been descriptively delineated in previous studies of these disorders in the retarded.[12] In the present study, the criterion for this diagnosis was evidence of an organic brain syndrome by mental status and physical-neurological examinations and/or a personal-clinical history of etiologically significant factors. The diagnosis of *OBS with behavioral reaction* was utilized for the subgroup who displayed inappropriate acting-out behaviors against a backdrop of delayed/disorganized personality figures (e.g., emotional lability, impulsivity, and frequent tantrums, but no psychotic symptoms). The subgroup with evidence of *OBS and psychotic reactions* presented a clinical picture different from schizophrenia because (1) the underlying *OBS* signs and symptoms of the disorder were prominent; (2) their out-of-contact behaviors—though the diagnostic hallmark of their presenting picture—were not the type commonly seen in schizophrenia (e.g., no hallucinatory experiences); and (3) their personality structures did not show the progressive involvement of multiple segments of functioning that is characteristic of schizophrenia. Based on these criteria, 20% of the study group was found to have OBS with behavioral or psychotic reactions.

10.2.3. Personality Disorders

Personality disorders are characterized by chronically maladaptive patterns of behavior (e.g., antisocial personality and passive-aggressive personality), which are qualitatively different from psychotic or neurotic disorders (DSM-III, 1980). Studies reported in the early history of retardation tended indiscriminately to view antisocial behavior as an expected behavioral accompaniment to mental retardation.[13] The antisocial personality designation continues to receive much attention and is frequently overrepresented in mildly retarded individuals. It would appear that behavioral problems of an antisocial nature are more frequently seen in this group because the same poverty of interpersonal relationships during childhood that leads to many cases of retardation tends also to lead to impaired object relations and poorly internalized controls.[14] Likewise, it leads to a reduced frequency of consistent parental and societal expectations and to a higher frequency of poor role models. The diminished coping skills of this group often necessitate their performing deviant acts simply to exist, and reduced judgment makes the acts more ego-syntonic. Finally, this group is most likely to be released from institutional settings in young adulthood and to illustrate graphically the effects of institutional detachment on the development of early personality structure.

It is interesting to note that although other personality disorders (e.g., schizoid personality) have been reported in the retarded, we noted this disorder in only four patients. Another personality disorder in the retarded that has received much attention is the "inadequate personality," even though the application of exact diagnostic criteria would exclude this disorder as a primary diagnosis in mental retardation. In our experience, these personality disorders occur in mentally retarded individuals whose behavior is based primarily on extrinsic factors and has no distinct etiological relationship(s) to the symptoms of mental retardation. The presence of personality disorders in 9% of our sample suggests that this group of disorders is not an infrequent accompanying psychiatric handicap for mentally retarded citizens.

10.2.4. Neurotic Disorders (Anxiety Disorders)

Earlier reviews[15] on this type of mental illness in the retarded suggested that its frequency was quite low. Interestingly, these reports suggest that neurotic disorders are more common in individuals in the high-moderate and mild levels of mental retardation and have prompted speculation as to whether the relative complexity of psychoneurotic transaction is beyond the adaptive limits of the more severely retarded. However, recent studies[12,16] disputing the concept of incompatability between the neuroses and retardation are quite explicit with respect to diagnostic criteria and attribute the neurotic phenomena to factors associated with atypical developmental patterns in conjunction with disturbed family functioning. For example, neurotic disorders in retarded children clearly link symptoms of anxiety (e.g., fear of failure and insecurity) to exogenous factors such as chronic frustration, unrealistic family expectations, and persistent interpersonal deprivation. These reported findings are not consistent with our experience of noting only seven mentally retarded individuals with neurosis.

10.2.5. Adjustment Disorders (of Childhood, Adolescence, or Adulthood)

Although this category of psychiatric disorders is perhaps overutilized in the assessment of the nonretarded, it is only infrequently employed during the clinical assessment of mental illness in the retarded population. In one study, one of the highest frequencies of psychiatric disorders was noted to be the adjustment disorders: 16.3% of the total sample. Mentally retarded individuals, because of their frequency of organic predisposition to overreacting to stimuli and their limited understanding of social-interpersonal expectations, are highly "at risk" for personality disorganization secondary to minimal interpersonal stress. In our experience, these adjustment reactions are most frequently caused by continuing inappropriate social-adaptive expectations or unexpected and frequent changes in externally imposed life patterns. Clinically, they respond rapidly to environmental adjustment (when coupled with specific counseling to realign the parental or the residential and educational personnel's unrealistic expectations or goals) and to supportive psychotherapy.

As more retarded persons remain in or return to the community, adjustment problems are appearing at a higher frequency than previously noted. Their presence in the community reveals a tendency for some retarded persons to have extreme difficulty in life changes. With the more severely retarded, even changes in classroom or teacher, movements from one group home to another, staff turnover, and so on can elicit serious adjustment problems.

10.3. The Dual Diagnosis

10.3.1. Levels of Mental Retardation

All levels of mental retardation were seen in this study group—from severe-profound retardation to mild retardation. Although the presence of the previously noted range of psychiatric disorders in the nonretarded population presents multiple clinical and programmatic challenges, these challenges are compounded when occurring in the mentally retarded. Table 2 depicts the incidence of psychiatric disorders as found in the different levels of retardation in our sample.

Table 2. Level of Mental Retardation in Mentally Retarded–
Mentally Ill Population Sample ($N = 305$)

Mild	55.7%
Moderate	25.3%
Severe-profound	19.0%

Each level of mental retardation presents special challenges in the diagnosis and treatment of the mentally retarded-mentally ill. The study group represented not only the entire range of psychiatric disorders, but also all levels of retardation. Whereas previous studies have focused on institutionalized retarded persons, who are generally in the more severe range of retardation, our study represents the entire spectrum of mental retardation.

10.3.2. Severe-Profound Mental Retardation

The severely retarded are characterized by gross CNS impairment and a high frequency of multiple handicaps, especially sensory impairments and seizure disorders. This population has a high vulnerability to psychiatric disorders.[17] The moderately retarded likewise present marked vulnerabilities for adequate personality development because of their slower rate of development and their need to problem-solve through concrete approaches. Webster[18] viewed the personality vulnerabilities of the moderately retarded as stemming from the interpersonal postures that the moderately retarded tend to use in their interpersonal transactions. These encompass selective isolation (benign autism), inflexibility and repetiousness, passivity, and a simplicity in their emotional life. The mildly retarded present other challenges because of their difficulty in understanding the symbolic abstractions of schoolwork and the complexities of the social-adaptive expectations of their family and peer groups.

Besides the vulnerability of the mentally retarded to mental health problems because of their level of mental retardation, other developmental disorders often cause breakdowns in their ability to participate in ongoing interpersonal and social transactions. A major allied developmental problem centers on the inability of the retarded person to process information from the world around him or her and the inability to express basic needs and emotions. Nearly all of the mentally retarded-mentally ill persons cited in Table 1 had severe language and communication disorders—in terms of both receptive and expressive language.

A major cause of the vulnerability of the retarded, especially the more severely retarded, to mental illness is their inability to process information from the world around them. Persons with more severe retardation are often overstimulated by external stimuli and react to this overstimulation through a range of primitive behaviors that can take the form of self-abusive, aggressive, or self-stimulatory behaviors. In a sense, these behaviors are forms of communication—nonverbal ways of responding to an otherwise confusing world.

Table 3. Other Developmental Disabilities in Mentally Retarded–
Mentally Ill Population Sample

Associated medical or developmental disabilities	
Cerebral palsy	12
Grand mal epilepsy	42
Psychomotor epilepsy	8
Petit mal epilepsy (minor form)	8
Petit mal epilepsy (major; myoclonic)	10
Acute otitis media	11
Congenital deafness	8
Diabetes mellitus	6
Hypothyroidism	8

The moderately and mildly retarded also present allied challenges in the area of language and communication—however, in a more subtle manner. They typically possess language and are able to verbalize their needs and emotions. Yet, these verbalizations are often deceptive in that they can mask the full depth of interpersonal and intrapersonal distress.

It is crucial to take into account the impact of these communication disorders in assessing the needs of the mentally retarded-mentally ill. The observed behavioral disorders of the mentally retarded should be considered in light of their likely communication and language disorders.

Another crucial factor to consider is the range of allied medical disorders often found in this population. Table 3 outlines the major allied medical disorders found in the aforementioned study of mentally retarded-mentally ill patients at the Nebraska Psychiatric Institute. Thirty-seven percent had major medical disorders on admission for treatment.

The major allied medical problem stemmed from seizure disorders: over 22 percent of the persons studied had ongoing seizure disorders (i.e., their disorders included petit mal, grand mal, Jacksonian, and psychomotor types of seizure disorders). These disorders tend to compound and exacerbate the problems inherent in both mental retardation and mental illness and often leave the person in a frequent postseizure confused state and thus periodically incapable of interpersonal and intrapersonal transactions.

10.3.3. Conclusion

The mentally retarded are vulnerable to the entire range of psychiatric disorders. Mental retardation itself, at its various levels, presents unique problems in terms of the person's ability to process information and to respond to and cope with stress. Furthermore, the occurrence of allied medical problems, especially seizure disorders, further compounds the treatment challenges.

Because of the nature of the dual diagnosis, it is necessary to define and provide a continuum of care to meet the chronic and acute needs of the mentally

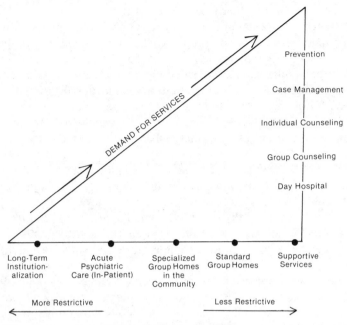

Figure 1. Continuum of care.

retarded-mentally ill during their lives. In the next section of this chapter, we outline such a continuum of programs and services.

10.4. A Continuum of Care

The mentally retarded-mentally ill present a unique range of psychiatric and developmental needs across their life span—as indicated in the previous section. To determine the types of programs and services that this population requires, it is helpful to focus on the range of residential and developmental programs that can help the mentally retarded-mentally ill become integrated into the mainstream of community life. A continuum of care must be able to respond to the needs of the mentally retarded-mentally ill, at any given point in their lives, with whatever programs and services are necessary to maintain them in or to return them to the mainstream of family and community life. It is necessary to develop a range of direct services such as acute care and specialized group homes, as well as a range of supportive services such as counseling and case management. Figure 1 depicts a suggested continuum of the residental alternatives needed to meet the residential needs of this population.

10.4.1. Long-Term Institutionalization

A very small percentage of mentally retarded-mentally ill persons require long-term hospitalization. The primary criterion for such a placement is that the person poses a chronic threat to himself or herself or to others. In the data in Table 1, there are six patients who for the above reasons were institutionalized. The specific reasons for such hospitalization centered around unpredictable aggressive behaviors and/or self-injurious behaviors, as well as in sexually deviant behaviors such as repeated child molestation. Of the six persons represented in Table 1 for whom long-term institutionalization was recommended, the following were the primary reasons: suicide attempts, child molestation, and violently aggressive behaviors. It should be kept in mind that these disorders represent an extremely small percentage of the population, 6 out of 305 persons.

Besides these person-specific reasons, institutions play a sociopolitical role in meeting the developmental and emotional needs of other retarded persons. Because it is only recently that communities have started to develop programs and services for the mentally retarded-mentally ill, many communities can serve this population in terms of neither the quantity nor the quality of services required. In the foreseeable future, some retarded persons with mental illness will remain institutionalized or will be admitted to institutions.

Whether these people are institutionalized for clinical or sociopolitical reasons, institutions can play a significant role in meeting their needs through the structure they provide and the preparation of each person for her or his eventual integration into community life. The rate and speed of this integration will depend largely on the development of adequate and appropriate community alternatives.

10.4.2. Acute Psychiatric Care—Inpatient

A vital issue in the continuum of care is the ability to meet the acute psychiatric needs of the mentally retarded, for example, treating persons with acute psychiatric symptomatology such as aggressive or self-injurious behaviors, withdrawal, or hallucinatory behaviors. In the proposed continuum, this service is provided through an inpatient, acute psychiatric care with services capable of treating psychotic symptomatology and behaviors such as hyperactivity, self-abusive, aggressive acts, and withdrawal. The mentally retarded, like any other citizen, should have access to acute psychiatric care. At the same time, this service should be specialized to meet the unique needs of retarded persons.

10.4.3. The Nebraska Psychiatric Institute Model

An example of an acute-care psychiatric service is the Mental Retardation Unit[19] of the Nebraska Psychiatric Institute (NPI), which serves as Nebraska's primary acute-care facility for the mentally retarded-mentally ill. In 1979, NPI established a six-bed inpatient unit to focus on this population. In 1981, NPI expanded its services to the mentally retarded-mentally ill by opening an adjacent specialized unit—increasing the total bed commitment to 15 (out of NPI's 85-bed facility). The primary purpose of this unit is to meet the acute psychiatric needs of the mentally retarded-mentally ill. A special team of professionals and paraprofessionals was identified to focus on the population to provide treatment and to act as a backup support for this population.

During the retarded patient's hospitalization in NPI (which lasts an average of 35 days), the primary treatment goal consists of decreasing interfering behaviors to a level where each person can be integrated back into appropriate residential, vocational, educational, and leisure activities in the community. There is an intense focus on redirecting and then substituting appropriate behaviors for the presenting abnormal, atypical, or premature behaviors through a closely scheduled, active, and developmentally oriented treatment day. Individual psychotherapy, educational therapy, individualized occupational and recreational therapy—all are utilized in conjunction with active family (or alternative caretaker) involvement. Concurrent with this central treatment approach is the judicious utilization of psychoactive medications as a treatment adjunct for initially assisting each person to become more actively engaged in appropriate psychosocial and developmental activities. Rather than focusing unduly on the role of psychoactive medications—a professional posture for which psychiatry has been frequently criticized—the *adjunctive* role of these medications is stressed in the overall treatment approach.

The careful selection, training, and attention to the administration of the programmatic personnel on this special unit is important. Primary professional personnel include (1) a clinical psychiatrist with a long history of involvement in the psychiatric aspects of mental retardation; (2) a part-time clinical psychopharmacologist; (3) a charge nurse; (4) three shift nurses; (5) a consistent paraprofessional-to-patient staffing with the capacity for one-to-one staffing when necessary; (6) an on-staff community liaison person; (7) a part-time social worker; and (8) a part-time psychologist. Specially trained personnel, as well as any other necessary resources, are utilized on a daily scheduled basis.

An important aspect of an acute care service is to define its role as a backup support to other programs and services. This role primarily consists of (1) acute psychiatric care; (2) crisis intervention; (3) parent training; (4) staff training; (5) program monitoring; (6) medication monitoring; and (7) public education. Though these foci are *not* "new" in the contemporary treatment–management approaches for the mentally ill, they *are* rarely utilized for the mentally retarded-mentally ill population.

10.4.4. Specialized Group Homes

Once a retarded person's acute needs are met, it is necessary to provide a transition for the person into community living, through specialized, community-based group homes. For most persons, these specialized group homes can be short-term (three to six months); for some, they are long-term (two to three years).

A specialized group home for the mentally retarded-mentally ill has as its goals the stabilization of the person's behaviors in a community setting and the gradual integration of the person into community life. A specialized group home is characterized by the following features.

10.4.4.1. Structure

The group home structures the person's day based on his or her current ability to attend to appropriate tasks and interactions. It utilizes the normal flow of the day (self-care and independent-living skills) as the mechanism for redirecting and reinforcing the person toward appropriate tasks and interactions.

10.4.4.2. Staffing Intensity and Flexibility

The group home provides a staffing pattern sufficient to meet the developmental-behavioral needs of each person. Initially, some persons may require one-to-one staffing. This is provided and then faded down to a three-to-one ratio as soon as possible.

10.4.4.3. Client Mix

The group home is careful to match the small group (three to six persons) living together so that the group is as compatible as possible. Even though all the residents are mentally retarded-mentally ill, the individualized mix of clients prevents inappropriate grouping such as a disproportionate mix of nonverbal clients, acting-out clients, self-injurious clients, and so on.

10.4.4.4. Developmental Orientation

The group home provides a teaching atmosphere. It is recognized that each person, regardless of the severity of the dual diagnosis, is capable of change over time. Each person has an individualized program plan. The initial goal is to gain instructional control over maladaptive behaviors (e.g., self-abusive, self-stimulatory, aggressive, or avoidant behaviors) through a constant and consistent redirection of those behaviors and a subsequent reinforcement of appropriate behaviors and interactions.

10.4.4.5. Behavioral Analysis Orientation

The group home bases itself primarily on the technology of applied behavioral analysis, especially with a particular focus on the gaining of appropriate behaviors. Behavioral procedures focus on the acquisition of appropriate behaviors rather than on the elimination of maladaptive behaviors.

10.4.4.6. Balanced Use of Psychoactive Medications

The group home uses psychoactive medications as an adjunct to developmental-behavioral programming. Medications are used only as a means to initially bring the person's interfering behaviors to the point where developmental programming can take over. As this occurs, medications are reduced or eliminated.

10.4.4.7. Comprehensiveness

The group home is part of a continuum of services that enable movement into less restrictive, less structured residential alternatives, as well as movement into acute care when necessary.

10.4.4.8. Consistency with Day Programs

The group home functions in coordination with educational and vocational day programs so that each person is assured of a full developmentally oriented program. All day programs are outside the group home.

10.4.4.9. Stability

The group home generally is short-term (three to six months). Most clients then move into less structured residential alternatives. However, for some persons, the group home may become a more long-term placement (up to two or three years) in order to provide the stability, the relationship building, and the time that the person needs to acquire the skills necessary to live in a less structured setting.

10.4.5. Other Community-Based Alternatives

Once the mentally retarded-mentally ill person's acute and subacute psychiatric needs are controlled and stabilized, a community should be able to respond to his or her needs with a range of less restrictive and less structured alternatives. These should take the form of group homes that serve the general retarded population, foster homes, support for the person in his or her natural family, and so on. As this movement occurs, the continuum of care should ensure that adequate supportive services will exist in the community so that the person's mental-health needs are met on an ongoing basis. Supportive services consist of (1) day hospitals that are capable of assisting the retarded person in his or her transition back into and maintenance in the mainstream of community life[20]; individual and group counseling to deal with ongoing behavioral-emotional problems[20-22]; and (3) case management services to ensure appropriate program planning, coordination, and monitoring.[23]

An emerging trend on the part of mental health programs is the provision of day hospital services for the mentally retarded-mentally ill. Fletcher[20] described one such day-treatment program as a specialized treatment program within a community health center. Its goal is to provide an opportunity for mentally ill-mentally retarded adults to participate in a combination of clinical, prevocational, social, and recreational services. This particular day-treatment program meets the needs of its clients in a part-time program (one or two days per week) while the clients continue in their vocational and residential community-based mental-retardation programs. Support to the clients is provided through a series of structured group activities: group therapy, horticultural therapy, community meetings, music therapy, educational support, and so on. Fletcher[20] reported measured increases in positive feelings about the self, more involvement in socialization activities, improved impulse control, and more effective problem-solving.

Along with the aforementioned supportive services, it is necessary to have a continuum of supportive educational services and leisure-time activities so that the person is as engaged as possible in family and community life. The residential alternatives need to work in close coordination with the person's public school, a sheltered workshop, or other vocational placement. Likewise, they need to involve the person as much as possible in the community's social-recreational life.

10.4.6. An Example of a Comprehensive Community-Based Service System

The Eastern Nebraska Community Office of Retardation (ENCOR) is a community-based mental-retardation program located in eastern Nebraska within a rural-urban population base of approximately 500,000 inhabitants.[12] It provides an array of residential, educational, vocational, and support services to 1,045 mentally retarded persons. Its residential alternatives include over 25 group homes (with no more than six residents per home) and over 200 foster homes. All school-aged children are in local public schools. Retarded adults are served in a range of vocational training alternatives, including a prevocational training center, five sheltered workshops, six work-stations-in-industry, and independent employment. There is also a variety of social-recreational activities through the use of community agencies such as churches, camps and the YMCA.

ENCOR serves the general retarded population as well as persons with the dual diagnosis of mental retardation and mental illness. Its clients represent all levels of mental retardation from mild to severe, as well as the entire range of psychiatric disorders. The population includes clients who have been institutionalized and those who have never been institutionalized. ENCOR, like most other community-based service systems, serves the vast majority of the mentally retarded–emotionally disturbed in nonspecialized services, for they do not require extraordinary programmatic services and supports. However, a certain percentage require specialized supports and services because of the severity and the complexity of their dual diagnosis.

In April 1982, the authors examined the records of the 1,045 ENCOR clients to determine the number of mentally retarded persons who presented significant programmatic challenges. This survey classified ENCOR clients into three levels:

1. Level 1—Clients who presented daily high-frequency behavioral-management problems such as the inability to attend to tasks, self-abusive behaviors, aggressive behaviors, and hyperactivity.

Table 4. Mentally Retarded–Mentally Ill Persons Requiring Specialized Services in ENCOR

Service	Number	Ages				Types of services				
		0–5	6–21	22–50	50+	School	Vocational training	Group home	Residential Foster home	Family
Urban areas	55	2	14	34	5	13	42	37	10	8
Rural areas	26	0	1	24	1	1	25	22	4	0
Total	81	2	15	58	6	14	67	59	14	8

   2. Level 2—Clients who presented occasional behavioral problems per month.
   3. Level 3—Clients who presented behavioral problems on several occasions throughout the year.

This study identified 81 ENCOR clients within these three levels who presented programmatic challenges significant enough to warrant specialized supports and services. These specialized supports and services included the type of personnel treating this population, staffing patterns and intensity, the need for backup supports such as special consultants, and the availability of acute psychiatric-care services. Table 4 shows the number of persons with these special needs by level and by service catchment areas (divided into urban or rural areas).

This population of 81 mentally retarded-mentally ill clients within the ENCOR service system is capable of being served in community-based settings if given adequate treatment supports. Table 4 also displays the types of residential, educational, and vocational services that these 81 persons receive. They are rather evenly dispersed across the five-county urban-rural ENCOR catchment area.

It is important to note that mentally retarded-mentally ill persons of all ages and levels of mental illness can be served in a community-based service system. The 81 persons served in the ENCOR program represent the entire range of psychiatric disorders and present a myriad of programmatic and treatment challenges. Table 5 outlines the primary symptom clusters and etiologies represented in this identified group.

Different programmatic and treatment modalities are based on the intensity and types of behavioral-emotional problems presented. For example, a client who displays high-intensity self-abusive behavior requires a service modality distinct from a mildly retarded person who displays aggressive behaviors only a few times per year. The self-abusive person might require acute psychiatric care to rapidly decrease such behaviors, followed by a specialized transactional group-home setting. The person with occasional aggressive behaviors might require only a highly structured group-home setting with well-trained paraprofessional staff and periodic psychiatric follow-along.

Table 5. Cluster of Acute, Subacute, and Chronic Psychiatric Needs

Symptom cluster	Etiology
1. Tense, insomnia, and fearful of any interpersonal changes.	Adjustment disorders of adolescence.
2. Hyperkinetic, impulsive, increased irritability, excessive focus on self, many instances of self-stimulatory behaviors (e.g., head banging) and primitive behaviors (e.g., pica). Out-of-control behaviors are noted on minimal stress.	Organic brain syndrome with psychotic reactions.
3. Withdrawn, passive and excessively sensitive to others.	Personality trait disorder.
4. Periodically delusional with minimal stress with paranoid features.	Personality pattern disorder.
5. Hallucinations, bizarre behaviors, out of contact with reality.	Functional psychoses (e.g., schizophrenia).
6. Insensitivity to the needs of others, manipulative, demanding, and extremely self-centered.	Antisocial personality.

In the ENCOR program, the following specific factors aid in serving this challenging population:

1. Acute psychiatric care is available for the small percentage of clients who require it on any given day. Out of the 1,045 mentally retarded persons in ENCOR, two to four persons require acute psychiatric care in a hospital setting for an average of 35 days. This service need is met through the use of generic psychiatric hospitals in the community.

2. Specialized group homes are designed to provide a transition for persons with subacute behavioral needs into less intensive residential settings. These group homes serve no more than six persons. Care is taken to ensure a compatible mixture of persons within each group. Staff are specially trained to deal with the behavioral needs of the residents. Essential backup support is available, as well as follow-up services from professionals in generic agencies in the community.

3. All clients are served in community-based day programs, that is, public schools and sheltered workshops with necessary supportive services.

4. Practicum training is provided to all paraprofessional staff and/or parents in the area of behavior management as needed. Staffing patterns are higher in these programs (typically one staff for every two clients) until behaviors are brought under control. All staff are regarded as teachers—with the primary responsibility of gaining control over the behaviors through nonaversive techniques.

The types of programs in which these persons participate are the same as those available to all other retarded persons: group homes, public schools, sheltered workshops, and so on. Staff are specifically trained to deal with high aggressive or self-abusive behaviors. Individualized services are well monitored by ENCOR caseworkers, and where necessary, secondary support services are called upon, such as special consultative services or hospitalization for acute care. These services typically cost nearly half of the amount of long-term institutionalization and at the same time provide maximum developmental benefits such as dramatic decreases in maladaptive behaviors, the acquisition of appropriate behaviors, and the integration of persons with these special needs into the mainstreams of family and community life.

The ENCOR model demonstrates that (1) the mentally retarded-mentally ill can be served in dispersed residential, educational, and vocational settings; (2) there is a need to specialize staff and programs to meet the unique needs of this population; (3) it is important to have a range of services and backup supports available; (4) initial staffing patterns need to be flexible; and (5) the availability of inpatient, acute psychiatric care is an important dimension in the continuum of care.

10.5. Treatment Issues

10.5.1. Introduction

Within the framework of the continuum of care, it is important to define a general treatment approach that will enable the mentally retarded-mentally ill to enter into or to remain in the mainstream of community life to the maximum extent possible. The general treatment approach recommended for this population encompasses several factors:

1. The professionals' postures toward this population.
2. A nonpunitive behavioral analysis orientation.
3. A total educational-vocational-communication approach.
4. A balanced approach between the use of psychoactive medications and the use of behavioral programming.
5. Programmatic flexibility.

10.5.2. Professional Posture

Community programs can adequately, appropriately, and developmentally serve even the most severely involved mentally retarded children and adults. The ENCOR program demonstrates this.[7] Services for the dual-diagnosis population can be characterized in the following manner: (1) they are concrete, comprehensive, replicable, development-oriented programs; (2) they are ensured across the person's lifespan based on the degree and intensity of services required by each individual; (3) they are small, no more than six persons being housed in any given setting; (4) the various programs and services are dispersed throughout the community in a well-managed service-delivery system; and (5) personnel resources are derived from and trained in the local community with adequate medical and psychiatric backup.

Community-based alternatives must be able to ensure mentally retarded persons and their families that there will be (1) a variety of community-based, less restrictive options utilizing modern treatment and programmatic techniques in small, dispersed residential, educational, vocational, and leisure-time services; (2) maximum parental input while still ensuring the individual client's rights; (3) ongoing internal and external monitoring of the quality of services; (4) a realistic cost per person for services and assurance that program financing will be continued across time; and (5) prudent risk for all mentally retarded citizens as they live, work, and play in communities, while at the same time safeguarding each person as much as necessary.

Professionals must first review and redefine their posture toward these children and adults—a posture built on developmental hopefulness, gentleness, and warmth. It is helpful for the professional to consider the creation of an *initial* passively dependent (or at least physically tolerant) relationship with each person. More severely retarded persons with severe behavior problems need to develop an initial passive-dependent relationship with the professional, which then tends to usher in an increasingly dynamic relationship between the professional and the person served. As this relationship develops, the secondary purpose becomes one of sequentially leading the person to a variety of learning-readiness opportunities, which we term the *threshold of learning*. This initial receptivity to developmental interactions gradually, but invariably, leads to control over the person's behaviors (self-abuse, aggression, self-stimulation, avoidance) and hence expands opportunities for advanced interactions within ever-increasing circles of interpersonal transactions. The professional needs to develop, in a persistent and stepwise fashion, a sequential (i.e., from obtaining eye contact to focusing attention on tasks) and a directional (i.e., from simple to more complex tasks) series of developmental interactions over a six- to eight-week period of time. In the beginning, these complex mentally retarded persons tend to "win" most of the interpersonal transactions via obstinacy, refusal to sit, screaming, striking self or others, running away, or indiscriminately throwing objects. The person initially attempts to maintain and even increase the barriers between himself or herself and the interacting professional, who represents an intrusion of the chaotic external world. The professional must understand this initial stage of rebellion against "outside" interference and must energetically continue to attempt to engage the person in a series of concrete, specific developmental activities. At the same time, the professional needs to tolerate—in a passively supportive, but firm, professional posture—the initial barrage of heightened inappropriate behaviors. These heightened maladaptive behaviors, rather than representing volitionally destructive or aggressive acts, are the mentally retarded person's basic protective mechanisms for coping with a world that has, prior to active treatment intervention, presented itself as quite meaningless and unresponsive. This initial interactive relationship (i.e., making initial meaningful contact) can best be achieved through a constant and sincere display of warmth, tolerance, and uncritical acceptance on the part of the caregiver.[24]

Behavioral specialists often tend to apply the principles of behavioral analysis in both a lock step and a negative fashion. This population requires flexibility and gentleness in all treatment procedures. If one is to maintain the aforementioned positive interpersonal posture and to create a dynamic relationship of predictability and trust with the retarded person, aversive behavioral modification techniques should be avoided. Rather than punishing this population for behaviors that are not of their own volition, a threefold, gentle technique should be employed when persistently inappropriate behaviors occur: (1) ignore; (2) redirect; and (3) positively reinforce (see Chapter 7). All three of these steps are needed simultaneously. For example, while ignoring fidgetiness and concomitant screaming, the professional should redirect the child by gently taking the person's hand and performing the requested task hand-over-hand with the person. This technique allows the professional an ongoing opportunity to positively reinforce the child. This does not mean that professionals completely ignore the maladaptive behaviors. Rather it means the focus is on the acquisition of appropriate skills and interactions. The person gradually learns that he or she will gain attention (i.e., positive rewards) for appropriate behaviors and interactions and, conversely, will regularly be ignored for maladaptive behaviors or interactions.

10.5.3. Programmatic Flexibility

The overall posture of uncritical acceptance and use of redirecting techniques must also be reflected in the type of general program in which the child or adult is served. Generally, these persons require six to eight weeks of intensive developmental programming before behavioral control is achieved to the extent necessary to integrate these children or adolescents into a less structured, normalizing program. The goal mechanism for accomplishing this aim is to develop a highly structured program (i.e., utilizing one-to-one staffing for at least 200 minutes per day) for the initial treatment-intervention time period.[24] This intense treatment programming gains control over the offending behaviors and progressively leads the person to the threshold of learning. Professionals need to divide the person's day into time modules ranging from 10 to 30 minutes, depending on the retarded person's ability to attend. Within these time modules, a series of developmental tasks is programmed. These minitime modules can be fairly normalizing in that they follow the normal flow of the day: self-care skills, academic skills, prevocational skills, communication skills, eating skills, and so on. This program structuring becomes the framework for the professional's ability to ignore, redirect, and reinforce the ongoing set of behaviors of the complex retarded person.

Another important variable in terms of programmatic flexibility is the control of the physical environment, especially for persons with aggressive or self-abusive behaviors. Professionals must be able to control the physical environment in order to accommodate the redirecting process in as inconspicuous a manner as possible.[25] At times, it is necessary to gain control in an environment that still permits the person to move in and out of the physical space where treatment is occurring.

In the beginning, the responsibility for a maximum degree of structure falls on the professional. There are a number of specific techniques that greatly help in initiating and obtaining treatment goals with this population.[26–29] Typically, these techniques require that the professional specifically plan all teaching approaches toward obtaining small initial graduations of behavioral control.

The posture and the programmatic flexibility do not necessarily lead to the meaningful engagement of the severely mentally retarded child or adult with coexisting mental illness in ongoing educational, vocational, and residential training programs. Treatment objectives, to be both useful and generalizable (i.e., to the living environment), must consistently focus on dampening (or redirecting) inappropriate behaviors so as to increase the probability that competing desirable behaviors will occur.[24] That is, if the professional knows that a person will inconsistently attend to a developmental task, or will not attend at all, the professional needs to arrange the learning environment in such a manner as to increase the probability that the person will attend.[26] A useful technique is to employ errorless learning.[30–32] When the person has persistent difficulty in performing a task and the professional is not able to focus on reinforcing the person for the acquisition of appropriate skills, the professional must arrange the treatment situation in such a way as to increase the probability that errors will not be made. Errorless learning can be accomplished by specifically analyzing desired tasks and interactions and then arranging these in a sequential manner and directly providing whatever physical or verbal assistance is necessary to successfully accomplish the task.[26,32–34]

10.5.4. Total Communication

One developmental technique that helps professionals gain control over inappropriate behaviors is to teach in silence[26] while simultaneously using signs and/or gestures. These children and adults frequently have major primary communication disorders, which appear to create many of the behavior problems that they display. Communicaton overstimulation from the *interpersonal* environment often leads to *intrapersonal* confusion. The intrapersonal confusion often becomes compounded and rapidly accelerates into behavioral outbursts. Because of this frequently noted mechanism for initiating personality explosion in these persons, it is helpful to teach *in silence* by the use of gestures, physical prompts, and environmental engineering. As the person becomes accustomed to the required task, verbal input can slowly be introduced. A secondary result of this technique is that it allows the caregiver to use verbal communication only for verbal reinforcements, thereby reducing possible sensory-input confusion for the person.

The issue of reinforcement for this population is frequently poorly applied by behavioral specialists. Typically, only two options are incorporated: either punish the person for inappropriate behaviors or use primary reinforcement. In our experience, the first option is harmful and counterproductive, and the second is generally unnecessary. It is better to decrease the probability that inappropriate behaviors will occur and direct the person toward appropriate behaviors. There is no reason whatsoever to provoke a child or an adult into an escalation of a behavioral outburst in the name of punishment. Indeed, punishment should be eliminated from the repertoire of treatment techniques of any caregiver. The aforementioned technique of ignoring, redirecting, and reinforcing is the basic intervention procedure. The end result is that inappropriate behaviors are deflected, and the person is continuously redirected toward appropriate behaviors. This treatment approach permits the caregiver to use positive, tactile, and social reinforcement.

10.5.5. Behavioral and Psychoactive Medical Treatment Balance

Another important dimension of the treatment with a dual-diagnosis person is the use of psychoactive medications as a tool to assist in leading the person to the threshold of learning.[35] A delicate balance must be struck between the use of psychoactive medications and an ongoing behavioral-intervention approach. Both psychoactive medications and behavioral management are essentially neutral tools. As such, either can be used to assist a person to move toward appropriate human engagement or toward human disengagement. They are both subject to abuse. Although excellent reviews of the clinical utilization of psychopharmacological agents in mentally ill-mentally retarded persons are available,[36,37] there are relatively few objective studies. The balance has little to do with an "either-or" posture toward the exclusive use of either psychoactive medication or behavioral management approaches. Instead, the focus should be on a balanced use of both of these approaches—always maintaining the goal of assisting the person to move toward meaningful engagements.

An initial consideration in this professional treatment balance is to briefly examine the clinical rationales for the use of psychoactive medications. The three basic rationales for utilizing medications are (1) to aid persons who display marked motoric overactivity; (2) to aid persons who display marked motoric underactivity; and (3) to aid persons whose overall behavior is slowly (or rapidly) escalating into "out-of-contact" behaviors (e.g., psychosis).

All ot these symptom configurations can produce serious interference with the person's ability to learn or to interact appropriately. Putting aside the extensive list of psychiatric syndromes, we find it important to objectively analyze the behaviors that are significantly interfering with the disconnected person's ability to learn and live in normalizing environments. This process involves (1) pinpointing in objective terms the major current interfering behaviors; (2) measuring and recording their extent and frequency; and (3) arriving at an objective conclusion about whether the observed behaviors are sufficiently disruptive to prevent ongoing learning experiences or maintenance of the person in the normalizing social-educational-work-recreational routines of community life.

This population requires a true interdisciplinary approach. For example, an adolescent may be hitting, running away, and biting himself at high frequencies. This pattern of behaviors obviously presents many major barriers to the initiation of *any* teaching or training process. Any medication prescribed in a balanced treatment approach should reduce these behaviors sufficiently so that program staff can safely work on the acquisition of appropriate skills and behaviors and so that initial behavioral redirection can occur. Thus, the use of psychoactive medications ideally serves the purpose of reducing the inappropriate and disruptive behaviors to a manageable level—just enough to enable the treatment process to take hold and move the disconnected person toward the threshold of learning.

The initiation of the use of psychotropic medications requires close monitoring by the psychiatrist, with frequent and ongoing descriptive input by the programmatic staff. Adjustments in the type of medications, the dosage, and the schedule are made on the basis of ongoing relevant programmatic inputs. All concerned persons should understand the basic process involved in this balancing of the use of psychotropic medications with intensive ongoing developmental programming. In the balanced treatment regime (i.e., the combined utilization of psychoactive medications and behavioral programs), the following basic processes typically occur.

10.5.5.1. Initiation Phase

There is noted the gradual effect of the psychoactive medication's dampening of the excessive amounts of inappropriate behaviors to the point where programming efforts can "take hold." This initial dampening effect of the psychoactive medication must be closely and sensitively monitored so as to prevent sedative effects; behavioral availability is the goal, not the disorganization or the depression of cognitive processes.

10.5.5.2. Catching-On Phase

As the initial dampening effect of the psychoactive medication joins forces with the intensive developmental programming (i.e., energetic one-to-one efforts to establish the threshold of learning), the acquisition of appropriate behaviors and skills begins to accelerate, multiplying by its own power—and the inappropriate behaviors begin to decelerate, usually in inverse proportion to the accelerating rate of appropriate learning acquisitions.

10.5.5.3. Reduction Phase

Once the second phase begins to stabilize, it is time to focus on the slow reduction and/or the elimination of the psychoactive medications utilized in the previous two phases. Concomitantly, intensive developmental programming must continue and extend further into extrinsic interpersonal transactions that permit the recently acquired behavioral improvement both to stabilize and to begin to generalize across a multitude of environments and situations.

10.6. Conclusion

In conclusion, it is clear that persons with the dual diagnosis of mental retardation and mental illness present a persistent challenge to community-based programs, and that they require specialized service models if they are to have their needs met appropriately.

Mentally retarded persons with severe behavioral and emotional problems can be served in community-based settings if a range of educational, vocational, and residential services and supports is available. On the surface, the components of care for this population appears to be no different from those types that are utilized for the mentally retarded population in general. However, they differ in their treatment intensity relative to staffing competency, staffing patterns, and the availability of backup supports such as acute psychiatric care and follow-up. There are concerns that must be dealt with in relation to the quality of the services that this population requires as well as to how their services impact on other clients in the service delivery system. Once clients are placed in a continuum of care, professionals need to develop a warm, accepting posture toward them and to apply a range of gentle treatment techniques to ensure optimal integration into community life.

References

1. Menolascino FJ: Emotional disturbances in mentally retarded children. *Am J Psychiatr* 126;54–62, 1969.
2. Chess S, Hassibi S: Behavior deviations in mentally retarded children. *J Am Acad Child Psychiatr* 9(2);282–297, 1970.
3. Donoghue EC, Abbas KA: Unstable behavior in severely subnormal children. *Dev Med Child Neurol* 13;512–519, 1971.
4. Philips I, Williams N: Psychopathology and mental retardation: A study of 100 mentally retarded children. *Am J Psychiatr* 132;1265–1271, 1975.
5. Groden G, Domingue D, Pueschel S, *et al*: Behavioral/emotional problems in mentally retarded children and youth. *Psychol Rep* 51;143–146, 1982.
6. Eaton LF, Menolascino FJ: Psychiatric disorders in the mentally retarded: Types, problems, and challenges. *Am J Psychiatr* 139;10, 1982.
7. Menolascino FJ, McGee JJ: The new institutions: Last ditch arguments. *Ment Retard* 19(5);215–220, 1981.
8. Menolascino FJ: *Schizophrenia in the Mentally Retarded. A Comparative Study of Thioridazine and Thiothixene in Retarded and Non-Retarded Scizhophrenic Adults.* New York, Impact Medical Communications, Inc., 1983.
9. Kanner L: Autistic disturbances of affective contact. *Nerv Child* 2;217–250, 1943.
10. Menolascino FJ, Eaton LF: Psychosis of childhood: A five year follow-up of experiences in a mental retardation clinic, in Chess S, Thomas A (eds): *Annual Progress in Child Psychiatry and Child Development*. New York, Brunner/Mazel, 1967.
11. Rutter M, Schopler A: *Autism: A Reappraisal of Concepts and Treatment*. New York, Plenum Press, 1978.
12. Menolascino FJ: *Challenges in Mental Retardation: Progressive Ideology and Services*. New York, Human Sciences Press, 1977.
13. Barr W: *Mental Defectives: Their History, Treatment and Training*. Philadelphia, Blakiston, 1904.

14. Menolascino FJ, Strider F: Advances in the prevention and treatment of mental retardation, in Arieti S (ed): *American Handbook of Psychiatry*, ed. 7. New York, Basic Books, 1981.

15. Beier D: Behavioral disturbances in the mentally retarded, in Stevens H, Heber R (eds): *Mental Retardation: A Review of Research*. Chicago, Chicago University Press, 1964.

16. May J, May J: *Overview of Emotional Disturbances in Mentally Retarded Individuals*. Presented at the Annual Convention of the National Association for Retarded Citizens, Atlanta, 1979.

17. Chess S, Horn S, Fernandez P: *Psychiatric Disorders of Children with Congenital Rubella*. New York, Brunner/Mazel, 1971.

18. Webster TB: Unique aspects of emotional development in mentally retarded children, in Menolascino FJ (ed): *Psychiatric Approaches to Mental Retardation*. New York, Basic Books, 1970.

19. Levie CA, Roberts BD, Menolascino FJ: Providing psychiatric services for clients of community-based mental retardation programs. *Hosp Comm Psychiatr* 30;383–384, 1979.

20. Fletcher RJ: *A Model Day Treatment Service for the Mentally Retarded/Mentally Ill*. Kingston, NY, Beacon House, 1982 (unpublished manuscript).

21. Baron FN: Group therapy improves mental retardate behavior. *Hosp Comm Psychiatr* 23;7–11, 1972.

22. Berkovitz IH, Sugar M: *Indications and Contraindications for Adolescents in Group and Family Therapy*. New York, Brunner/Mazel, 1975.

23. Baucom LD, Bensberg GJ: *Advocacy Systems for Persons with Severe Disabilities: Context, Components, and Resources*. Lubbock, Texas Tech University, 1976.

24. Greenspan S: *A Unifying Framework for Educating Caregivers about Discipline*. Omaha, NE, Boys Town Center for the Study of Youth Development, 1980.

25. Hewitt FM: Educational engineering with mentally disturbed children. *Excep Child* 33;459–467, 1967.

26. Gold M: Research in the vocational habilitation of the retarded: The present, the future, in Ellis N (ed): *International Review of Research on Mental Retardation*, vol 6. New York, Academic Press, 1973.

27. Horner RH, Bellamy GT: A conceptual analysis of vocational training with the severely retarded, in Snell M (ed): *Systematic Instruction of the Moderately, Severely, and Profoundly Handicapped*. Columbus, Charles E. Merrill, 1978.

28. Irvin LK, Bellamy GT: Manipulation of stimulus features in vocational skill training of the severely retarded: Relative efficacy. *Am J Ment Defic* 81;486–491, 1977.

29. Fisher MA, Zeaman D: An attention-retention theory of retardate discrimination, in Ellis N (ed): *International Review of Research on Mental Retardation*. New York, Academic Press, 1973.

30. Terrace HS: Discrimination learning with and without "errors." *J Exp Med* 6(1);1–27, 1963.

31. Irvin LK: General utility of easy to hard discrimination training procedures with the severely retarded. *Educ Training Ment Retard* 11;247–250, 1976.

32. Crosson JE: *The Experimental Analysis of Vocational Behavior in Severely Retarded Males*. Final report (Grant No. OEG32-47-0230-6024). Washington, D.C., U.S. Department of Health, Education, and Welfare, 1967.

33. Crosson JE: The functional analysis of behavior. A technology for special education practices. *Ment Retard* 7(4);15–19, 1969.

34. Bellamy GT, Horner RH, Inman D: *Vocational Habilitation of Severely Retarded Adults: A Direct Service Technology*. Baltimore, University Park Press, 1979.

35. Wilson J: Psychopharmacological agents in mental retardation. Issues and challenges, in Menolascino F, McCann B (eds): *Bridging the Gap: Mental Health Needs of Mentally Retarded Persons*. New York, Wiley, 1982.

36. Freeman RD: Psychopharmacological approaches and issues, in Menolascino FJ (ed): *Psychiatric Approaches to Mental Retardation*. New York, Basic Books, 1970.

37. Lipman RS: The use of psychopharmacological agents in residential facilities for the retarded, in Menolascino FJ (ed): *Psychiatric Approaches to Mental Retardation*. New York, Basic Books, 1970.

A Plan Designed to Deliver Services to the Multiply Mentally Handicapped

Helen Houston

11.1. Introduction

In February 1982, I established at the Middletown Psychiatric Center (an 850-bed state psychiatric center located some 75 miles northwest of New York City) a separate *treatment unit* for the group of patients I describe as being "multiply mentally handicapped." The multiply mentally handicapped are those individuals carrying an established medical diagnosis of mental retardation plus an established medical diagnosis of one of the mental illnesses. Either the mental retardation or the mental illness may be the primary diagnosis. Or the diagnoses may be deemed to coexist with other handicaps with neither area as the "primary" diagnosis; or they may be cyclical: one diagnosis and then the other is seen as being the major clinical concern.

I established the treatment unit for one critical reason: individuals with a dual diagnosis literally had no place to go for treatment at a time in New York State's history when treatment for mental illness and mental retardation has become generally accessible. The multiply mentally handicapped are often shunted back and forth from mental retardation centers to mental institutions, with neither institutional setting being equipped to cope with mental illness *and* mental retardation. "We have no appropriate means for treating this person" is the typical response when a multiply mentally handicapped individual appears for admission at either a mental institution or a mental retardation center. This is a legitimate response because institutions have long been structured to treat retardation *or* mental illness, but no institution was designed in New York State to cope with patients who have both afflictions.

Clearly, these complex individuals are square pegs in the world of mental hygiene, where treatment plans are designed for individuals who fit into round holes. My knowledge of the plight of patients with the dual diagnosis is not totally a conceptual one. On the contrary, as the director of Middletown Psychiatric Center, I have repeatedly (and directly) observed the plight of the multiply mentally handicapped. Briefly, the multiply mentally handicapped are not treated because psychiatric centers are not geared to dealing with the men-

Helen Houston • Chief Executive Officer, Middletown Psychiatric Center, New York State Office of Mental Health, Middletown, New York 10940.

tally retarded condition, and the developmental centers are not equipped to handle the mental illness dimension of the mentally retarded. Two natural consequences arise from this situation:

1. Both the psychiatric centers and the developmental centers often work quite hard at not accepting a multiply mentally handicapped person. Consequently, at critical times, when it becomes necessary to place such a patient, special meetings are called to mediate differences of opinion on which facility *must* take the multiply mentally handicapped person. Usually, such mediations wind up with a higher authority ordering either a psychiatric center or a developmental center to take the patient. Once the arguments have subsided and a decision has been reached, the multiply mentally handicapped patient is transferred to the "lucky" facility.

2. No matter which way the placement problem of the multiply mentally handicapped patient is resolved, the individual patient tends to receive less than adequate treatment. For example, whenever the multiply mentally handicapped patient is ordered to a developmental center for the mentally retarded because of his or her disruptive behavior secondary to a function in psychosis, he or she often disrupts the programs in progress at the developmental center for the clients who are "just mentally retarded." Such disruptions are predictable, and some staff members are forced to work independently with that one multiply mentally handicapped patient and thereby shortchange the other "just retarded" clients.

On the other hand, when the multiply mentally handicapped patient is sent to an institution for the mentally ill, he or she is placed on a psychiatric service that is not equipped to deal with mentally retarded individuals. One might ask: Is *either* of these specific placements significant to treatment outcome? In my direct clinical experience, prior to setting up a specific treatment unit for these dual-diagnosis individuals, they *did* live lives of not-so-quiet frustration. In a psychiatric service, retarded patients cannot keep up—intellectually—with the rest of the patients; for example, they have limited arithmetic skills, so money becomes a problem for them; they have limited reading and writing skills, so signs mean nothing in their lives. Frustration gives way to temper tantrums, which often brings forth extended periods in a camisole or in a seclusion room. Accordingly, the need for a special treatment unit, designed exclusively for the dual-diagnosis patient, becomes a high-priority consideration if specific treatment is to be provided for these complex individuals.

The establishment of a specialized treatment unit at the Middletown Psychiatric Center for the treatment of the multiply mentally handicapped actually began in my mind while I completed research concerning patients with this dual diagnosis as part of my studies for a doctorate in public administration. A somewhat startling fact emerged following my extensive search of the literature (both domestic and international), coupled with my personal visits to agencies in the metropolitan New York City area: I did not find anyone treating *adult* dual-diagnosis patients. I did note two agencies with programs for the multiply mentally handicapped: one had a very limiting criterion for treating those who are multiply mentally handicapped and worked exclusively with individuals living in Putnam (New York) County, a sparsely inhabited area just north of Westchester County. The other agency, the Jewish Guild for the Blind, treated only those with a dual diagnosis who were *blind*. Blindness was the main consideration; the guild treated only children and adolescents, and its focus was primarily an educational one.

I cannot state categorically that programs for treating the *adult* multiply mentally handicapped do not exist in the United States. However, if those programs do exist, they are not being written about in the professional journals. If one searches for the reasons for such a lack of concern for the adult multiply mentally handicapped, one can note several explanations: the younger multiply mentally handicapped patients are seen, from the professional's point of view, as being easier to deal with than adults with the dual diagnosis. For example, professionals tend to get very upset when adults insert their fingers in electrical outlets, put inappropriate objects in their mouths, take off their clothes in public, rummage through garbage, or have major temper tantrums. Yet, those same symptoms are taken as being of less consequence when young patients (i.e., children) with a dual diagnosis engage in the same behavior. These symptoms are not viewed objectively. Staff is repulsed by the adult, sympathetic to the child.

11.2. Goals

The treatment unit for dual-diagnosis individuals at the Middletown Psychiatric Center had the following three goals:

1. To search the center's medical records for those with a mental retardation diagnosis so they could be grouped together in one or two wards. Forty-nine such patients were discovered. (Of course, everyone in the center had a mental illness diagnosis.)

2. To gain new knowledge about multiply mentally handicapped individuals, who present one of the most difficult of all diagnostic and treatment problems facing mental health clinics and psychiatric inpatient services. Grouping all patients with a dual diagnosis was deemed necessary so that new knowledge concerning these patients might be systematically gathered.

3. To develop treatment strategies and methods that would enable the center to care for the multiply mentally handicapped as effectively and appropriately as clinically possible, yet as inexpensively as possible. It was up to the center not only to utilize existing resources and develop new resources but also to provide coordinated treatment for such individuals.

11.3. Establishment of the Treatment Unit

What follows now are the details of how the treatment unit was established, along with the many practical, nontheoretical considerations that influenced its structuring for the care of the multiply mentally handicapped.

Work on setting up the treatment unit was begun in January of 1982 with three fundamental purposes uppermost in my mind: (1) ending *at once* the crisis approach employed in the treatment of the multiply mentally handicapped (an approach that shunts those patients from pillar to post and back again); (2) setting up a service for the care of individuals with a dual diagnosis; and (3) monitoring the quality and the quantity of services provided.

In light of my desire to end as quickly as possible the shunting back and forth of the multiply mentally handicapped, a "Let's start now and put things in place as they evolve" approach was taken. That approach was not taken without closely weighing the two basic approaches to launching new programs in the mental health field. The first approach may be called, for lack of a better descriptive title, "We won't start until every item and every dollar is in place!" The second, the one I chose, can best be called, "We'll begin with what we have, and we'll put things in place as they come!" Each of those approaches to launching new programs has its benefits and drawbacks. The major benefit of the first approach is obvious: there is little or no anxiety surrounding the program because there are no unknowns. As to drawbacks, there are several, and they are critical. First, this approach delays the starting of a program for an inordinately long time. Second, the few staff members initially hired to help put the program together become accustomed to small work loads, pleasant hours spent "training," and little or no pressure. Consequently, their productivity suffers, and these staff members become quite elitist and seldom lose that attitude once the program is actively in progress.

A major benefit of the second approach is obvious: a service gets delivered about as fast as humanly possible. Other benefits are that the staff members work at full speed (full productivity) from the outset and develop an *esprit de corps* as they help patients, despite the hectic initial administrative and service-delivery environments. It is that very hectic set of environments that comprises one of the major drawbacks to this second approach: because the program has begun before everything is in place, the staff is forced at times to work with catch-as-catch-can equipment, limited office space, and construction noises as walls are rearranged and painted, telephones are installed, and so on. Also, authorities who have promised funding are sometimes reluctant to dispense those promised funds when they see that the program is "Already under way and doing OK." Counterbalancing that drawback, however, is the fact that an ongoing program (even if it is piecemeal) can sometimes develop a loyal, vocal constituency that will help keep the pressure on those agencies that have promised funds and are now teetering on the fence.

11.4. Setting Up a Separately Staffed and Programmed Service

I established an inpatient program for 49 dual-diagnosis patients on two adjacent coed wards, thereby creating a separate functional unit. Because approximately one third of these multiply mentally handicapped individuals were already residing on two adjacent wards, those two wards were selected as the "home" for the treatment unit. It made sense in that fewer patients would have to be moved from one ward to another ward. Moreover, because one of those two wards had been a coed ward for over a year, with positive results, it was decided to make both wards—the entire unit—coeducational in composition.

The age range in these 27 males and 22 females was 19–65 years (the mean age was 43 years for the females and 46 years for the males). All 49 patients had long histories of hospitalization, with an average length of stay of 18 years. It should be noted that this figure may underrepresent the length of hospitalization as it was the average length of stay for the *current* hospitalization and does not represent time previously spent in other hospitals and institutions. Approximately one half of this population required a constantly supervised level of activity, and the other half was on an independent level and able to go to programs and activities on their own or with another patient.

11.5. Problems in Development the Treatment Unit

In identifying these patients, it became apparent, in virtually every instance, that those with the dual diagnosis were very difficult patients with special needs. Previously, there had simply not been either the professional time or the capacity of staff members to concentrate on the special needs of this population when it was housed with patients whose major problems were psychoses. As one staff member with a U.S. Navy background explained it, "Meeting the special needs of those with a dual diagnosis would have been like polishing brass while the ship was sinking."

An initial challenge was the large variety of neglected physical ailments that were initially identified by the staff; this was a major treatment concern and resulted in intensive efforts to obtain appropriate medical services. Examples of medical problems requiring both immediate and long-range attention included dental services, a wide variety of surgical interventions (such as vein stripping, ankle-pin removal, and urogenital problems), and the discovery of additional physical illnesses such as cancer, diabetes, and epilepsy. The patients were also evaluated for special services such as speech therapy. Considering the poor physical condition of these patients, one might well ask, "How could such illnesses be overlooked—even given the fact that staff had little time for patients with mental retardation?" This valid question points up once again that there *are* difficult patients with a vital need for special attention. They frequently cannot express themselves well. They either do not admit that they are in pain or react so intensely to small bumps and slight bruises that their complaints become easy to overlook as just "another one of Sally's acts." Unless there are such obvious signs as bleeding or fainting, they indeed do get overlooked by the staff working with a mixed population.

Extensive polypharmacy was yet another pressing issue as the staff evaluated the patients in this treatment unit. For example, there was the need to withdraw one patient from the Valium he had been taking on a constant dosage level for seven years. Each person's drug profile was reviewed, and recommendations followed from psychiatric and pharmacology consultants to this unit.

11.6. Aberrant Behavior

As might be expected within this dual-diagnosis population, there was a large variety of aberrant behavior. While assessing the prospective patients for the unit, it appeared that aggressive-assaultive behavior was the most prevalent type of aberrant behavior: the patients had low frustration tolerance and poor impulse control; they were easily exploited or they exploited others; they had poor reality testing; and so on.

11.7. Resistance

When the unit was initially planned and discussed, there were some forms of resistance from the patients, their relatives, and the staff. (Staff resistance will be dealt with in Section 11.10.) The relatives were the most vocal in expressing their opposition to the coed wards. The parents of two females were especially concerned about the sexual "opportunities" of a coed ward. The problem of parental dissatisfaction with coed wards did not disappear once the treatment unit was in operation: it has been an ongoing concern that gets raised in the relatives' meetings (a monthly meeting of relatives to discuss any questions or concerns that they have about the unit). Interestingly, the most support for the coed wards came from relatives who had patients on the initial coed ward before this unit was established.

The patients, prior to the formation of this unit, expressed some mild reservations about being with "dumb" people and also about the coed wards. Some of the female patients were concerned that they would not have bathrooms for women only. Other females wondered about the sleeping arrangements. Concern was so strong in some patients that they visited me in my office; in each instance, the patients and I visited the wards to see how they were organized, and I explained that life would be a bit easier now because they would not have to strive to keep up with other patients: everyone on the treatment unit would be going along at essentially the same rate. These preplacement visits to the wards with staff members, along with the conversations with the author, seemed to remove the major resistances of the patients.

There was another type of resistance on the part of both patients with staff about patient participation in programs and the role of the therapy aide in that activity to which they were assigned. Most of the staff understood their roles in a rehabilitation framework as opposed to a more traditional custodial approach. Unfortunately, there were some staff members who still found it difficult to *allow* the patients to do a task (e.g., make their beds or dress themselves, rather than making the beds or dress the patients themselves). Part of this resistance was related to the staff's being more comfortable with a more traditional approach, but there was also the variable that much more staff time is taken up if one permits the patients to struggle with making their beds. Obviously, it is easier and far less aggravating for a staff member to do the task himself or herself rather than to wait "all day" for a mentally retarded patient to figure out which is the bottom sheet, which is the top sheet, and then get them both on the bed properly.

11.8. Life on the Unit

Every patient has a full schedule of activities for each day, and the schedule is individual to that person's needs, skills, and attention span. Trying to develop the full capacity of each person entailed, at times, the taking of calculated risks. For example, a patient whose lifestyle on the treatment unit consisted of chiefly ripping off his clothes and persistently digging in the garbage and ashtrays was asked to come to a seder service some three months after his arrival. He arrived wearing a jacket and tie, accompanied by a staff member who regularly rewarded his appropriate behavior with cookies. The patient stayed for the entire program and went back to the treatment unit still wearing his tie and jacket properly. Progressive growth and development were expected.

Initially, the program was developed with the purposes of providing structure and routinization and of giving staff the opportunity to observe each patient's capabilities and deficits. The program, in the intervening 18 months, has gone through major revisions and, at this point, is by no means a finished product. There is now a need for the development of more programs in the basic activity of daily living skills, socialization, and normalization. Throughout the program, there has been intertwined a variety of special programs, such as community outings and celebrations of holidays and birthdays. There are van trips twice per week, monthly bus trips, and picnics.

A camping program was initiated this past summer that, from all indications, has met with great success. By *success*, I mean that the patients enjoyed the trips and are looking forward to future trips; the staff that volunteered to go on the first camping trip have asked to go again; and finally, the patients appear to have gained self-confidence as a result of having gone on—for them—such an adventure. Other special trips thus far have included taking the patients for boat rides up the Hudson River on the "Day Liner." These programs have proved very beneficial in giving patients the opportunity to dress and behave in an appropriate manner outside the facility.

11.9. Management of Major Behavior Problems

The primary means of dealing with behavior problems is through an alert, well-trained staff who are well acquainted with the patients and who can react in an anticipatory manner to aberrant behaviors, which are frequently triggered by subtle signs. As one staff member stated, "We are always looking, frequently talking (diverting), listening, and sometimes steering someone out of range." As one patient explained, "I like George. [George is a staff member.] He listens to me. Not many people listen to me. They got orders for me to do this, do that. I like listening. I don't like orders."

We have incorporated in the treatment unit several approaches to creating a warm and nonthreatening atmosphere. For example, the nonnursing professionals have their offices on the wards. Thus, they are instantly accessible when needed, and the knowledge that help is only a few feet away tends to reduce the threatened feeling that patients might harbor. Furthermore, having an office *on* the ward makes those professionals committed to the ward and not to some social worker's or psychologist's department off in an administration building. Finally, having their offices on the wards helps make what happens on the ward as much their own responsibility as it is the responsibility of the nursing staff.

When the unit was established, decision was made that seclusion rooms would not be used. Instead, two rooms (one on each ward) were designated as "time-out" or "quiet" rooms. These rooms do not have locks on the doors. The rooms are used to provide a place for individuals who feel that they want to get away or who feel that they are losing control and want to get out of the general hum of the ward for a while. These rooms are also used at those infrequent (and becoming even less frequent) times when a patient requires a camisole. At such a time, the person is removed from the rest of the patients and put in the quiet room. An employee remains with the patient at all times until the camisole is removed and the patient is ready to rejoin ward life.

From the outset, this system of helping patients regain control of themselves and eliminating outside stimulation has proved to be beneficial to both the patients and the staff. It is beneficial to the patients because their dignity is maintained and their behavioral control is usually regained in a very short time. It is beneficial to the staff because it is clear that the quiet room—and the camisole, if needed—is used to help the patient regain self-control and not for punishment. That approach helps the staff control themselves and helps the patients not to panic and thereby add to the other problems that they may be experiencing.

Restraints (limited to the camisole) within the unit have been used with decreasing frequency. Most recently, there have been two patients, both on the same ward, who have had to be placed in the camisole, usually during the evening shift. The timing of these occurrences has led us to believe that, rather than patient needs, we may be identifying staff issues. Indeed, with that discovery, a camisole has not been used for a month. Surprisingly, in terms of assault, there have been very few incidents. Early in the history of the unit, given the background of these patients, this was an area of concern. In general, assaultive kinds of behavior have been at a minimum and are on the decrease.

Visitors to the unit usually express surprise at the cheerful colors and the good-looking, intact furniture, drapes, and plants that are a part of each ward. This situation reflects both administrative and direct staff interest in creating and maintaining a pleasant, homey atmosphere.

In a unit beset by controversy merely because of its existence, one could well ask, "Why risk the wrath of the gods by adding another dimension of controversy, a coed ward?" The answer is at once simple and complex. I have run coed wards for several years. Our basic unit of living as a society is the family, and certainly, the family is a coed unit. Indeed, one of the greatest societal concerns of this generation is the relatively new "one-parent families." Years ago, the division of patients and staff in an institution along sexual lines was not only by wards and by buildings but by roads as well: no efforts were spared to keep the men from the women. And woe to the patient found, quite literally, on the wrong side of the road. That rigid and unnatural division of the sexes appears to me to be an enforcement of institutional habits that are not functional anywhere else. Consequently, if we adopt as a working premise the belief that we will normalize as much as humanly possible the living patterns in an institution, we must create a coed living situation with coed staff as well. Other benefits to this coed approach appear to have accrued, once we had established a coed living pattern. For example, female staff are frequently able to handle potentially violent males *without* force. Male staff are frequently able to do the same with female patients. Patients appear to be less violent and to show more care about their general appearances and activities in coed environments.

11.10. Staff Dimensions

To congregate the future staff for this unit, I surveyed everyone in the hospital via a written questionnaire: "Would you like to work with the multiply mentally handicapped?" Staff members who agreed would, in some instances, have been able to change their working hours—from day shift to night shift or evening shift, for example. The response to the initial request was extremely poor: nobody volunteered! However, and fortunately, the staff members who had been working on the two wards that would now become the treatment unit agreed to "stay on and give the unit a try." For the most part, those staff members have stayed and have enjoyed their new patients. Quite understandably, other staff members hav found it difficult to relate to this unusual patient population.

Realistically speaking, the unit was established with little more enriched staffing than was found on any other ward at the center. Interestingly enough, however, the staff's perceptions of enrichment are somewhat different. Although the accomplishments of the staff and the resulting gain of the patients are many, a survey of the staff reveals that they uniformly acknowledge that, although it appears that the unit is richly staffed, it is not. Indeed, say the staff, they become quite frustrated about providing appropriate programming; meeting rigorous schedules for clinics, especially in view of the physical needs of the population; and, at some times, ensuring (particularly on the evening shift) that employees will get their well-deserved breaks and mealtimes.

Recently, a local psychiatrist and psychologist (who had run an equivalent unit in another state psychiatric center that was short-lived) have told me that my unit is unusually well staffed with personnel and could probably use more nonnursing professionals. The administrative personnel at Middletown Psychiatric Center see these two wards for patients with a dual diagnosis as needing a full, steady, and well-trained staff.

These staffing challenges are consistent with what can be done in other regional or state planning efforts. For example, the central office (at Albany) and the regional office (at Poughkeepsie) in New York State plan to set up one multiply mentally handicapped treatment unit in each of five regions throughout New York. In my region, a 20-bed unit will be established to accommodate the multiply mentally handicapped. That unit will serve five New York State psychiatric centers.

11.11. Training

In the early development of the unit, one of the biggest doubts expressed by staff members, relatives, the center's board of visitors, and the Mental Health Information Service was the concern that the author and the staff "did not know what they were doing" with this dual-diagnosis population. Rather than argue that position, my acting unit chief and I took great pains to agree. Virtually no one has written about experiences in working with the multiply mentally handicapped. As a consequence, my staff and I believe that we are not further behind or less informed than most others working in this unchartered land.

To help overcome this serious deficiency, the staff and I have attempted to train in specific skills areas and then either to use or to modify and adapt the skills for working with these patients. Obviously, the success of the treatment unit reviewed here depends on the achievements of those people working in the program. It is easy to fall into the trap of believing that success is ensured by the administrator's intellectual brilliance, innovative program development, grantsmanship, and ingenuity. Although those qualities are necessary, they are not sufficient; in the final analysis, all mental-health treatment depends on the staff's skill and performance.[1] Working as we do at Middletown Psychiatric Center, a matrix organization with interdisciplinary teams, we find additional staff issues that are not unique to the multiply mentally handicapped unit but are true of all staff at the center. The concept of the harmonious mental-health team that has "jelled" must be considered and understood in the light of the conflict and the competition inevitable among various professional groups. In addition to the differences of personalities and personal strengths and skills of the various team members, the relationship among professions and the specific responsibilities of each group are very much in flux. Each professional group is feeling its way, and the relationships among them are sensitive and changing. Professions such as psychiatry and social work are undergoing tremendous internal change, and others, such as recreational therapy, are searching for an appropriate role. Moreover, each of the groups not only is responsive to the circumstances of its work situation but is also sensitive to the definitions of prestige and activity within its own professional structure.[2]

No discussion of a plan and its implementation can be considered complete until one explores the very real issue of the costs of setting up an entity such as the treatment unit. Start-up costs for this treatment model are modest: initially, the services are housed in sites that already exist (e.g., wards in Middletown Psychiatric Center) or can be initiated at state-run sites in the community and at sites available at existing local provider programs.

Minimal remodeling was a necessity in order to have separate bathrooms for men and women on each ward. There was also a small expense for the wallpaper that acted as a "sign" for those who might not be able to read the labels "Men" and "Women." Because the staff members were already employees of the center, special staffing was not a cost consideration. Clearly, had the patients not been in the dual-diagnosis unit, they would have been elsewhere throughout the center and would have been cared for by those same staff workers.

11.12. Systematic Continuing Study of the Effectiveness of the Treatment Unit

The carrying out of the program for the treatment of those patients with a dual diagnosis is only one side of the coin. How effective is the program being conducted? Are the patients better off? Is the institution providing all that it can? Answers to such questions call for a systematic study of the program through periodic evaluations. Thus, evaluation becomes an integral, important, and continuing part of the functioning of the unit.

When the need for services is so pressing, it sometimes seems necessary to administer and to justify programs without providing any formal or systematic evaluation of accomplishments. Perhaps, too, there is a reluctance even to attempt evaluations because the requirements in terms of personnel, equipment, and design sophistication seem too formidable. As a result, many mental-health programs feel that evaluation is simply beyond their means. Many organizations do not have the facilities even to efficiently collect and retrieve the kinds of information needed to monitor and evaluate a program, although most generate a great deal of the necessary data during the normal course of their work. The unwillingness of most funding sources to pay for the development of more adequate evaluation systems has made it easy for this situation to persist.

However true these observations are, the fact nonetheless remains that evaluation is one of the core responsibilities of the program or unit manager. With few resources and no universally accepted guidelines on how to proceed in treating this population, we must find ways to discharge this obligation if we are to manage successfully. To complicate matters further, evaluation can mean many different things. Sometimes it means "Are you doing what you said you were going to do?'' Sometimes the questions become more difficult, like ''How much are you accomplishing?'' Or ''Are your accomplishments worth the effort?'' These are all legitimate questions.[3]

The following evaluation system answers those questions satisfactorily. The system calls for (1) training observers; (2) designing the instruments; (3) utilizing the professional staff already employed; and (4) making records accessible to meet the needs not only of this evaluation but of several other evaluation groups such as the Joint Commission on Accreditation of Hopsitals (JCAH).[4]

Peer evaluation is the key approach to evaluating a service. Unfortunately, peer evaluation has typically been rejected for reasons that are not explicitly stated in the literature. However, one gets the implicit message from reading the literature that most mental-health professionals believe that peer evaluation simply cannot be done effectively. Their reasoning would appear to be as follows: because staff resistance to evaluation performed by an outside expert is unusually high, staff resistance would just naturally reach the ''boiling point'' if and when peers and not outsiders were used to monitor the services.[5-17] Pressing external constraints, which have already been described, and my positive experience with peer evaluation (despite the gloomy literature) led to the election of peer evaluation rather than retaining an outside expert to monitor the treatment unit. Peer evaluation, of course, is just one of several official critiques of the program for the patient with a dual diagnosis. There are evaluations conducted by Utilization Review, Medicare, and JCAH. Additionally, for ease of monitoring, the medical records are kept in the uniform case-record style—a style adopted statewide that is a goal-oriented system of recordkeeping.

Research comprises the second part of the evaluative process. Research is critical to this program because so little empirical study has been done by the mental health industry on treatment *per se*. Nobody knows for certain what results the treatment will bring about. (Some clinical observers—such as Lanzkron[18]—have been entirely pessimistic about treatment outcome.) It is possible that the results of treatment might be no more than physical: a more tractable, manageable patient. On the other hand, it might just be possible, with medication and modern teaching techniques and appropriate therapy, to help at least some patients achieve a life outside an institution at some level of independent functioning that is stable. That is the issue that our research is attempting to take on boldly.

The treatment-unit model described here for delivering services has been developed with a great concern that it not duplicate other existing services. Thus, an important ingredient in this plan is the utilization of and a linkage with existing services. Clearly, this model for the care and treatment of the multiply mentally handicapped in Middletown is neither a cure for nor a prevention of the dual diagnosis. Realistically, the model is a system of thoughtful, appropriate supports that will allow the multiply mentally handicapped to function at their highest level. The plan is a system for caring for the individual with a dual diagnosis that has been offered at a time when no comparable plan exists. *Caring* is the key word in this treatment plan. Clearly, the mental health professional cannot magically take away retardation or mental illness from a person with a dual diagnosis. The professional can, however, teach that person many basic and vital social skills: how to shop, how to cook, how to deal with money, how to use community resources such as buses and generic services, and so on. Such rehabilitation approaches and beliefs may be the only currently realistic ways to deal with such patients. It is unfortunate that the knowledge needed to reverse the basic conditions of psychiatric illness is frequently lacking, but rehabilitation efforts devoted to helping the individual live with his or her condition are sometimes criticized as "defeatist." Until we have a better understanding of the etiology, the course, and the treatment of most mental illnesses, it appears to be more practical and more reasonable to attempt to limit the *extent* of the disabilities that are present.

Another aspect of "caring" concerns teaching the multiply mentally handicapped not only how to get along in society at a very basic level but also how to avail themselves of the community's resources. Successful social functioning depends on a person's ability to mobilize effort when such effort is necessary, on the manner in which he or she organizes and applies such efforts, on his or her psychological and instrumental skills and abilities, and on supports in his or her social environment. Although social support is well developed within most community-care programs, the other facets of social functioning have been relatively neglected.[2]

11.13. Discussion

The model for the treatment unit for the multiply mentally handicapped may sound fluid. It was purposely designed that way. The following paradigm for planning this unit was used:

1. *Planning is not a simple act.* Rather, it is a process consisting of a series of interrelated steps or phases. Furthermore, the planning process is continuous and interactive. That is, the plan converges on a desired state through several repetitions of the planning cycle.

2. *Planning is hierarchical in nature.* In general, the manager designs a system of plans, rather than an individual plan.

3. *Planning must allow for flexibility.* That is so because planning premises, internal requirements, and external influences all are capable of changing in the months—even days—ahead.

4. *The plan must be a strategic one that includes a focus on the public opinion factor.* It must set the basic purpose and direction of the organization, one that is broad and that is concerned with both ends and means as well as with tactics. Plans that cope only with the short term are narrow, are more detailed, and are concerned chiefly with the means of implementation while ignoring the ends are almost certainly doomed to fail. For example, strategic planning concerns itself with the location and the construction of a new unit, the degree of interinstitutional affiliation, and the scope of services of the unit.

On the other hand, tactical planning includes such considerations as patient scheduling, purchasing, inventory control, and maintenance.[19]

Based on my experiences, it is possible to reallocate inpatient resources to treat and identify already-existing populations, provided consultation and planning take place within the formal hierarchy as well as with community leaders—leaders such as elected officials and lay board members. Such consultation must take place before the initiation of implementation. To launch any mental health endeavor successfully, it is necessary to identify accurately the leaders in each community, then meet with them (informally at first, later on a formal basis) to discuss *planned* mental-health programs. In this way, those leaders learn what is about to happen *before* it happens. Such an approach to the community's leaders also gives them the opportunity to modify the proposed program. Basically, those leaders do not appreciate surprises: one day no program in the community; the next day, constituents banging on the leaders' doors demanding to know the what, the when, and the how-come of a proposed program.

The public opinion vis-à-vis the mentally ill and the mentally retarded is a divided one that makes it difficult to establish a successful plan. Such divisions in thinking set up a "damned if you do and damned if you don't" situation. Consider the following. On the one hand, there are major court decisions that establish quite neatly the distinct rights of patients, including their right to treatment (i.e., the landmark court decisions are *Wyatt* v. *Stickney*,[20] the Donaldson decision,[21] and the Willowbrook Consent Decree[22]). The patients' right-to-treatment decision means not only that patients cannot be held in institutions so as to be kept, "off the streets and out of the community's hair," but also that any patient who is mentally ill must be treated. Consequently, the multiply mentally handicapped have the right to be treated *not* as social outcasts, but as another legitimate group in need of mental health treatment.

On the other hand, however, there are large groups of individuals within almost all U.S. communities who fear having the "crazies" situated in halfway houses in *their* neighborhoods. Such groups tend to be vehement and vocal, and in constant touch with their local legislators, whenever the "threat" of such an "invasion" emerges. The elected officials representing such groups are quite sensitive to and responsive to the needs and wishes of those vocal communities. As a result, it is often difficult to place clients in the community—despite the rights of such patients to sound treatment.

The institutions involved are, quite naturally, pulled in two different directions simultaneously. For instance, it is expected that the institution will conform to all legal requirements pertaining to their patients, including seeing that the patients' civil rights are protected (rights such as the right to vote); seeing that patients are placed in the least restrictive setting appropriate to their condition; and seeing that the patients are treated as patients and not as members of a cheap labor force who can help out in the institution's kitchen, in the laundry, or on the grounds, picking up litter. But, and it is a big *but*, those same institutions must also "protect" society from these "undesirables," who may be dangerous to both themselves and others.

11.14. Summary

The challenge of meeting the services needs of the multiply mentally handicapped may at first seem overwhelming. The purpose of this chapter has been to provide the reader with a unique opportunity to share in and understand how such challenges can be met in the initial planning, implementation, and monitoring of a comprehensive inpatient program.

I have presented the major goals, necessary in my opinion, to assuring a successful program. First, it is important to initiate the program and end the current crisis-treatment situation that exists for this population. Second, in establishing the program, there are numerous problems that need to be addressed, such as space, medication, staff selection and training, treatment of problem behaviors, and the development of a solid philosophical base. And third, the monitoring of such a program demands a rigorous evaluation to measure the effectiveness of the treatment model while paying close attention to those externable variables (e.g., funding and politics) that can impact on its success.

In short, it is my hope that the reader has been able to share in and profit from our experience and that such efforts will prove useful in serving the multiply mentally handicapped while advancing, in some small way, this area of research and service.

References

1. Whittington HG: People make programs: Personnel management, in Feldman S (ed): *The Administration of Mental Health Services*. Springfield, IL, Charles C. Thomas, 1973.
2. Mechanic D: *Mental Health and Social Policy*. Englewood Cliffs, NJ, Prentice-Hall, 19.
3. Binner P: Program evaluation, in Feldman S (ed): *The Administration of Mental Health Services*. Springfield, IL, C. C. Thomas, 1973.
4. Roemer MI: Evaluation of health service programs and levels of measurement, in Levey S, Loomba PN (eds): *Health Care Administration*. Philadelphia, Lippincott, 1973.
5. Zusman J, Levine M: Program evaluation: An introduction. *Int J Ment Health* 2;2–5, 1973.
6. Levine M, Gelsomino J, Joss RH, et al: The consumer's perspective of rehabilitative services in a county penitentiary. *Int J Ment Health* 2;94–110, 1973.
7. Holmes D: Day care for the aged: Problems in start-up evaluation design. *Gerontologist* 13;97, 1973.
8. Mannino FV, Shore MF: Demonstrating effectiveness in an aftercare program. *Social Work* 19(3);351–357, 1974.
9. Jacobs AM, Nicyols G, Larsen JK: Critical nursing behaviors in the care of the mentally retarded. *Int Nursing Rev* 20(4);117–122, 1973.
10. Miller S, Helmick E, Berg L, et al: Alcoholism: A statewide program evaluation. *Am J Psychiatr* 131(2);210–214, 1974.
11. Levin S, Bishop D: An evaluation tool for feedback and leverage of mental health delivery systems. *Can Psychiatr Assoc J* 17(6);437–442, 1972.
12. Winn RJ, Rich C, Dolby J, et al: Program evaluation of Texas mental health and mental retardation centers. *Hosp Comm Psychiatry* 26(1);36–38, 1975.
13. Pierce CH: Recreation for the elderly: Activity participation at a senior citizen center. *Gerontologist* 15;202–205, 1975.
14. Miller PM: Behavioral assessment in alcoholism research and treatment: Current techniques. *Int J Addic* 8(15);831–837, 1973.

15. Zusman J, Bissonette R: The case against evaluation (with some suggestions for improvement). *Int J Ment Health* 2;111–125, 1973.
16. Weber CA: Evaluating a multiphasic consultation program in a large urban setting. *Exchange* 2(5);29–39, 1974.
17. Koret S: *Evaluation of Children's Mental Health Services.* Final report, NIMH Grant MH-22997, 1974.
18. Lanzkron J: The concept of pfropf-schizophrenia and its prognosis. *Am J Ment Defic* 61;544–547, 1957.
19. Levey S, Loomba PN: *Health Care Administration.* Philadelphia, Lippincott, 1973.
20. *Wyatt v Stickney:* (District Court of Alabama) 344 Federal Supplement, p. 387. Modified on appeal by 5th Circuit Court of Appeals, 503 Federal Supplement, p. 1305.
21. *Donaldson* v. *O'Connor:* (Court of Appeals of Florida) 493 Federal Supplement, p. 507. See also: *Psychiatric News* 10;14 (July 16, 1975); and *The New York Times*, 1 June 1975, Section 4, p. 20.
22. *Willowbrook Consent Decree:* A private agreement—simply supervised by the court—between Willowbrook's relatives' group and New York State.

A Model Day-Treatment Service for the Mentally Retarded-Mentally Ill Population

Robert J. Fletcher

12.1. Introduction

Persons of normal intelligence who experience psychiatric problems can avail themselves of clinical services from a variety of resources within the mental-health delivery system. Mentally retarded persons, on the other hand, who experience similar psychiatric problems do not have easy access to mental health services either within the mental-health delivery system or within the mental retardation system. These persons, although in need of multiple services because of their double handicap, are frequently without the necessary support systems. Historically, neither the mental health nor the mental retardation systems have adequately addressed the mental health needs of this population. Because these individuals are not appropriately categorized and directed into one or the other delivery-care system, their unique mental-health problems have largely been neglected. Persons in this population who are typically unidentified as doubly handicapped either "fall through the cracks" or are programmed into a system in which their needs are only partially addressed.

Many professionals in the mental health field are vulnerable to cultural biases, misconceptions, and ignorance regarding this dually diagnosed population. Ignorance and the associated lack of training greatly contribute to the problem. Many professionals have little or no training in the field of mental retardation. Leaverton and Van Der Heida[1] found that only 51% of child-psychiatry training programs included any material on mental retardation in the curriculum. It has been pointed out by Menolascino and Bernstein[2] that the first prerequisite for psychiatric interviewing in the area of mental retardation is that the examiner have interest in and a positive attitude toward the client.

Walker[3] contended that mentally retarded persons are often denied adequate mental-health services because of the negative attitudes of mental health professionals. These negative attitudes are associated with both ignorance and bias. Ignorance plays a major role in the formulation of attitudes toward the mentally retarded and are frequently based on misunderstandings, myths, and

Robert J. Fletcher • Founder and Executive Director, National Association for the Dually Diagnosed and Director, Dual Diagnosed Day Treatment Program, Beacon House, Ulster County Mental Health Services, Kingston, New York 12401.

unfounded beliefs. Phillips[4] called attention to three related misconceptions about maladaptive behavior in the retarded person. First, it is often thought that the maladaptive behavior of the retarded is a function of their retardation. However, the disturbed behavior in the retarded is not primarily the result of limited intellectual capacities but is related to delayed, disordered personality functions and interpersonal relationships with meaningful people in the environment. Second, it is assumed that emotional disorders in the retarded are different from those seen in persons with normal intellectual endowment. Actually, the gamut of psychopathology seen in normally intellectually endowed people are also seen in the retarded. The third misconception is that certain symptoms complexes and maladaptive behaviors in the retarded are a result of organic brain damage that produces these particular symptoms. Symptoms such as hyperactivity, short attention, distractibility, and impulsive irrational behavior are frequently associated with organicity. However, these symptoms are also manifested in children with low or high IQ and with or without organic involvement. These three misconceptions add to the previously noted professional ignorance and are particularly important with regard to the clinical understanding of, and attitude toward, the mentally retarded–mentally ill population. Any treatment program utilizing an interdisciplinary team approach needs to have a staff that is not only knowledgeable, but that has a positive attitude toward the clientele that the agency serves.

This chapter is concerned with the description of an innovative day-treatment program designed to meet the mental health needs of a neglected population: those who are multiply disabled with both mild retardation and mental illness. A highly structured small-group method, which is described in the following pages, has been demonstrated to be effective in improving the psychosocial function of this special population.

Prior to the establishment of this specialized program, there was a day-treatment facility that accepted individuals who were mentally retarded and psychiatrically disabled. However, these individuals, because of characteristic problems associated with impulse control, high distractibility, and need for direction as well as attention, did not adjust well to the general therapeutic program. The treatment activities in the therapeutic milieu needed to be operationalized in small groups and with a staff-intensive program. In recognition of the special needs of this population, I developed a program designed to address the specific mental-health needs of individuals who are both mentally retarded and psychiatrically disabled.

12.2. Overview of Beacon House

Because this specialized program resides within the context of a larger therapeutic milieu, an overview of the philosophy and programs of Beacon House is presented first. Beacon House is located in Kingston, New York; it is a psychosocial rehabilitation center that serves a mentally disabled adult population. The center is part of the Ulster County Mental Health Services and is licensed as a day-treatment program under the New York State Department of Mental Health.

The functional operation and philosophy of the program follows that of a psychosocial club model. Beacon House offers a wide range of diversified treatment and program services in milieu-therapeutic environments in which members are encouraged to take an active role in the milieu community. The term *member* is used rather than *patient*, as the emphasis in the milieu reflects human potential, rather than pathology and illness. Members have an opportunity, within a communitylike atmosphere, to participate in a combination of clinical, prevocational, social, recreational, and educational services.

As an extension of the therapeutic community, a large community meeting is held each week in which staff and members discuss and work together to resolve "house" concerns, such as program planning, problems, trips, or recognition and celebration of special events or persons.

Similar to the community meeting, the workshops begin with a half-hour meeting in which staff and members discuss issues pertinent to their workshop. There are four workshops—each of which is designed to help members sharpen prevocational skills and skill development. Each workshop produces for the club either clerical services, food preparation, maintenance, or items for sale. The workshops provide not only a meaningful work experience with associated personal gratification, but also vehicles wherein members, as a group, plan and initiate action.

Specific therapy approaches are available, such as individual and group psychotherapy, medication therapy, sexuality groups, age-peer groups, and a wide range of creative arts therapy, which includes music, art, and movement therapies.

The utilization of socialization and recreation completes the necessary ingredients for a functioning community. Interest groups, clubs, committees, and recreational opportunities are means for meeting many of the social and recreational needs of our members. Play, friendships, and socializing are essential ingredients in everyone's life. Experimental learning, role modeling, and encouragement by and for members in planning these activities are an integral part of our methodology.

Within the three treatment-focus areas—workshops, therapy, and socialization-recreation—Beacon House provides the individual with a meaningful set of program experiences that facilitate maximum psychosocial functioning.

Beacon House serves three distinct subpopulations of the mentally disabled. One group consists of members who, after a varying length of time, will be capable of returning to the community. Many of these individuals have experienced a reactive or episodic decompensation, have had brief psychiatric hospitalizations, and need supportive and treatment services for a limited period. Others in this category, especially those with a long history of mental illness, need this service for an extended period. The age range is from 18 years to 50 years, and there are approximately 80 members who attend three days a week. These people reside in various living environments, including community residences, boarding homes, privately maintained apartments, or with their families.

The second group can be referred to as the chronic mentally ill population who have a long history of psychiatric hospitalizations. The level of psychosocial functioning of this category is lower than that of the above-mentioned group. The age range is from 50 years to 90 years, and there are approximately 100 members who attend two days a week. Most of the members of this population reside in state-supported family-care homes, although some live in community residences.

The third group that Beacon House serves consists of persons who are handicapped with both mental illness and mental retardation. The program involves a number of highly structured clinical, social, and educational groups designed to address the mental health needs of this population. Unlike the other two groups, this one is not involved in a workshop activity. The age range is from 19 years to 46 years, and there are 10 members. It is this last group, the Independent Living Group, that is the focus of this chapter.

12.3. Clinical Profile

All 10 of the individuals in the program have a dual diagnosis: mental illness and mental retardation. The mean IQ is 64. The diagnostic classifications are on Axis I of the *Diagnostic and Statistical Manual* of the *American Psychiatric Association.*[5]

Table 1 lists the diagnostic categories represented in this group.

There are 7 males and 3 females in the program; the mean age is 31 years. With respect to living environments, 5 live with their families, 4 live in supportive living arrangement, and 1 lives independently. Of the 10 individuals, 4 have had organic brain damage; the etiology of the mental retardation in the remaining 6 is unknown. Of these 10 members, 5 have had multiple psychiatric hospitalizations; 4 have been in residential treatment facilities; and only 1 individual in the program has not been in either a psychiatric hospital or a residential program.

Common threads throughout the case histories of these individuals are rejection by peers, failure in schools, and disappointed families who find it

Table 1. Diagnostic Categories

Diagnosis	Number of members
Major depression	2
Bipolar disorder	1
Passive-aggressive personality disorder	1
Intermittent explosive disorder	2
Atypical psychosis	2
Schizophrenia	2
Total	10

difficult to give the emotional nurturing and support needed for healthy personality development. In addition, all have had difficulty in establishing or maintaining healthy interpersonal relationships.

The members have been attending the Beacon House program for an average of 14 months.

12.4. Program Organization

Referrals to Beacon House come from a variety of sources. These referrals are processed through the intake unit, and an assessment is made with regard to the appropriate program, to which the individual is recommended. If a candidate is suspected of having a dual diagnosis of both mild mental retardation and mental illness, then he or she is referred to the coordinator of the Independent Living Program for further evaluation as well as for the purpose of facilitating a transition into the program.

Members who are screened into the Independent Living Program attend on Tuesdays and Thursdays and are involved in vocational training at a community-based sheltered workshop for the remaining three days. The Independent Living Program consists of various therapeutic groups: (1) community meeting; (2) movement therapy; (3) music therapy; (4) remedial education; (5) arts and crafts; (6) group therapy; (7) sensory integration therapy; (8) horticulture therapy; and (9) cooking. Except for the community meeting, held once a week, sessions are 45 minutes in length with a 15-minute break between each session. This time frame provides a maximization of concentrated effort during group sessions and allows for frequent and necessary respite.

The day begins with a half-hour coffee break. This is a time, along with an hour for lunch, in which the members of the program assimilate and interact with members of the other programs at Beacon House. Social interactions occur, and relationships develop during these essentially unstructured and important times. Other occasions that encourage the members to feel an integral part of the larger Beacon House community are picnics, parties, and trips. The culmination of this social integration process takes place when the entire house goes on "vacation" for five full days at a sleep-over camp during the summer. Some special functions, such as the celebration of a member's birthday, afford the opportunity both to socialize and to receive recognition of individuality and self-worth.

Each member is assigned to a counselor, whose function it is to be an advocate, a case manager, and a therapist. The role of the counselor is an essential part of the treatment process. Case reviews at interdisciplinary treatment-team meetings are held quarterly, and input from collateral agency and family contacts are welcome so that a comprehensive psychosocial assessment can be developed. Psychiatric assessments, consultations, and prescriptions for medications are available through the staff psychiatrist, who is an integral part of the treatment team.

The following is a typical daily program schedule in the Independent Living Program:

Tuesday		Thursday	
9:00–9:30	Arrival	9:00–9:30	Arrival
9:30–10:00	Coffee Break (Socialization)	9:30–10:00	Coffee Break (Socialization)
10:00–10:15	Community Meeting	10:00–11:00	Group Psychotherapy (Rap Group)
10:15–11:00	Movement Therapy	11:15–12:00	Sensory Integration Group
11:15–12:00	Music Therapy	12:00–1:00	Lunch
12:00–1:00	Lunch	1:00–1:40	Horticulture Group
1:00–1:40	Education	1:45–2:30	Arts-and-Crafts Group
1:50–2:30	Cooking Group		

12.5. Group Psychotherapy

Group psychotherapy with the emotionally disturbed population has long been recognized as an effective therapeutic approach. However, mental health professionals usually are reluctant to use this approach with the retarded population. Few studies have been cited in the literature regarding the use of group psychotherapy with the emotionally disturbed–mentally retarded population. Among these are Wilcox and Guthrie,[6] Rosen and Rosen,[7] and Gorlow *et al.*[8] Paradoxically, most studies are from the 1950s and 1960s with a few from the 1970s, including Baron[9] and Richards and Lee.[10] Most studies were accomplished in institutional settings with children, and few employed control groups or stabilized rating scales. These studies have suggested that group psychotherapy with the retarded population can be successful and that the results point toward a positive change in personality characteristics.

Group psychotherapy sessions, or "rap" groups, as we call them at Beacon House, are a central component in the treatment process. The group has its own set of norms and values, which help shape a positive attitude in the members and make the group a cohesive and supportive one. The following is a sample of a typical psychotherapy group, through which it is hoped the reader will be able to sense the strengths, the limitations, and the striving for mutual support that characterize the interactions.

The session typically begins with either the therapist or the members saying, "Who is not here today?" This question emphasizes the feeling of group concern and illustrates the importance of each member as noted by their absence. Then, sufficient time is allowed for the discussion of problems of immediate concern to the members. For example, a member who lives in a community residence says, "I am mad at my roommate because he's been smoking in our room after supper and this is against the rules." The member has an opportunity to express his anger, which in itself produces a cathartic therapeutic effect. The discussion continues by utilizing the group process as a therapeutic tool. The member is given recognition by either the therapist or others in the group for being able to identify a problem and being willing to bring the problem to the group. This recognition is given verbally and generally is followed by group applause.

Then, one of a wide range of clinical issues is discussed. The utilization of the group process is again employed, and the members are encouraged to be actively involved. Discussions of handicaps and associated functional limitations occasionally arise from comments such as "Why can't I get a job?" and "Why do they call me a retard?" These issues, when handled with the necessary reassurance, have been demonstrated to be therapeutic in enabling the individual to understand and accept himself or herself as a worthy human being. Other concerns, such as object loss, separation, and problems in interpersonal relationships, are a few of the many clinical issues that are addressed. The group also discusses individual goals as they relate to program objectives. Issues such as impulse control, problem solving, self-esteem, peer relationships, and alternatives to "acting out" are meaningful, identifiable, and clinically relevant to all group members.

The therapist begins the last phase of the group therapy session by asking the members to review the sequential order of the activities for the day—because this is the first group on Thursday morning. This review reinforces structure and individual involvement in the group. The group therapy session ends with holding hands in a circle, and then a member is asked by the therapist to lead a brief, nonstrenuous physical exercise. Spontaneous applause generally follows, which provides a positive tone for the day as well as group recognition, support, and celebration of and for itself.

It is worth noting that the group therapist plays an active leadership role. The therapist frequently needs to provide group structure and movement in the group. At times, the leader needs to generate topics for discussion and facilitate members' related experiences. Some individuals need to be reminded to listen and to be helped to acknowledge the feelings of others in the group. The group leader periodically checks for the group's understanding not only of the therapist's language but of the communication among group members. This particular role, as noted above, is in agreement with Berkovitz and Sugar.[11] According to Jacob,[12] the clinical problems of the mentally retarded are not different from those of people of normal intelligence, and their problems are just as amenable to treatment through group psychotherapy. The group therapy differences lie in the fact that those whose intellect is limited require a group leader who takes a more active role and supplies strong direction and guidance. Understanding and insight take longer, and thus, the therapist needs a great deal of patience.

Substantial gains have been made with the dually diagnosed population in using a group psychotherapy approach as an important and integral part of the treatment process. The group fosters increased social interaction, increases problem-solving skills, and has a positive effect on decreasing feelings of isolation, rejection, and defeat.

12.6. Sensory Integration Therapy

Sensory integration can be described as the ability to organize and process the sensory functions of the central nervous system, which are reflected in motor behavior and patterns of learning. A disruption of the information-gathering and -processing functions can lead to sensory integration dysfunction. The health field of occupational therapy has greatly stimulated the development of sensory integration therapy. Occupational therapy for sensory integration dysfunction involves the active participation of a person in a series of prescribed purposeful activities directed toward improving sensory processing, facilitating sensory integration, and making possible affective and appropriate interaction with the environment. The theoretical principles for sensory integration began in the early 1960s, when Jean Ayres[13] began research that laid the foundation for a neurobehavioral orientation in the field of psychiatric occupational therapy. Sensory integration therapy, according to Ayres, is based on the premise that the brain is a self-organizing system that integrates or coordinates "Two or more functions or processes in a manner which enhances the adaptiveness of the brain responses; one of the most powerful organizers of sensory input is movement which is adaptive to the organism" (p. 221).

One's ability to organize, integrate, and interpret internal and external stimuli is based on the perceptual process. The perceptual process is developmental and begins with the early experiences of infancy and develops throughout adulthood. Tiffany[14] has indicated that if the process is interrupted or if the central nervous system is in some way dysfunctional, then the perceptual distortions may prevent normal interactions between the individual and her or his environment. The result may be major difficulties in reality testing, as well as lack of development of functional cognitive and motor abilities.

Recent research has pointed out that the mentally retarded and the mentally ill are high-risk groups for developing and manifesting sensory integration dysfunctions. Molnar[15] found that mentally retarded infants have significantly delayed motor development, and McCracken[16] noted that retarded children are significantly inferior in manual forms, finger identification, graphesthesia, and perception of spontaneous stimuli. Therapeutically, Resman[17] found positive changes in eye contact in the retarded population when a sensory integration approach was used, and Clark et al.[18] reported relative effectiveness with sensory integration approaches in retarded populations. Norton[19] and Kantner[20] have demonstrated in separate, but similar, studies that vestibular input is a therapeutic modality aide in the development of improved postural reactions in the retarded population. A number of researchers have found a relationship between emotional disturbances and the vestibular system. Fish[21] reported that early neurological deviations were more characteristic of severely impaired schizophrenic children with IQs under 70 and that more than half of such children demonstrated irregular and delayed postural development. Erway[22] contended that there is an impaired vestibular function in schizophrenic patients and that adequate vestibular function is basic to emotional stability. King,[23] building on the early research of Ayres, has developed a body of knowledge about sensory integration dysfunction and schizophrenics. She believes that schizophrenics have defects in proprioceptive mechanisms that result in sensory integration dysfunctions such as a lack of perceptual constancy, poor body image, inadequate motor planning, and fatigue-producing postural patterns. These neurophysiological impairments, it is hypothesized, lead to severe emotional problems. King has found validated success in employing sensory-integration therapeutic approaches to neurophysiological dysfunctions. The sensory-integration remediation approach utilized at Beacon House is based on King's methods.

At Beacon House, activities are selected on the basis of two criteria: first, conscious attention is on the outcome, not on the motor process; and second, the activity must be pleasurable. The treatment process uses purposeful activities that provide selected sensory input primarily through vestibular, proprioceptive, and tactile channels. The treatment goals are to provide sensory stimulation, to promote socialization, to enhance body awareness, and to increase self-esteem. Individual goals are further specified according to individual needs. Examples of specific treatment activities are described in the following paragraphs.

Games using a nylon parachute are especially useful in stimulating proprioceptive and vestibular functioning. While some members lift the balloon over their heads, other individuals attempt to move under it to the other side before it floats down. Another technique utilizes balloons that are bounced on top of fabric or rolled around on fabric, the object being to keep them in motion while not allowing them to fall to the ground. Ball games, involving tossing a ball into a basket, passing it from one to another over the head or between the legs, and so on, are excellent eye–hand exercises that enhance coordination and directionality. Jumping exercises also enhance the sense of balance and timing. Other specific activities are used to facilitate the development of color, texture, hearing, visual, and smell discrimination. These involve games in which the players experience different sensory stimulations.

The ability to process sensory information is fundamental if a person is to effectively function in his or her environment. The theories in research related to sensory integration have provided a basis for the utilization of sensory integration theory by our occupational therapists at Beacon House for this multidisabled population.

12.7. Horticulture Therapy

Gardening was employed as preventive medicine centuries before the field of psychiatry was developed. Olszowy[24] has reported that in 1768 Benjamin Rush believed that digging in the soil had a curative effect in the mentally ill, and by 1806, hospitals in Spain were emphasizing the benefits of agricultural and horticultural activities for their mentally ill patients. By the turn of the century, programs had been developed in many hospitals and institutions making use of grounds and farms. Veterans' hospitals have used garden therapy for the treatment and rehabilitation of disabled soldiers. There have been a number of citings in the literature indicating that plants have a positive effect on human behavior, including studies by Beatty,[25] Carew,[26] Kaplan,[27] and Menninger.[28] The pioneer work from the Menninger Clinic during the 1950s added to the credibility of horticulture as a bona fide therapy. The emergence of college-level programs in horticulture therapy during the 1970s reflected this acceptance.

Beacon House has long recognized the therapeutic value of working with plants as exemplified by having a horticulture therapist on staff since its inception. The horticulture program that was developed for the Independent Living Group is provided in a nonthreatening milieu in which both verbal and nonverbal communication takes place. The verbal interaction is involved in group planning; the activity itself is essentially nonverbal and is frequently done on an individual basis. This year, each member has made his or her own terrarium using recycled bottles. In the summer, a large garden supplies most of the vegetables used in the Beacon House lunch program. Another special project is the maintenance of landscaping around the City Hall in Kingston, and an indoor greenhouse enables projects to be continued during the winter months.

Mentally retarded and mentally ill persons frequently misinterpret sensory impulses, and working with plants activates sensory awareness. The stimulation of the senses that working with plants evokes facilitates the development of sensory awareness and integration. Also, working with plants aids in the development of fine and gross motor skills. Working with plants also involves the acceptance of responsibility and the realistic expectation of a successful experience. Specific clinical issues, such as motivation, delayed gratification, object loss, and social interaction, are addressed with plants as the medium. Horticulture therapy enables the members to develop these skills, for example, motivation to plant the seeds, patience in watching their slow growth, understanding and acceptance of a plant's death, and interactional skills in group planning. Additionally, caring for plants provides a socially acceptable means through which one's need to nurture can be met. Plants are nonthreatening and respond in a demonstrative way to care and attention.

Horticulture therapy in our Independent Living Program provides a vehicle for group planning, a means to achieve individual success, and a channel in which plants serve as clinical prototypes.

12.8. Cooking Group

The cooking group is a "here-and-now," action-oriented group activity with an emphasis on both interactional and skill development. Learning new skills and learning appropriate interactional behaviors are interdependent variables and are incorporated into the learning process of the cooking group.

The planning phase is a group endeavor. The members, along with two staff members, plan four weeks in advance what the group will make. This planning is necessary for administrative ordering of the food, but more important, it provides the group with planning responsibility, which, in turn, establishes internal structure and organization.

The second phase is the actual preparation and cooking. This part of the process also begins with a short group meeting to decide on who will do what in the process. The members are encouraged to make decisions in terms of individual contributions to the cooking group. Choice, physical limitations, and skill level are considered when tasks are divided among the participants. The normative standard is that all members be involved at one task or another.

The cooking process is usually gratifying, enhances self-esteem, and fosters a sense of responsibility and accomplishment. Verbal praise for active involvement is frequent and is made public. For instance, one member who has poor gross-motor skills because of cerebral palsy elected to mix a large cake batter. This willingness to risk received a round of applause. Staff and members stopped what they were doing and gave recognition—not for accomplishing a task—but for willingness to try something that was obviously difficult for this individual.

The third phase of the cooking group is the actual consumption of the selected delectable. This is an obvious reward for the labor.

The cooking group is designed to teach members practical cooking skills and is geared to promote mental health. The learning of food preparation and cooking facilitates further independent-skill-level functioning, which contributes to increased feelings of self-worth, self-esteem, and self-satisfaction.

12.9. Community Meeting

The community meeting, which is the first group meeting of the week, is short, but it serves a variety of functions. One function is to provide a forum for members to express feelings or concerns. Like the psychotherapy or "rap" group, this opportunity for ventilation serves the purpose of cartharsis. The community meeting also serves to foster individual decision-making with respect to special group activities such as field trips. It promotes a sense of responsibility for making decisions, and these decisions foster a sense of autonomy and self-control. Like the psychotherapy group, the community meeting begins with, "Who is not here today?" I am the group leader for both the psychotherapy group and the community meeting.

12.10. Dance/Movement Therapy

The field of dance/movement therapy emerged during the 1940s and is traced to the great influx of mental patients into psychiatric hospitals after

World War II. The field has been gaining increased acceptance in the mental health arena as a viable therapeutic approach to treating mentally ill and mentally retarded populations. The American Dance Therapy Association (ADTA), which was formed in 1964, defines dance therapy as a psychotherapeutic use of movement to further the emotional and physical motivation of the individual.

Wilhelm Reich[29] wrote about the interdependent relationships of the physical and mental states. He pointed out that physiological behavior determines psychic behavior, as the psyche equally determines physiological behavior. This formulation has become the basic theoretical construct of dance/movement therapy. Pioneers in the field, like Marian Chace, [30] have applied this principle in utilizing the therapeutic medium of dance/movement.

All persons express themselves nonverbally: they scratch their heads when they are thinking, or they yawn when tired. Such physical language is difficult to control at best, and being partly beyond conscious control, it enables the dance/movement therapist to probe beneath the surface to reveal clinical and diagnostic material and thus to make appropriate assessments and interventions.

Mentally retarded people typically display muscular control difficulty, tend to imitate rather than initiate movements, and characteristically perserverate in their body movements. Schizophrenics, on the other hand, whose body image fantasies often center on the loss of body boundaries, may have an unrealistic sense of body limits and distorted body images.

There has been some descriptive evidence found in the literature indicating a correlation between the nonverbal therapy of dance/movement and subsequent improvement in functioning. At present, the research is scarce and generally has been observational or descriptive. For example, Dryansky[31] has reported an increased verbal interaction with peers and staff by a hospitalized schizophrenic young woman in a long-range dance-therapy program.

The dance/movement therapy program for the Independent Living Group meets once a week for a 45-minute session. The dance/movement therapist uses the techniques prescribed by Marian Chace,[30] who is one of the founders of dance/movement therapy. A primary goal of this therapy is for the expansion of a movement vocabulary to increase the ability of the individual to express attitudes, feelings, and ideas.

In applying the Chace method to the group, the members guide themselves, and the role of the therapist is to support the individuals in the group. The therapist works at the same level at which the member is functioning. For example, the group had been doing a psychodrama experiential exercise. A member whose psychopathology is characterized by childlike behavior began to withdraw from the group and began to lie on the floor in a fetal-like position that stimulated the member's verbal and nonverbal behaviors. From this interaction, member and therapist were able to identify at the same functioning level, and this identification initiated a meaningful therapeutic contact. There was a nonverbal acknowledgment in which the member was aware that the therapist was there at that moment for support and reassurance. After reflecting his image, through her body language, the therapist proceeded to sit up; the member then followed. She moved to a standing position, and he continued to mirror her posture. The member was asked to rejoin the group and a group discussion was then initiated by the therapist to process the feelings of this experience. Closure was precipitated by the group's doing a grounding exercise to reaffirm adult stance and posture. The movement therapist's first intervention was to mirror the member's body; intervention was initiated via a more assertive posture and was designed to be used as a role model; it was effective in enabling the member to redirect his focus, to be more adultlike, and to actively join the group.

The above illustration demonstrates that the mentally retarded–mentally ill population can use their bodies to convey emotions with dance/movement therapy as a medium. The therapist was able to connect with a regressed, socially isolated individual; to communicate at his level; and then to bring him into active group involvement. One objective that applies to all members of this group is to help develop an accurate body image, which is indispensable for building a positive self-image. Dance/movement therapy has the secondary benefit of working on fine and gross motor skills, at the same time aiding in the development of sensory integration. It is important to note that movement therapy is especially useful in the case of those individuals who, because of cognitive limitations, have poor verbal communication skills. Even when such skills are intact, verbal communication can be perceived as threatening.

This modality of therapy is a resourceful treatment technique that is particularly useful with this group in that contact, relationship, motivation, and prescribed treatment outcomes can be achieved in a nonthreatening verbal, as well as a nonverbal, expressive treatment approach.

12.11. Music Therapy

Music as a medium for therapy emerged during the 1940s in response to the growing number of patients who did not respond to a verbal therapy approach in veterans' hospitals during World War II. During the 1950s, a number of colleges and universities established a specialized curriculum designed to train music therapists. The National Association of Music Therapy (NAMT) was established in 1950 and has provided greater unity in educational standards, clinical practice, research, and certification. During the 1950s, there was a considerable amount of investigation that began to probe the relationship between music and behavioral changes. The use of music therapy in working with mentally retarded individuals has grown more rapidly than any other use of music therapy.[32] This trend is largely a result of increased professional awareness of the therapeutic effects of music therapy with this population. Michael-Smith[33] described a study in which music therapy resulted in progress in group relatedness and in verbal and kinesthetic self-expressions. At the same time, the parents of his subjects reported increased initiative and self-expression in the home. Gaston[34] has stated, with reference to the mentally retarded population, "Music offers an excellent situation for the operation of group dynamics. Thus, music operates as an integrating and socializing agency by providing a situation for the adaptation of suitable behavior to group function" (p. 43).

The music therapy techniques employed in the Independent Living Program are based on the theories of Gaston,[34] Marti-Ibanez,[35] and Diekurs and Crocker.[36] The objective is to employ music as a therapeutic means of illiciting appropriate emotional responses from individuals who generally exhibit few or no appropriate responses. This is accomplished by matching the music to the prevailing mood as closely as possible, and then gradually altering the music in the desired direction. For example, as the group was sitting in a circle, the music therapist asked, "How are you feeling today?" One member yawned, and then the therapist yawned, followed by other members yawning. The therapist used the response to help the group create and sing a song in slow tempo about being tired. Beginning at the members' energy level, the therapist slowly increased the tempo, and the members responded by singing louder and with more alertness. The mood of the group moved from lethargy to enthusiasm. By integrating gestalt psychotherapy principles of the here and now with music therapy techniques, the music therapist incorporated approaches to resistance and other behavioral responses into the music activities to bring about the desired change in affect. The ability of music to be soothing can create an environment that is relaxing and that therefore can significantly lower anxiety. Furthermore, the verbal content of music is effective in dealing with personal issues. Encouraging the group of individuals to make up words to their own original piece is a way of illiciting information from the members that might otherwise be resisted. The music therapist at Beacon House utilizes this approach to bring the group to a common point of focus. Participation in a music group provides a form of feedback for the individual's own identity and accomplishments. It also promotes a sense of self-worth and group contribution. In addition, music instills focus, organization, and structure in a manner that is experienced as fun. Lastly, the structure provided by a music activity responds to the need for repetition and familiarity.

The value of music as a medium in group therapy helps to enhance appropriate affect, self-esteem, and socialization. The deficit of appropriate communicative ability, which handicaps the members of the Independent Living Program, necessitates initiating satisfying, socially acceptable means of communicating feelings. Music therapy is a viable vehicle for this expression because it provides a nonthreatening verbal, as well as nonverbal, milieu experience in which trusting therapeutic relationships can develop.

12.12. Education

Although concern about treatment for the mentally retarded has varied widely over the centuries, the actual education of mentally retarded people was not a matter of interest until the early nineteenth century. A host of different philosophies concerning how best to educate the mentally retarded was developed during the twentieth century. An emphasis on emotional and social variables preempted the earlier physiological and multisensory orientation to education. In the early 1950s, social scientists began to have a persuasive and pervasive influence on the special-education curricula and methodology for teaching the mentally retarded. The influence of the principles of behavior analysis became an important part of the special-education process during the 1960s.

A psychoeducational approach is employed as the key remedial educational focus in the Independent Living Program. The program encompasses the traditional learning skills of education in a supportive therapeutic environment. There are three staff members assigned to the group. Experience has indicated that small groups consisting of two or three members with a staff instructor are necessary in order to maintain interest and motivation in the learning process. Another factor involved in this staff-to-member ratio is the wide range of educational experiences, interests, abilities, and learning potentials within the membership.

The educational program is divided into three subgroups on the basis of academic ability. One group learns basic skills, such as number identification, shape discrimination, and writing name, phone number, and address. Another group works on coin identification, money exchange, and financial management; this group follows a sequence dealing with money and will later work on understanding and managing bank accounts. The third group works on reading comprehension and the writing of compositions.

Each group changes focus and subject matter about every three months. This periodic change helps to maintain interest and motivation for both members and staff. In the past, Beacon House has covered various psychoeducational areas. Last year, a consultant from the Planned Parenthood League conducted an eight-week sexuality seminar, which was a valuable experience both educationally and therapeutically. Initially, it was difficult for some of the members to talk about their bodies and sexuality. However, by the end of the eight weeks, it was quite obvious that each person had learned a great deal and was able to contribute to the seminar. The group uses a wide variety of audiovisual equipment, such as films, tapes, records, and educational workbooks.

As many of our members felt unsuccessful and defeated during their former education years, this program is designed to provide each member with a sense of accomplishment and success, thus having a positive and influential effect on self-esteem and self-worth. The members receive a great deal of individual attention and are praised at every step in the educational therapeutic process. A successful step does not necessarily mean attaining competency in a particular academic area. Involvement in the group process by sharing feelings and information with others is a key element in maintaining enthusiasm and interest.

12.13. Arts-and-Crafts Therapy

Ann Mosey[37] offered three principles associated with activity therapy. One of the principles of this approach comes from the concept of milieu therapy and characterizes the everyday interactions of people as a way of facilitating individual growth, development, and the acquisition of new skills. A second principle is that the dynamics of group interaction can be used to foster change. The support of a cohesive group can help shape behavior in a way that is more satisfying to the individual and to the group. A third principle in activity therapy is based on the concept that psychosocial dysfunction results, in part, from not having learned to function in the macrocommunity. These three principles are applied to the arts-and-crafts therapy program and fully capitalize on the current knowledge about the teaching–learning process to develop needed behavioral and interactional skills.

The members, as a group, decide on the types of projects to be considered. Individuals work on their own individual projects but work at one table and share supplies such as glue, paper, and paints. Three staff members—consisting of an occupational therapist, a student in the same field, and a program aide— act as group facilitators. Three staff members are needed because many of the members require one-to-one guidance. Even a simple one- or two-step activity requires an integration of the motor, cognitive, perceptual, and emotional systems. Because these are the maladaptive and dysfunctional behavioral systems characteristic of this dual-diagnosis population, careful guidance and support are important prerequisites for a successful arts-and-crafts therapy program.

Group process is employed to facilitate interactional skills, decision making, and responsibility. To illustrate, recently the group decided to make wind chimes out of clay (in a multiple-step process). The first step involves throwing clay to make it pliable. A member of the group was unable, at first, to take a handful of clay and throw it on the table. The person said, "I can't do it." A group therapist stood behind her, held her arm, and physically helped her throw the clay. As this was happening, the therapist, acting as the member's alter ego, said, "I can do it, I can do it." Support was provided by other group members who were encouraging her to throw the clay. Another member said, "Do it, it really feels good." After this support provided by staff and members, she made progress and gradually began to throw the clay with much more fluidity of movement. The following week, when the project was completed, she appeared more relaxed with the activity, less restricted, and pleased with the result.

Arts and crafts as an approach to activity therapy provide a means by which individuals can gain a sense of accomplishment, self-worth, and success in a way that promotes interaction and group relatedness. This modality is also a vehicle for addressing the needs of neurobehavioral dysfunctions in areas of perception, bilaterality, directionality, and motor skills. A trained occupational therapist can assess emotional and physical impairments and thus prescribe appropriate interventions as they relate to individual needs to promote optimal functioning.

12.14. Research Study

In order to test the effectiveness of the Independent Living Program, I did the following research study.

The 10 subjects were evaluated by six different counselors as they appeared on admission, and again after an average of 14 months in the program. The evaluation consisted of rating each of the 10 subjects on a scale from 1 ("poor") to 7 ("high") in six different categories. The categories included (1) self-esteem (i.e., favorable opinion of oneself as observed in verbal and non-verbal behaviors); (2) socialization (i.e., ability to socialize and interact with others); (3) problem solving (i.e., the resourcefulness with which a member responded to a situation of difficulty or conflict); (4) impulse control (i.e., the behavioral management of, or appropriate response to, a sudden influence of feelings, thoughts, or actions); (5) meeting program criteria (i.e., ability to be at a group or a function at the scheduled time or place); and (6) program participation (i.e., degree of the member's involvement in the Independent Living Program).

For each counselor, the mean of the admission scores for all of the subjects for each of the categories was computed. The same procedure was conducted after an average of 14 months in the program. Each counselor had a total of 12 means—6 means in each category before the treatment and 6 means for each category after the treatment. The following is an analysis of the differences of those means in each of the six categories.

The means representing evaluations on admission to the program are referred to as the *prescores*; those following attendance in the program are referred to as the *postscores*. The six counselors are designated by the letters A through F.

12.14.1. Methodology

The objective of the following statistical tests was to determine if there were any significant differences between each of the means before and after the program was administered in each of the six categories. The 10 subjects served as their own control group. The randomization test for matched pairs was used to determine if the means in each category differed significantly. For each of the six tests (one for each category), the following null-hypothesis format applied: The set of mean scores given by the evaluators before the program do not significantly differ from the set of scores given after the program. The alternate hypothesis was: The set of means scores given after the treatment program is significantly higher than the scores given before the program.

Let alpha equal .05. $N = 6$, the number of counselors evaluating the subjects. The alpha error is the probability that the conclusions of this report are incorrect. The randomization test for matched pairs[38] is a nonparametric test that is a variation of the sign test, which examines the binomial distribution of the signs of the differences between two sets of data. This test actually weighs the value of the differences, which makes it more powerful than the standard sign test.

The sampling distribution consisted of the permutation of the signed differences that occurred between the prescores program and the postscores. In this case, this included a possible 64 different permutations on six differences. Because the hypotheses (the null and the alternate) were clearly stated in this study, a one-tailed test is appropriate. The region of rejection consists of the top three outcomes in the list of permuted sums of sign differences, which are listed for each experiment.

TEST NO. 1
CATEGORY: SELF-ESTEEM

COUNSELOR	PRESCORES	POSTSCORES	DIFFERENCES
A	1.3	2.5	+ 1.2
B	2.6	2.9	+ 0.3
C	2.0	2.7	+ 0.7
D	2.8	3.5	+ 0.7
E	2.0	3.2	+ 1.2
F	2.8	3.1	+ 0.4

Conclusion: The number of extreme permutations greater than or equal to the above outcome is 1. The probability of this occurrence is .016. Because this is less than alpha, our decision is to reject the null hypothesis. The differences are significant ones.

TEST NO. 2
CATEGORY: SOCIALIZATION

COUNSELOR	PRESCORES	POSTSCORES	DIFFERENCES
A	1.8	2.7	+ 0.9
B	2.3	2.3	0.0
C	1.8	3.4	+ 1.6
D	3.2	4.1	+ 0.9
E	2.8	4.0	+ 1.2
F	1.8	2.4	+ 0.6

Conclusion: The number of extreme permutations greater than or equal to the above outcome is 1. The probability of this occurrence is .016. Because this is less than alpha, our decision is to reject the null hypothesis. Again, the differences are significant.

TEST NO. 3
CATEGORY: PROBLEM SOLVING

COUNSELOR	PRESCORES	POSTSCORES	DIFFERENCES
A	2.0	3.1	+ 1.1
B	2.6	2.7	+ 0.1
C	2.4	2.7	+ 0.3
D	3.6	4.2	+ 0.6
E	2.4	3.4	+ 1.0
F	2.1	2.3	+ 0.2

Conclusion: The number of extreme permutations greater than or equal to the above outcome is 1. The probability of this occurrence is .016. Because this is less than alpha, our decision is to reject the null hypothesis. The differences are significant.

TEST NO. 4
CATEGORY: IMPULSE CONTROL

COUNSELOR	PRESCORES	POSTSCORES	DIFFERENCES
A	2.5	3.8	+ 1.3
B	2.6	2.7	+ 0.1
C	2.5	2.6	+ 0.1
D	3.8	4.4	+ 0.6
E	4.8	5.7	+ 0.9
F	2.5	2.8	+ 0.3

Conclusion: The number of extreme permutations greater than or equal to the above outcome is 1. The probability of this occurrence is .016. Because this is less than alpha, our decision is to reject the null hypothesis. Again, the differences are significant.

TEST NO. 5
CATEGORY: MEETING PROGRAM CRITERIA

COUNSELOR	PRESCORES	POSTSCORES	DIFFERENCES
A	2.1	3.0	+ 0.9
B	2.3	2.4	+ 0.1
C	3.1	3.9	+ 0.8
D	3.5	4.2	+ 0.7
E	3.3	4.7	+ 1.4
F	2.5	3.1	+ 0.6

Conclusion: The number of extreme permutations greater than or equal to the above outcome is 1. The probability of this occurrence is .016. Because this is less than alpha, our decision is to reject the null hypothesis. The differences are significant.

TEST NO. 6
CATEGORY: PARTICIPATION

COUNSELOR	PRESCORES	POSTSCORES	DIFFERENCES
A	1.9	3.1	+ 1.2
B	2.4	2.5	+ 0.1
C	3.4	3.6	+ 0.2
D	3.8	4.8	+ 1.0
E	3.6	4.1	+ 0.5
F	2.2	3.2	+ 1.0

Conclusion: The number of extreme permutations greater than or equal to the above outcome is 1. The probability of this occurrence is .016. Because this is less than alpha, our decision is to reject the null hypothesis. The differences are significant.

12.14.2. Interpretation of Overall Results

Each of the six tests showed that the counselors as a group rated the subjects with mean scores that were significantly higher *after* attendance in the Independent Living Program than *before* their attendance in the program in every category. The effectiveness of the program, in categories from most effective to least effective, was (1) socialization; (2) meeting program criteria;

(3) self-esteem; (4) participation in program; (5) impulse control; and lastly, (6) problem solving. Clearly, the Independent Living Program has been of value to these 10 dual-diagnosis individuals. The results of this objective research study have prompted us to want to extend the number of individuals served by the program.

12.15. Recommendations

It is unfortunate that many clinicians have historically perceived that traditional treatment for the psychiatric problems of the mentally retarded is a futile and unwarranted exercise. Much of this prejudice is based on ignorance, lack of training, or a client population preference. It is time for professionals to reevaluate their values and attitudes on this topic and to assess their interference with the quality and the quantity of psychiatric care that can be provided to this neglected population.

It is imperative that professional schools that prepare practitioners for the mental health field include in their curriculum a section that addresses the psychiatric problems of the retarded. For those already in the field, courses through continuing-education workshops, in-service education, and the like would be beneficial. These learning experiences would not only impart knowledge but would have a positive effect on the attitudes and values of professionals, which, in turn, would result in better quality mental-health services for the retarded.

Just as individuals in the mental health profession need to reexamine their roles, the mental-health and mental-retardation delivery systems need to reevaluate the bureaucratic structure. The systems for mental health and mental retardation have been so rigidly regulated that the need for interdigitation of services has been inhibited and difficult to achieve.

The present bureaucratic structure makes it difficult to clearly identify the psychiatric problems of the retarded and to provide adequate help. Funding problems and the need to set priorities result in each agency focusing on its own client population. Therefore, the dually handicapped remain largely undiagnosed, largely untreated, and largely neglected. The fundamental dilemma is that the psychiatric problems of the mentally retarded are not identified. Clinicians need to be more aware of the fact that a mentally retarded person may also have a psychiatric disorder. Once this fact is recognized, the next step is to plan a comprehensive rehabilitation program; such a program requires systematic and cooperative efforts by both the mental health and the mental retardation systems.

American culture is very work-oriented, and the ability to earn money through one's own effort is highly valued. As a member of this society, the dually diagnosed individual also adheres to this work ethic. The ability to produce and earn enhances one's self-esteem and one's perception of his or her position in society. For this reason it is recommended that a vocational program such as a sheltered workshop be included in the rehabilitation–treatment program.

It is not difficult for existing psychiatric treatment centers to expand their service to include a program similar to the one just described. The establishment of the Independent Living Program did not expand the budget of Beacon House. The program was developed and still exists without any additional funds or salaried staff. Creative use of internal professional and paraprofessional staff, graduate students, and shared staff from other agencies constitutes our present staffing pattern. We are now in the process of developing a volunteer program to augment our staff, which will include high functioning members from other sections of Beacon House.

A day-treatment center can replicate the milieu treatment model as described in this paper, or it can modify one to address the needs and resources of a particular agency. The first step is to identify those individuals within a service agency who may have the dual diagnosis of mental retardation and mental illness. A careful screening, including a psychiatric evaluation, psychological testing, a neurological examination, a psychosocial assessment, and a developmentally oriented case history, can be a cogent aid in this process. Once the population has been identified, a staffing pattern can be developed and coordinated. As in Beacon House, this did not require new staff; rather, it utilized the strengths of existing internal staff augmented by other resources in the community.

12.16. Conclusion

The program at Beacon House has been demonstrated to be effective in addressing some of the critical mental-health needs of the mentally ill–retarded population. Small and highly structured groups, in a supportive environment, have provided a viable method for effecting positive and lasting changes in psychosocial functioning.

The members have formed a cohesive group with a corresponding strong and positive group identity. A considerable amount of support and encouragement is demonstrated by one member to another. This type of interaction has been modeled by the members of the staff. Also, the sense of belonging to a peer group counteracts the pervasive feelings of isolation and inadequacy that are characteristic of these individuals.

It is important to note that, through the description of the Beacon House program, the emphasis has been primarily on the process rather than on the content of each group transaction. One's active involvement in the process is, indeed, the treatment. In the model just described, the therapist must keep this focus constantly in mind. The role of the groups is to effect change through personal involvement. The end result in terms of concrete skills is secondary. The success of the program is measured by an increase in positive feelings about the self, more involvement in socialization activities, enhancement of impulse control, and more effective problem-solving. The research reported here has clearly indicated that these improvements have, indeed, occurred at Beacon House.

In conclusion, the size and scope of the mentally retarded population at risk for mental illness have important theoretical and practical implications for the delivery of mental health services. Traditionally, the population that is affected with the multiple disability of mental retardation and mental illness has not been significantly identified; therefore, the needed mental-health services have not been made available. The mental health professionals and the organizations with which they are affiliated need to take a more active role in providing services to this neglected population.

In the 1980s, with shrinking financial resources, agencies need to explore nontraditional methods of providing mental health services. Maintaining existing services may not be enough. The care delivery system must continue to identify those in need of services and actively advocate services for those least able to speak for themselves. Agencies need to build bridges with other agencies, explore resources, and develop creative methods and ideas of programming and funding.

References

1. Leaverton DR, Van der Heida C: *Lip Service No Longer.* Paper presented at the American Association on Mental Deficiency Annual Meeting, Portland, OR, 1975.
2. Menolascino FJ, Bernstein N: Psychiatric assessment of the mentally retarded child, in Bernstein NR (ed): *Diminished People—Problems and Care of the Mentally Retarded.* Boston, Little, Brown, 1970.
3. Walker, P: Recognizing the mental health needs of developmentally disabled people. *Social Work,* MASW;293–297, 1980.
4. Phillips I: Children, mentally retarded, and emotional disorder, in Phillips I (ed): *Prevention and Treatment of Mental Retardation.* New York, Basic Books, 1966.
5. American Psychiatric Association: *Diagnostic and Statistical Manual,* ed 3. Washington, D.C., Author, 1980.
6. Wilcox GT, Guthrie GM: Changes in adjustment of institutionalized female defectives following group psychotherapy. *J Clin Psychol* 13;9–13, 1957.
7. Rosen HB, Rosen S: Group therapy as an instrument to develop a concept of self-worth in the adolescent and young adult mentally retarded. *Ment Retard* 7;52–55, 1969.
8. Gorlow L, Butler A, Einig K: An appraisal of self attitude and behavior following group psychotherapy with retarded young adults. *Am J Ment Defic* 67;893–898, 1963.
9. Baron FN: Group therapy improves mental retardate behavior. *Hosp Commun Psychiatr* 23;7–11, 1972.
10. Richards LD, Lee KA: Group process in social rehabilitation of the retarded. *Social Casework* 53;30–38, 1972.
11. Berkovitz IH, Sugar M: Indications and contraindications for adolescent group psychotherapy, in Sugar M (ed): *The Adolescent in Group and Family Therapy.* New York, Brunner/Mazel, 1975.
12. Jacob I: Psychotherapy of the mentally retarded child, in Bernstein NR (ed): *Diminished People—Problems and Care of the Mentally Retarded.* Boston, Little, Brown, 1970.
13. Ayres AJ: The development of perceptual motor abilities: A Theoretical basis for treatment of dysfunction. *Am J Occup Ther* 17;221–223, 1963.
14. Tiffany EG: Elements of the psychiatric therapy process, in Hopkins HL, Smith HD (eds): *Williard & Spackman O.T.,* ed. 5. Philadelphia, Lippincott, 1978.

15. Molnar G: Motor deficit of retarded infants and young children. *Arch Phys Med Rehab* 55;393–398, 1974.
16. McCracken A: Tactile function of educable mentally retarded children. *Am J Occupl Ther* 17;397–402, 1975.
17. Resman MH: Effect of sensory stimulation on eye contact in a profoundly retarded adult. *Am J Occup Ther* 35;31–35, 1981.
18. Clark F, Miller L, Thomas J: A comparison of operant and sensory integrative methods on developmental parameter in profoundly retarded adults. *Am J Occup Ther* 32;86–93, 1978.
19. Norton Y: Neuro-development and sensory integration for the profoundly retarded and multiply handicapped child. *Am J Occup Ther* 29;93–100, 1975.
20. Kantner R: Effects of vestibular stimulation on systems response and motor performance in the developmentally delayed infants. *Phys Ther* 56;414–421, 1976.
21. Fish B: The creator of schizophrenia in infancy: A ten year follow-up report of neurological and psychological development. *J Am Psychiatr Assoc* 21;768–775, 1965.
22. Erway L: Otolith formulation and trace elements of schizophrenic behavior. *J Otolith Psychiatr* 4;16–26, 1975.
23. King LJ: A sensory integrative approach to schizophrenia. *Am J Occupl Ther* 28;529–535, 1974.
24. Olszowy DR: Principles of horticulture therapy, in *Horticulture for the Disabled and Disadvantaged*. Springfield, Mass., Charles G. Thanes, 1978.
25. Beatty VL: Highrise horticulture. *Amer Hort* 53;42–46, 1974.
26. Carew HJ: *The Composition of Horticulturists*. Proceedings of the Seventeenth International Horticultural Congress 2;89, 1966.
27. Kaplan R: Some psychological benefits of gardening. *Envir Behav* 5;145–161, 1973.
28. Menninger CF: Recreation and moral: I. *Hort Bul Menninger Clin* 6;65–67, 1972.
29. Reich W: *Character Analysis*. New York, Simon and Schuster, 1945.
30. Chace M: Autobiography, in Chaikline H (ed): *Marian Chace: Her Papers*. Baltimore, American Dance Therapy Association, 1975.
31. Dryansky V: *A Case Study of Chronic Paranoid Schizophrenic in Dance Therapy*, in Monograph No. 3. New York, American Dance Therapy Association, 1973.
32. Howery B: Overview, in *Music in Therapy*. New York, Macmillian, 1973.
33. Michael-Smith H: Psychotherapy in the mentally retarded, in Michael-Smith H, Kastein S (eds): *The Special Child*. Seattle, New School for the Special Child, 1962.
34. Gaston T: Dynamic music factors in mood changes. *Music Educators Journal* 37;42–44, 1951.
35. Marti-Ibanez F: Psychic muse: music, the dance, and medicine. Medical News Magazine, 20;14–15, 1976.
36. Diekurs R, Crocker E: Music therapy with psychotic children, in Gaston ET (ed): *Music Therapy*. London, Allen Press, 1955.
37. Mosey AC: The teaching-learning process. *Activities Therapy*, 4th ed. New York, Raven Press Books, 1973.
38. Siegel L: *Nonparametric Statistics for the Behavioral Sciences*. New York, McGraw-Hill, 1956.

13

A Home Intervention Program for Mentally Retarded-Emotionally Disturbed Individuals and Their Families

Robert B. Allin and Diana W. Allin

13.1. Introduction

The present project, entitled the Home Intervention Program (HIP), is an attempt to help fill the gap in services offered to individuals with mental retardation and emotional disturbance. The program model represents the unique combination of several distinct components: (1) services provided in the natural environment; (2) a husband–wife therapist team; (3) an eclectic approach to treatment; and (4) flexible time scheduling (i.e., time of day and amount of time).

The purpose of this chapter is to present an account of our work with this program model, including a brief review of the research studies and basic assumptions that have stimulated and supported its design, a description of program methodology, and a presentation of project findings highlighted by individual case examples. In addition, discussions are provided that focus on the population and the treatment and on the advantages and the limitations of the HIP model.

13.2. Literature Review

With the relatively recent trends toward deinstitutionalization and normalization of the mentally retarded, as well as the subsequent demands for alternative modes of services at the community level, parents have been the focus of much attention. Strategies for therapeutic intervention with parents

A cooperative venture between the Mental Health and Mental Retardation Services of the Community Services Board in Chesterfield County, Virginia, the Home Intervention Program began its research and design phases in late 1978. Program implementation and data collection commenced in mid-1979, and evaluative findings early in 1982 supported the continuation of HIP services. The project has been encouraged and funded by the Virginia Department of Mental Health and Mental Retardation, and the Chesterfield County Board of Supervisors.

Robert B. Allin and Diana W. Allin • Chesterfield Mental Health and Mental Retardation Services, Lucy Corr Court, Chesterfield, Virginia 23832.

and families of retarded or developmentally delayed individuals tend to fall into three general categories: (1) the psychiatric or psychodynamic approach; (2) the didactic approach; and (3) the behavior modification approach.[1,2]

The *psychodynamic approach*, in assuming that intrapsychic data are of paramount importance, generally places an emphasis on the parents' emotional reactions toward their offspring. These reactions have been variously characterized as chronic sorrow, grief, guilt, shame, denial, withdrawal, and rejection.[3-5] The goal of this approach is for parents to "work through" their feelings toward their retarded child in order to gain an acceptance of the child and his or her disordered behavior.

As a single intervention strategy, the psychodynamic approach has received much criticism. The tendencies for dynamically oriented professionals to stereotype parents' reactions to having a mentally retarded child are seen as destructive by Roos.[6] Dynamic practitioners often ignore the wishes of the parents by giving them therapy when they want counseling on behavior management and facts about mental retardation.[1,7] The appropriateness of applying this approach to all or most parents rather than only in cases in which there is an implicit need for it has also been questioned.[8,9] Furthermore, even if parents acquire some degree of acceptance of their mentally retarded child, their handling of the child may not really be changed, and his or her potential may not be fully realized.[2]

The *didactic approach* to working with parents of retarded offspring involves the dissemination to parents of factual information about retardation and the effects of that retardation on their child's development.[1] Such information may relate to a broad range of topics, including the causes of retardation, the diagnostic process, the prognosis and treatments, the effects of the child on the family, home management, normal child development and its relevance to retardation, the feelings and needs of the retarded child, the interpretation of retardation to relatives and friends, a review of the available community services, and information on existing national and state laws. Tymchuck[2] stated that parents need reliable information in order to overcome the deficits often created by an "accurate information vacuum." Such a vacuum may be filled with inaccurate other information that hampers the parents' accurate assessment of their child's potential future. Also, the inaccurate and often unrealistic expectations that parents may have in regard to their retarded offspring place pressure not only on him or her, but on the parents and the family as well. The effectiveness of the didactic approach has received support.[9]

The *behavior modification approach* has received much attention in the literature as an intervention strategy for teaching parents to alter the behavior of their offspring. Reviews by Berkowitz and Graziano[10] and by O'Dell[11] attesting to the growth of interest in this area substantiate its potential effectiveness in teaching parents to more successfully manage the behavior of offspring noted as retarded, psychotic, and brain-damaged, as well as others with a variety of disruptive or abusive behaviors. Behavioral management counseling with parents emphasizes actual observable behavior and the environmental variables that maintain certain behavior patterns. The counseling procedures focus on teaching parents how to apply the principles of learning theory to their specific child-rearing problems.[12]

Two major assumptions appear to underlie the use of the behavior modification approach with parents.[1,10] First, maladaptive behavior has been acquired by the child in his or her natural environment and can best be changed by modifying that environment. Parents, as primary social agents within the child's environment, are in an excellent position to accomplish this task. Indeed, as noted by Hawkins,[13] the issue is not whether they will unconsciously use such techniques with an unknown, unchosen, and unhappy result; rather, the choice is that they will use them consciously, efficiently, and consistently to develop the qualitites that they choose for their offspring. The second assumption underlying this approach involves the maintenance of newly acquired behaviors. Such maintenance depends also on the successful modification of the child's natural environment and again implies a consideration of parent–child interactional patterns.

Although research on the effectiveness of the behavioral approach with parents is encouraging, the number of weak areas has made an accurate evaluation difficult. O'Dell[11] reported that most studies have had the tendency to focus on the parents' implementing changes in the child, while neglecting to obtain data on producing and maintaining changes in parental behavior. There have also been insufficient data on parents' abilities to generalize their changes to different situations, and on whether or not the subsequent quality of parent–child interactions has been altered. Although there has been evidence that parents use operant techniques in a laboratory situation, their conscious use of these techniques in the child's natural environment has been questioned.[1,10,14]

Despite these criticisms, the rapidly expanding literature on parent training in behavior modification has evolved to the point where behavioral training specifically for the parents of retarded children would appear to hold great promise.[8,10,15]

Despite the criticisms and the apparent weaknesses of the psychodynamic, didactic, and behavioral approaches, as well as the lack of research on their comparative effectiveness, it seemed safe to conclude that each has had great utility and value as an intervention strategy. Further, it seemed obvious to us that the choice of which strategy to use would depend heavily on the diverse, and often complex, needs of each individual family unit and its particular situation. It also appeared likely that any particular family would benefit from more than one type of approach. The manner in which services have been offered has not, however, always followed these assumptions, as parents too frequently have received only the particular service approach provided by helping professionals simply because it was their orientation and the only service they offered.

In developing the HIP model, the treatment approach issue was of great concern. A reasonable and potentially effective service equipped for intervention with the parents and families of retarded individuals appeared to be an *eclectic orientation*, that is, a program highly sensitive to situational demands and able to provide a particular approach, or combination of approaches, to effectively meet individual needs. The feasibility of, and support for, a combined approach orientation has been addressed in the literature.[2,16–18]

13.3. Utilization of the Home Setting

Although the typical settings for therapeutic assessment and intervention have been the office, the clinic, or "institutional" situations, a small body of research indicates that the home, or the "natural environment," could provide an excellent and even superior medium in which to assess and implement various treatment modalities.[7,19–21] From these studies, several advantages of *in vivo* intervention can be highlighted: therapists are able to observe, assess, and more fully understand problem situations as they occur in the settings in which they most frequently occur; clients feel that therapists are better able to understand their situation; treatment modalities that take into consideration specific need areas are more accurately indicated and can be plugged directly into the natural setting; the family can learn to apply newly learned techniques, acquired knowledge, and insights to their own situation; and therapists are available to give immediate feedback on parent–family efforts, to shape their skills in applying techniques, and to alter the treatment plan if necessary.

Studies of home intervention also report positive results as a function of home-oriented programs. Perhaps one of the most important results is the prevention of unnecessary institutionalization. Home intervention programs have been reported as successful in changing parents' attitudes toward institutionalizing their children[19,22] and in avoiding large expenditures of money per client for placement outside the home.[21] Problem behaviors of children at home have been effectively eliminated as a result of home intervention.[23] Home visits have also been noted to increase the parents' level of confidence in handling their children,[8] to increase the stimulus potential of the home, and to produce measured gains in tested intelligence.[24] Furthermore, home intervention has been reported to enhance the parents' overall effectiveness as behavioral change agents.[15,25]

13.4. The Home Intervention Program

13.4.1. Participants

Participants in the Home Intervention Program included families or acting families with a member (to be identified as the *client*) who was mentally retarded and who presented problem abusive and/or disruptive behavior at home. This behavior usually created, or was fostered by, problems in the home that made it difficult for the family to maintain the individual in that environment. Problem behavior typically overwhelmed family members to the point where they no longer felt able to cope, and outside placement was considered in some cases. Frequently, the behavior problems of these individuals carried over into other environments, such as work, school, and other community programs or services, which limited, and in some cases prohibited, continued participation.

Because program services were usually extended to a maximum of three families concurrently, a selection process was utilized that determined the next recipient. This process involved rating eligible candidates in the areas of (1) risk of institutionalization; (2) need for immediate intervention; (3) potential to benefit from treatments; and (4) client–family motivation to receive and participate in services. The cases with the highest ratings were the next to participate in the program.

A total of 12 families participated in the *evaluative component* of the Home Intervention Program. These included 13 individuals who were identified as clients (one family had mentally retarded twins) and 41 family or "acting family" members (a range of 2–7 per family) who were regarded as being actively involved in the treatment efforts. Thus, a total of 54 individuals participated in the program. They ranged in age from 19 months to 32 years, with a mean age of 14.2 years. The full-scale IQ scores of this client group, which included 3 females and 10 males, ranged from 14 to 79, with a mean IQ of 46.50. At the time of referral, 9 clients were living at home with the natural parents, 2 were in foster homes, and 2 were pending discharge from institutional settings. The mean family income was $18,830/year (range: $8,000–$30,000), and the mean educational level of the parents in years completed was 14.8 for the mothers and 16.2 for the fathers.

13.4.2. Staff

The program staff consisted of a husband-and-wife therapist team who usually worked together on each case. Occasionally, visits were made by one team member when the team approach was not necessary or clinically indicated.

13.4.3. Program Procedures

A planned aspect of the HIP was that the program procedures would remain flexible enough to meet the individual needs of the participants and to be responsive to situational demands. Although the treatments therefore were individualized in terms of design and implementation, several phases or program procedures were considered common to all cases. In temporal order, they were as follows:

1. Case preparation phase
   a. Introductory visit
   b. Preparation of data base
   c. "Preexperimental" evaluative questionnaire given
2. Intensive involvement phase
   a. Observation and problem assessment
   b. Development of treatment plan and Goal Attainment Scales
   c. Implementation of treatment
3. Supportive involvement phase
   a. Reduction in staff time
   b. Increased expectation for family to take full responsibility for implementation of techniques

    c. "Postexperimental" evaluative questionnaires given at outset
4. Termination phase
    a. Continued phasing-out of staff time
    b. Termination issues addressed
5. Follow-up support phase
    a. "Follow-up" evaluative questionnaire given
    b. Support given to families on an as-needed basis via occasional visits and/or phone contacts

The phases outlined above and the major aspects of each are discussed here in brief detail. Although these phases occurred in the temporal order listed, it is important to note that the time spent in any given phase was subject to a variance dictated by individual needs and situational demands.

13.4.3.1. Case Preparation Phase

An important part of this first phase of HIP involvement with cases was the introductory visit: face-to-face contact of the staff and family usually occurred in the home and served several useful purposes. Most important was the opportunity for program participants to meet staff and ask questions regarding having "outsiders" or "strangers" in their homes. Program details and examples of the techniques that could be expected were explained by staff. Family members were provided with an opportunity to discuss their specific problems and needs. This first contact occurred before any final agreement by the family or staff to begin treatment.

Once the final agreement to begin treatment was made, staff began to compile a data base. All preexperimental evaluative questionnaires were administered, and staff formulated a timetable for their task of observation and problem assessment, which was reviewed and finalized with the family.

13.4.3.2. Intensive Involvement Phase

A major focus of this phase was observation of the client in his or her natural environment. Staff observations typically occurred over a three- or four-day period and took place in a variety of settings, such as the home, the school, and the work or training center. Observation visits were planned during both "problem" and "no-problem" times and ranged in duration from one to five hours. In general, the role of staff during periods of observation was one of "casual observer." For example, it was explained to family members that their normal routine and responses to situations should continue and that staff would not make suggestions for handling problems differently at this time. Staff, in most cases, remained visible (e.g., in the same room or part of the house) so that clients and family members became more accustomed to their presence. The interactions of staff and family members during these observation sessions were limited by staff to the aims of (1) enabling staff to more clearly understand problems and (2) establishing increased levels of comfort and rapport between staff and family members.

Another major focus of this phase was the development of a treatment plan that was directly based on information previously gathered; it was individualized for each case. Planning sessions between staff and family took place to establish the problem areas to be targeted for treatment. Staff then drafted an initial treatment plan that was presented to the family and significant others to be involved for explanation, modification, and finalizing. A time schedule for the next several weeks was then discussed, and treatment goals (Goal Attainment Scales) for each problem area were established. Whenever possible the "client" was involved in the treatment-planning process.

The third major focus was on implementation of the treatment plan. This aspect of program procedures was the most crucial and required the greatest concentration of time and effort. It usually began with the teaching and explanation of the techniques that would be used in changing and coping with problem behaviors. Principles of behavior modification or effective communication, for example, were reviewed and discussed by staff during the initial sessions. No lengthy teaching of academic principles was attempted; emphasis was placed on the *application* of techniques: "teaching by doing" and modeling for parents were emphasized. As treatment progressed, staff increased their expectations that parents and other family members would take on more responsibility for implementing techniques with gradually decreasing staff assistance. Techniques were practiced in hypothetical situations when necessary, then gradually introduced into real problem situations. Practice (*fire drilling*, as we refer to it) was especially used in situations where the behavior targeted for change was low in its frequency of occurrence and high in its problem intensity.

Throughout the implementation of the treatment plan, staff used various methods of assisting, coaching, or reminding the parents to employ the techniques in the treatment plan. These methods ranged from verbal prompting to passing written messages. Frequently, information and reminders were posted on the refrigerator or in some other highly visible location. In situations where behavioral techniques were used, the recording of data was required to be done by one or two specific members of the family. These data records were also posted, and checks on their reliability were periodically made by staff. Also, in situations where the clients had reading skills, information such as responsibility schedules or point systems was posted in tactful locations for their observation.

Ideally, throughout the treatment plan implementation, the family members would be highly motivated and active in their follow-through. However, this was not true in the majority of cases. Issues contributing to resistance or difficulty in carrying through aspects of the treatment plan required, and received, special consideration from staff. Sometimes, the issue was easily identifiable and quickly dealt with. One set of parents, for example, were progressing nicely until the plan required that they ignore their daughter's crying in certain situations. The matter was explored with them, and it was found that both parents were feeling a sense of guilt for abandoning their child when the tantrum crying occurred. They were soon able to ignore this behavior, and consistently so, after discussing their feelings and receiving assurances from staff. In other cases, issues such as fear of being physically hurt by an offspring if the plan was implemented, unrealistically low expectations of client behavior, parental burnout, and overprotectiveness required considerably more time and attention.

13.4.3.3. Supportive Involvement Phase

This phase can be viewed as a continuation of the treatment plan implementation discussed above with two major changes. First, there was a reduction in staff–client contact time. Although visits occurred more frequently and were usually of longer duration during the period of intensive involvement (e.g., four visits per week; three to four hours per visit), both the number of visits and the time length of each visit were reduced during the supportive phase (e.g., two visits per week; one to two hours per visit). Second, there were increased expectations that family members would take more responsibility for implementing aspects of the treatment plan. The teaching and learning of techniques were considered completed, and family members during this phase were encouraged to adjust to following through with the techniques with considerably less staff assistance. The staff role was one of providing support by encouraging consistency in follow-through, sharpening the parents' ability to use the techniques, and generalizing their ability to use the techniques in similar or new problem situations. Factors that contributed to families' tendency to be dependent on staff for plan implementation were identified and dealt with during this period. At the outset of this phase, all "post" evaluations were administered.

13.4.3.4. Termination Phase

The final stages in the removal of regularly scheduled staff–case contact time occurred during the termination phase. This phase also involved a reduction in staff contact time: visits during this period usually occurred one time per week for a one- to two-hour period. The family was expected to carry through with all areas of the treatment plan for which they had responsibility. During this phase, the issue of termination was specifically addressed in terms of its impact on the family system and the ability of the family members to continue their use and application of the learned skills.

13.4.3.5. Follow-Up Phase

The final aspect of HIP involvement was the case follow-up. All evaluations were administered for the final time at the outset of this phase. Contacts via phone or actual visits to the natural environment were made on an "as-needed" basis. These contacts were initiated by both staff and family members for the purposes of giving and receiving further assistance in carrying out techniques, problem solving in new or crisis situations, monitoring the family's continued use of the program techniques, and checking on the extent to which the reduction or elimination of problem behavior had been sustained over time.

The amount of time spent with each case in any given phase of the program procedures varied in accordance with individual needs and situational demands. The major concentration of time and visits occurred during the intensive phase of the program procedures. During this phase, the cases received an average of 42 hours of direct contact over 16 visits, as compared to means of 19.5 hours over 9 visits, and 9 hours over 4 visits during the support and termination phases, respectively. Thus, as the program progressed in each case, the families were in a sense "weaned," with increasingly smaller amounts of time during the final phases. New cases were accepted as soon as current cases reached the support and termination phases. In this manner, the HIP provided regular program services for three families simultaneously, each in a different phase of involvement.

The total time spent with any individual case ranged from 16 to 130 hours, and the total number of visits per case ranged from 11 to 76. The average amount of total direct contact time per case was approximately 70 hours, and the mean number of total visits per case was 30. The mean length of time spent per visit was about 2 hours and 20 minutes.

In general, there was no established or rigid plan for coordinating the time when visits would occur. Although tentative schedules for contact were discussed for each phase of program involvement, staff typically set up final schedules with the families on a weekly or daily basis to maintain flexibility in responsiveness to client needs. Scheduling frequently became a rather complex piece of business that took into consideration such factors as the availability of the family members, "prime" problem times, and the schedules that staff had established with other cases concurrently receiving treatment.

13.5. Program Evaluation

An important aspect of the present project was the incorporation of an evaluative component to assess the effectiveness of the program model (i.e., services provided *in vivo*, husband–wife therapist team, eclectic approach, and flexible time scheduling) for the population served. Program implementation followed the delicate course of providing services to clients while also attempting to adhere closely to the standards of empirical investigation. Dependent measures were obtained from parents or significant others in the areas of knowledge of behavior modification principles (KBP), sensitivity to others (STO), and locus of control (LOC). Dependent measures pertaining to each client's level of developmental and adaptive functioning (ABS) were also obtained, in addition to data recorded on specific target behaviors. Goal Attainment Scales[26] were established for each case that made it possible to statistically determine degrees of success in accomplishing the goals that were set according to the unique problems and situations of each participant and family. All measures were obtained and rated on the "pre," "post," and "follow-up"

Table 1. The Service Delivery Objectives[a]

Objectives specific to the "client":
1. To decrease or eliminate presenting problem behaviors (GAS, ABS, behavioral data).
2. To increase independence skills such as self-help, leisure, and communication skills when applicable (GAS, ABS, behavioral data).
3. To increase self-control (GAS, behavioral data).
4. To increase self-esteem (GAS, behavioral data).
5. To increase positive, constructive behavior in general (GAS, ABS, behavioral data).
6. To increase acceptability to other family members.
7. To live in community.

Objectives specific to the parents or family:
1. To increase knowledge of behavior modification principles (KBPAC).
2. To increase the conscious and constructive application of behavioral skills with son or daughter (behavioral data, GAS).
3. To decrease "overwhelmed" feelings and increase feelings of personal control (GAS, LOC).
4. To decrease overprotective behavior and foster independence and responsibility in son or daughter (GAS, behavioral data, STO).
5. To increase overall quality of interaction with son or daughter (STO).
6. To increase awareness of, and ability to deal with, feelings and attitudes relative to son or daughter.
7. To increase knowledge of mental retardation, if necessary.
8. To increase knowledge and understanding of emotional-behavioral component of problems presented by son or daughter.
9. To formulate, if necessary, realistic expectations of offspring's potential.
10. To increase acceptance of son or daughter as family member.

[a] Key to dependent measures used to evaluate objectives:
ABS: American Association on Mental Deficiency Adaptive Behavior Scale
Behavioral data: Recording of specific behavioral information
GAS: Goal Attainment Scales
KBPAC: Knowledge of Behavior Principles questionnaire
LOC: Locus of control measure
STO: Sensitivity to Others questionnaire

basis described in Section 13.4.2. Consumer satisfaction was also determined at the end of all treatment phases.

Specifically, the Home Intervention Program itself was the main independent variable in the investigation. The main dependent variables were the behaviors of the client and his or her parents or family. Because the HIP focused on work with the parents and the family to effect change in client behavior, the behavior of the parents and the family served as an intervening variable that was both an independent and a dependent variable.

It was generally hypothesized that the Home Intervention Program model (independent variable), with its unique blend of approaches, as defined above, would promote achievement of the service delivery objectives outlined in Table 1. Achievement of these objectives would directly relate to changes in the behavior of the client and his or her family (dependent variable).

13.5.1. Case Examples

The following two case examples demonstrate the application of the Home Intervention Program procedures. The first case involves behavior problems that we have found to be quite typical of young adults who live at home and are referred to us for treatment. The second case is somewhat less detailed and presents problems indicative of more severe emotional difficulties. Brief descriptive data, basic aspects of the treatment, and a discussion of outcome are presented in each example.

13.5.1.1. Case 1

Allen was a Caucasian, partially blind, moderately retarded male who was 23 years of age at the time of his referral to the HIP. He was the youngest of four siblings and lived alone at home with his 59-year-old mother. He was a large-framed individual weighing approximately 195 pounds, and he wore a prothesis in his left eye socket. Allen was referred to HIP for services because of physical and verbal abuse to his mother, frequent abuse to property, and generally uncooperative, stubborn behaviors. These behaviors carried over to a vocational training program, where his attendance was poor. The referral to the HIP came during a "crisis" time for the family: Allen had recently pushed his mother to the ground, punched a hole in the wall, and damaged several household items.

Assessment observations in the home indicated that his mother was threatened and in a sense "controlled" by her physically large and demanding son. She typically would do things for Allen that he had the potential to do for himself or would "rearrange" the environment in an effort to avoid angry displays or to appease the situation. A strong hostile-dependent relationship with his mother obviously existed; Allen appeared to control and promote his dependency via physical threats and hostile actions. When he did not want to do something, or if things did not go the way he wanted them to, he would become angry and have a temper outburst. It was quite apparent that Allen had "learned" behaviors that effectively produced results that were "positive" for *him*. It was also our impression that his mother was somewhat predisposed to "do for Allen" as she assisted him in tasks that he could do independently with a minimum of training (e.g., toothbrushing, shaving, bathing, making his bed, and fixing simple meals). In fact, Allen would perform some of these tasks when he visited his sister, but his mother would do them for him at home. His mother attributed some of her tendency to "do for Allen" to her late husband's strong feeling that others in the family had everything, but Allen, because of his handicaps, had little, and family members should do whatever they could for him. She was aware that she did too much for him but was too threatened and scared to begin setting and enforcing limits. Allen had extremely low feelings of self-worth. He would complain that things were very hard for him and that he was "no good." After an outburst, it was typical for him to feel guilty and depressed. He talked frequently of leaving home and his mother, and of getting a place of his own.

Basic aspects of the HIP treatment intervention with Allen and his family focused on the following: eliminating/reducing destructive and/or harmful temper displays and replacing them with more appropriate coping behaviors; establishing methods to set limits in the home; increasing attendance at the vocational services program; increasing Allen's independence skills and behavior; increasing Allen's feelings of self-esteem; and supporting his mother in her efforts to set limits and to gradually assume less repsonsibility for Allen. The support and frequently active involvement of other members of the family—who lived away from home—were an asset and were utilized whenever possible throughout implementation of the treatment plan.

   a. Temper Outbursts. Treatment intervention in this problem area involved several aspects briefly listed as follows: (1) teaching Allen to identify and process feelings, especially those of frustration, hurt, and anger; (2) helping Allen to distinguish between "feelings and actions" in the sense that his feelings (e.g., of anger) were OK, but inappropriate (anger) displays were not; (3) rehearsing (repeatedly) in practice sessions alternative behaviors to being abusive or destructive; (4) learning to identify Allen's anger signals and dealing with them directly rather than avoiding or reinforcing problem situations; (5) teaching communication skills to family members in conjunction with problem-solving suggestions (e.g., reflect to Allen when he looks angry: "You look to me like you're feeling angry"; asking Allen what appropriate things he could do when he felt angry); (6) encouraging and supporting his mother in gradually taking less responsibility for altering the environment so that it was not less frustrating for Allen and not more frustrating for her; and (7) establishing with the family at home and the staff at the vocational program definite consequences and responses to temper outbursts (paying back, picking up, replacing items damaged) and positive reinforcement for appropriate behavior.

   b. Independence Skills. Allen could perform responsibility tasks alone if it was insisted that he do so, but prior to treatment, his mother assisted him extensively in doing them. Part of her reason for doing this was to speed things along in the morning so that Allen would not be late for work, but as we quickly found out in the early stages of intervention, any insistence that he perform these behaviors at home without his mother met with an angry display. The temper outburst was a typical response to newly set limits or changes in routine that required Allen to take on more responsibility. Therefore, work in the area of increasing independence behaviors was coordinated closely with work in the problem area of temper outbursts. Strategies outlined for treatment in this area focused on (1) establishing limits at home for the particular "independence" behaviors expected, and (2) establishing a routine and natural system of consequences and responses that would follow Allen's performance of these "expected" behaviors. For example, Allen needed to be dressed, ready (teeth brushed, shaved, and so on), and downstairs by 7:15 A.M. in order to get breakfast. He earned daily soda money by riding the vocational-training-center van to work, and he went on a weekend family outing if he attended for the entire week. He was expected to become increasingly responsible for getting ready in the morning and getting on the van without assistance from his mother. Thus, one "independence behavior" was expected at first, then two, then three, and so on. It was also established that his mother would not drive Allen into the vocational workshop should he fail to ride the van. Further, it was understood that being at home on a workday was "OK" only for people who were physically sick and that sick people would eat only very light meals like chicken broth and crackers and would need to stay in bed all day (this was usually aversive to Allen). Thus, Allen's failure to get to work on his own had implications throughout the day at home. This system of consequences was explained fully to Allen and reviewed repeatedly with him prior to implementation (and even several times daily at first). The system was explained as a series of "choices" that he was free to make (i.e., he could *choose* to eat breakfast by being dressed, ready, and downstairs by 7:15 A.M.). These choices and consequences were considered similar to those made by other young adults and thus were expected of Allen (i.e., if someone sleeps late or takes a long time getting ready, they may have to skip breakfast in order to get to work). In addition, the personal hygiene behaviors of toothbrushing, shaving, washing and drying hair, and bathing were all skills that Allen had but simply refused to use independently. Thus, a minimum of learning new skills was necessary, and the primary emphasis was on using the skills without dependence on, or assistance from, his mother.

   c. Self-Concept. It was apparent at the onset of treatment that Allen became overwhelmed with feelings of being "dumb and stupid," and that a "poor me" attitude would accompany periods of depression and lethargic behavior. This would most typically occur after a major temper display but also seemed to be evident after weekends spent with older siblings who had their own homes and spouses. Treatment in this area was integrated closely with work in the areas of temper outbursts and independence skills. By reducing or eliminating temper displays and increasing independent behavior, Allen could feel better about himself. In addition, he met one hour per week with the male team member in the HIP office in addition to the regular program time spent in the home. This "special time" was considered his only (without mother or family) and was used to help him to process feelings. Issues ranged from those such as what he wanted for his future to how he felt after a temper outburst.

   d. Family. Treatment also focused on the family, particularly his mother and her feelings of being overwhelmed and her tendency to overprotect. Whereas the practical or behavioral side of these areas were addressed in other aspects of treatment intervention, "cognitive" and "feelings" aspects of being overprotective and overwhelmed received specific attention via individual meetings often between only the female member of the HIP team and the mother. These sessions encouraged the mother to express and process her feelings, and to work through issues that might reduce or inhibit her ability to carry through aspects of the treatment plan with Allen. One issue, for example, was her fear of being physically hurt or having damaged property as a result of setting limits or saying "No." Another issue involved confrontation from HIP staff regarding her expectations and treatment of Allen as a "child" rather than a 23-year-old adult.

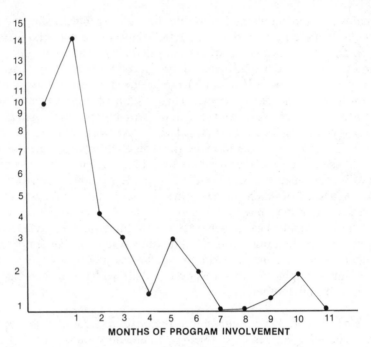

Figure 1. Temper outbursts per month of program involvement (Case 1); baseline 1 month prior to HIP involvement.

e. Outcome. Data recorded for temper outburst behavior at home and work per month of program involvement are presented in Figure 1. A great deal of progress was made as the outbursts decreased from the baseline rate of 10 per month to an average occurrence of 1 outburst per month for a five-month period. It was quite apparent that Allen was able to utilize the alternative and positive coping behavior of "taking a walk when angry." He would state, "I'm angry, I need to walk outside" and would then take a walk that lasted from 5 to 20 minutes. This newly learned response demonstrated an increased ability to identify feelings of anger and to exhibit increased "internal controls."

These internal controls may have resulted from several aspects related to treatment. First, as mentioned earlier, Allen was required to replace any property damaged during an outburst. This necessitated that he do extra chores at home, like taking out the trash or doing the dishes, for which he could earn money to pay for broken items. Another source of replacement cash was to forfeit the soda money he had earned for attending work the pervious day. During the course of HIP involvement Allen paid for a window, a hole in the den wall, a sweater belonging to a vocational-services staff person, an electric razor, a lamp, and a shirt belonging to an HIP staff person. Required repayment for items damaged seemed to establish for Allen a definite consequence pattern that he eventually sought to avoid. (He did not like giving up sodas to pay for the razor and so on.)

A second treatment aspect was the time spent in processing with him his feelings of guilt and "self-hate." The major emphasis was on helping him to make connections between negative behaviors and the negative self-feelings that followed them. Allen stated to staff that he would walk outside so he would not feel "stupid." By avoiding angry outbursts, he would avoid feeling bad about his behavior and himself.

Another important contribution to Allen's increased internal control was simply that angry displays did not produce the usual positive results for him. His mother was increasingly able to avoid "giving in." Thus, his outbursts were, in a sense, ignored. It is interesting that the recorded data on temper outbursts presented in Figure 1 are similar in pattern to graphs typical of behavior that undergoes extinction. As can be seen, outbursts during the first month of HIP involvement actually exceeded the baseline rate by 40% before decreasing over the following months. Identifying for the family and the vocational services staff that a temporary "worsening" of this problem would occur was an important treatment intervention.

Attendance data recorded by staff who worked with Allen at the vocational training center were used to measure progress in attending the program. Allen attended the program at the adult training center an average of 52% of possible days during a two-month baseline period. When this figure is compared with an average of 95% of possible days in attendance for a five-month follow-up period, a great deal of progress in this area is evident.

The use of Goal Attainment Scales provided additional outcome information. These scales were developed and rated on a "pre," "post," and "follow-up" basis with the family and are presented in Figure 2. Scales 1, 2, and 3 focused on treatment problem areas related to Allen: anger control, independence skills, and self-concept. The remaining scales, 4 and 5, dealt with treatment issues that focused on Allen's mother: overwhelmed feelings and overprotectiveness. Examination of the rating for all five scales indicates that progress was made in all areas as treatment continued. The improvement noted in Scales 1, anger control, and 2, independence, is supported by the behavioral data recordings for these areas discussed earlier.

The individual case data obtained for the family indicate a high degree of treatment success, particularly in the areas of reducing temper outbursts and increasing work attendance. Improvement in these areas is seen as a result of setting clear limits and attempting to consistently follow through with a system of "natural consequences" for both positive and negative behaviors. In addition, the staff time spent with Allen's mother, in our clinical judgment, was necessary and of extreme value in terms of dealing with resistance to her implementation of the treatment plan. This included individual time with his mother for the processing of feelings and also the many long and frequent early-morning (6:00 A.M.) hours spent in the family home during the first weeks of program implementation. Successful treatment was enhanced greatly by a high degree of motivation and active involvement by family members, especially Allen's mother, to carry through on the treatment plan. The coordination and communication between vocational services staff, HIP staff, and his mother

SCALE ATTAINMENT LEVELS	SCALE 1: Independence: related to personal skills & work attendance.	SCALE 2: Self-concept: self-confidence, positive self-image.	SCALE 3: Anger control (temper outbursts):	SCALE 4: Mother's feelings of being overwhelmed: Terrorized, unable to set limits, have own needs.	SCALE 5: Mother's overprotectiveness (expectation level at home):
Most unfavorable treatment outcome thought likely — 0	Takes on no personal responsibility for self-help skills or work attendance.	Is deeply depressed and frequently exhibits self-destructive behaviors.	Continuously demonstrates temper outbursts which are of both high frequency and high intensity.	Is overwhelmed that son cannot live at home. She feels constantly threatened and terrorized, unable to set any limits.	Consistently does for son, not allowing him to do for himself at all.
1		√	√	√	√
Less than expected success with treatment — 2	√ Takes on some personal responsibility for many self-help skills and work attendance.	√ Is depressed and is exhibiting many negative self-statements but few self-destructive behaviors.	Frequently demonstrates temper outbursts which are of high intensity.	√ Mother often feels overwhelmed but wants son to remain in home. She is only occasionally able to set limits. Frequently feels threatened.	Mother able to entertain idea of doing less for son. Allows son some increased independence with staff support.
3					√√
Expected level of treatment success — 4	Takes on responsibility for many self-help skills and work attendance.	Mood is variable. Is exhibiting no self-destructive behaviors and few negative self-statements.	√√ Occasionally demonstrates temper outbursts that are of moderate intensity. Uses appropriate coping behaviors when reminded.	√√ Mother able to set limits fairly regularly and feels threatened only occasionally.	Making effort to give son independence and such occurring most of the time.
5	√√	√√		√√√	√√√
More than expected success with treatment — 6	Takes on responsibility for most of self-help skills and work attendance.	Is usually in a positive mood and exhibits positive self-statements 85% of the time.	Rarely demonstrates temper outburst behavior. Will verbalize angry feelings and self-initiate appropriate coping behaviors most of the time.	Mother regularly able to set limits with minimal fear.	Mother only occasionally does for son when he is able to do for himself.
7	√√√		√√√		
Best anticipated success with treatment — 8	Takes on responsibility for all of self-help skills and work attendance within physical limitations.	√√ Is a happy, positive person and exhibits positive self-statements 95% of the time.	Does not exhibit temper outbursts. Handles anger appropriately at all times.	Mother not threatened at all by son and is able to set limits without any fear.	Mother always encourages son to be more independent and doesn't do for him if he can do for himself.
9					

Figure 2. Goal attainment scales for Case 1; (√) pre; (√√) post; (√√√) follow-up.

in regard to following through with treatment aspects greatly facilitated improvements by providing increased consistency and clear messages across environments. Finally, Allen's progress over the months was reflected by his being chosen as the first recipient of a newly started "Trainee of the Month" award, given by the vocational services facility to show recognition for his outstanding task performance, social skills, and work attendance!

13.5.1.2. Case 2

> Tom, a 22-year-old adopted Caucasian male with a tested IQ in the borderline range, was living at home on a 60-day "convalescent" leave from a state mental institution at the time of his referral to HIP. His mother, father, and brother (also adopted) were overwhelmed about the hospital's plan to discharge him. The family felt helpless in their tolerance of, and ability to effectively deal with, the problems and disruptive behaviors Tom had demonstrated prior to his hospitalization: suicidal threats, somatic complaints, fits of anger, bouts of depression, lack of cooperation, irresponsibility, and poor personal hygiene. They feared that their family could not cope with his reentry into the home unless some professional assistance could be received.

Initial assessment observations of the family at home revealed that many of Tom's disruptive behaviors had positive consequences for him, whereas the other family members frequently were left upset. His stating "I wish I were dead" typically earned him much attention and concern. The family did not push him to do chores or uphold responsibilities at such times. His somatic complaints and acting out of signs of physical ailments resulted in similar "rewarding" consequences. The mother, for example, frequently left her job to drive Tom home from the vocational workshop when he complained of, or acted out, symptoms of being "sick" (gagging) or "wanting to die" (lying in the roadway near the parking lot). He then would "recover" at home by watching TV and eating snacks. When confronted about this by his parents, he would withdraw and/or begin screaming that he "wanted to die," often outside in front of the neighbors. The parents would become embarrassed and angry and eventually would back off. An atmosphere of tension, hostility, and anger typically resulted.

The treatment plan with Tom and his family focused on five major areas: (1) temper outbursts and other behaviors classified as attention seeking (screaming "I wish I were dead" throughout the neighborhood, excessive somatic complaints, and exhibition of somatic behavior such as gagging); (2) responsibility and independence (completing daily chores and following through on planned activities such as attending the occupational workshop and the community-support day-treatment programs); (3) self-esteem; (4) the family's "overprotectiveness"; and (5) the parents' overwhelmed feelings. Joint planning between the family and several representatives of the county's mental-health and mental-retardation services programs was productive in terms of providing them with options for assistance. The family agreed to receive HIP services in combination with two programs that involved Tom during the daytime. Thus, the "services package" consisted of Tom's attending a vocational services program three days per week and a community support program two days per week, and the HIP focused on treatment with the family at home in addition to the coordination and extension of treatment between the home and all involved programs and staff. Interventions centered on breaking the behavior–consequence pattern that rewardingly released Tom from responsibility and resulted in upsetting others. Treatment also focused on shaping Tom's independent behaviors, teaching and practicing appropriate behaviors and language as alternatives to acting out, and building confidence to complete tasks on his own. The family was given support in letting him struggle with his own problems without assuming major responsibility for them. Although behavior modification was the primary "technique" employed in this case, parent training in "communication skills" and "problem ownership"[27] was also incorporated into the plan of treatment. Staff sensitivity and work in the areas of parent–client feelings and family dysfunction were also major aspects of the treatment.

Behavioral *intervention and outcome* in four identified problem areas can be briefly reported.

1. *Somatic complaints* were defined as any verbal or "acted-out" indications of being physically ill when it was obvious that no real physical illness or symptoms existed. A typical "somatic complaint" for Tom was gagging behavior: entering the bathroom and sounding as if he were vomiting without actual results. Tom's parents followed the procedure of "ignoring" (not attending to or "reinforcing") somatic complaining behavior, with one exception: when the behavior did occur, he was to be treated as actually physically sick in terms of being expected to remain in bed and receiving only chicken broth soup at the next meal. Recorded data indicated a decrease in the number of somatic complaints or gestures made at home from the week-long baseline rate of 5.6 per day (40 per week) to a mean of 0.6 complaints per day (4 per week) during the final 10 weeks of HIP involvement.

2. *Death-related statements* ("I wish I were dead"), which Tom made as typical responses to confrontation or not getting his own way, were observed by HIP staff as being highly manipulative. Family members and all program staff used a reflective listening technique after the first verbalization. Continued and excessive verbalizations were ignored. It was mutually agreed that such statements might at times convey serious feelings and that to totally ignore them would show poor clinical judgment; thus, the reflective or active listening technique was used to provide Tom with an outlet for his feelings. There was no success in reducing the number of death-related statements. In fact, as treatment progressed, the number of such statements actually increased.

3. *Refusal to follow through on activities* that Tom had previously agreed to attend was identified as a specific target behavior. These activities included work at the vocational workshop, attending the community support program,

and planned family outings that Tom had previously stated he would participate in. After a week-long baseline period, the family and the program staff began to react differently to Tom's refusals to attend in several ways. When refusals occurred, effective communication techniques were used as initial responses if appropriate in the situation (e.g., "I am angry that you have decided not to go to the baseball game with us. Now the money spent on your ticket is wasted!"). This reaction exposed Tom to the effect of his behavior on others. In addition, Tom was not permitted to remain at home during times when he had previously agreed to attend planned activities. (Shelter and bathroom facilities were available without actually being in the house.) The reinforcing factors of staying home (watching TV, eating snacks, and being very comfortable) were therefore eliminated until the time he would normally have returned. In addition, Tom's father made a contract with him under which he could earn 50 cents per day for attendance at the workshop, and his mother no longer took him home during activities when he complained of sickness or not wanting to be there. It was understood that if he wanted to leave, he would have to walk home; once home, of course, he was not permitted in the house. Recorded data indicated that the frequency of this problem decreased from occurring nine times during the week-long baseline period to an average occurrence of one time per week for the following 12 weeks of HIP involvement.

4. *Refusal to complete daily chores* by Tom left family members feeling angry and often in the position of doing these tasks for him. Treatment consisted of the entire family's establishing a "daily-routine responsibility schedule" with Tom, which was posted on the refrigerator next to the data-recording sheets. This schedule was a clear definition and reminder of what was expected each day. The use of TV, radio, and record player were now considered privileges to be earned through the completion of chores, so that watching TV in the evening, for example, was contingent on his completing all the required tasks on the responsibility schedule. Family members used specific communicative phrases when chores were or were not completed. Chores not completed by Tom were, whenever possible and reasonable, not completed by others. The completion of daily tasks increased from 51% at baseline to a mean of 91% for chores completed over the 12 weeks following baseline. Family members stated that the efforts they made to verbalize their feelings about tasks not done left them less angry and better able to interact positively with Tom.

Behavioral data indicated that very positive changes were made in particular problem areas. The most positive and lasting changes occurred in areas that involved definite consequences, rewards, or effects that could be directly "felt" by Tom. He would complete chores to watch TV and did not somatize, so that he could eat a full meal. Problem areas in the treatment plan that did not so directly or concretely affect him did not produce positive or lasting results (attempts to reflectively listen to or ignore verbalizations of "wanting to die" were apparently not successful in reducing that problem). Improvements in specified target behaviors represented only part of the outcome picture. An interesting aspect of this case was that the family's increased abilities to carry through on the treatment plan appeared to create a crisis for Tom. As the family and the staff got better at setting limits and following through on consequences, Tom presented new problem behaviors that were more difficult to deal with in the natural environment. These included defecating in inappropriate areas, an obsessive fear of the toilet, and walking in front of a car. Although in our clinical opinion the emergence of these behaviors reflected efforts on Tom's part to test limits, seek attention, and avoid responsibility, continued treatment within his home was not considered viable. The decision to rehospitalize him was based on the need for a more controlled environment at this point in treatment. It was obvious that Tom had, in a sense, tested the limits of home intervention in his natural environment. Rehospitalization occurred with the recommendation that Tom earn his way back into the community by demonstrating appropriate behaviors at the institution (he did not like hospitalization) and that, if necessary, HIP involvement would continue at that point. Although hospitalization was considered undesirable, it was necessary at this point in the treatment process. Positive changes had occurred as a result of program efforts, especially in the parents' increased skills in dealing with problems and the greatly reduced feelings of being overwhelmed by Tom's problem behaviors, which were tearing the family apart at the outset of the treatment. In addition, the intervention was successful in giving clear messages to Tom about the things expected of him at home.

13.6. Issues and Impressions

The clinical impressions and information that we have acquired seem to fall into two major categories. Information that strongly relates to characteristics of the population served, especially to the problems initially presented by individuals and families as a group, are addressed first. Second, factors that emerged throughout the process of providing treatment to program participants are discussed. These categories are not considered mutually exclusive.

13.6.1. Characteristics of the Population Served

A distinct impression was that the types of problems presented by the entire client–family group were surprisingly similar. Despite the uniqueness of each individual case and its specific demands for treatment, the same basic types of problems seemed to emerge from case to case. Comparison listings, inclusive of the range of major presenting problem areas and their prevalence from case to case, are presented in Table 2 for clients and Table 3 for parents and families. If it can be assumed that participants in the present program constituted a representative sample, then these problem areas would seem to be characteristic of the larger mentally retarded–emotionally disturbed population.

In addition to the prevalence, from case to case, of particular presenting problems, there were related factors that emerged that appeared to be char-

Table 2. Prevalence of Major Problem Areas Identified for Clients[a]

Problem area	# and % of clients with problems	Further description of problem area
Temper outbursts	9—70%	Major or violent outbursts usually involving physically abusive-destructive behavior to others or property.
Independence/self-help	9—70%	Skill deficits in areas where potential existed but was not realized; refusal or "inability" to take responsibility.
General behavior problems	7—54%	Wide range of disruptive behaviors that were not particularly abusive or destructive (i.e., getting into cabinets or refrigerator, wandering, verbal abuse, etc.).
Communication	6—46%	Deficits in ability to identify and verbalize thoughts or feelings to others; reluctance to communicate with others.
Self-esteem	4—30%	Low concept of self as evidenced from lack of confidence, shyness, misunderstanding of problems, fear of failure, statements degrading self, etc.
Self-abusive behavior	2—15%	Behavior harmful to self; may be a temper display or self-stimulatory.

[a] Based on total of 13 cases.

acteristic of the group served. One issue involved the expectations that parents had of their mentally retarded son or daughter. We found that parents typically had low levels of expectation, which contributed to their overprotective tendencies and the excessive dependence of their offspring. Associated with this parental overprotection, especially in cases involving older clients, was a tremendous amount of anger. Hostile-dependent relationships particularly seemed to be a problem between higher functioning (moderately mentally retarded or above) male offspring 22–35 years of age and their mothers. These individuals seemed to be caught between their desires to be independent and the frustrating realities of their dependence.

Another dynamic was the "exclusion" of the mentally retarded members by others in the family system. Motivated by parental tendencies to overprotect and avoid, exclusion took several behavioral forms. Some family members would purposely "talk in code" or discuss family issues in language too obscure to be understood by the retarded individual. This tack was initially taken to prevent tantrums or upset. Other parents or family members typically refrained from expressing their honest feelings to the mentally retarded member. Finally, interactions would be generally limited as if guided by an underlying family philosophy that their mentally retarded members "can't understand anyway so they don't need to know." Although serving its purpose in the family system to keep things running "smoothly," exclusion had a serious and detrimental impact on the individual who was retarded. Reluctance to share or to openly

Table 3. Prevalence of Major Problem Areas Identified for Parents and Families[a]

Problem area	# and % of clients with problem	Further description of problem area
Overwhelmed feelings	10—77%	A felt inability to cope with problem situation that manifests in many ways: anger, depression, guilt, exhaustion, hopelessness, helplessness, etc. At end of rope, on edge emotionally, etc.
Overprotectiveness	7—54%	Tendencies to take responsibility for behavior of son or daughter, to do for him or her when not necessary. Adjusting routine to avoid or prevent problems. Behavior that diminishes independence and encourages dependence.
Inability to set limits/inconsistency	6—46%	Difficulty in sending "clear messages" to son or daughter that results in behavior problems. Usually occurs because of not knowing what to do or what is right to do, or feelings of being overwhelmed or burned out.
Sibling rivalry	3—23%	Sibling of client "acting out" because of excessive attention required or demanded by client.
Intrafamily communication	1—8%	Reluctance of family members to communicate with HIP staff.

[a] Based on total of 13 cases.

discuss important family matters greatly reduced opportunities to learn about the realities of life. Failure to openly and effectively express honest feelings impacted on the sensitivity of the retarded members to others because of limited opportunities to make associations between their behavior and the effect it had on others. Finally, exclusion gave strong messages that the retarded member couldn't be trusted, was unloved, or was incapable. These effects often acted as causal agents for emotional-behavioral problems by fostering the confusion, frustration, insensitivity, and hostility that produced temper outbursts or contributed to feelings of low self-worth.

Another problem, common and meaningful in families where a higher functioning individual was involved, was that the issues of one's mental retardation and one's sexuality were typically unaddressed. Facts about retardation and the feelings, for example, associated with being in special-education classes had seldom, if ever, been discussed between the parents and their offspring. Similarly, information regarding sexual development and the client's sexuality had received little communication or attention, except, of course, when a "problem" such as masturbation surfaced. In one recent case, a client's inappropriate sexual behavior was greatly reduced after he was helpfully confronted in a single meeting by family members about his public masturbation and was given acceptable alternatives.

A final factor that emerged in our home intervention work with parents and families involved a universal concern about the impact of their problem situation on their neighbors. Parents typically felt embarrassed and under enormous pressure in regard to problem behavior that was exhibited in the neighborhood. Often, the assumptions that were made about neighbors' thoughts and reactions were more overwhelming to the parents than the actual problem behavior. HIP interventions in these situations focused on family–neighbor meetings for the purposes of exchanging information and, if possible, including neighbors in aspects of the treatment plan.

13.6.2. Resistance to Treatment

An extremely important issue in our work with program participants was resistance to treatment. The resistance to changing behavior or to carrying through with the plan of treatment occurred at various levels of intensity in every HIP case. Given that the parents and family were active in carrying out their responsibilities in the plan of treatment, the client may have demonstrated some "resistance" to change by intensifying current problem behavior or by presenting new dilemmas. This "limit testing," a form of client-based resistance, was usually regarded as a positive step in the course of treatment, indicating that we were "onto something" in the process of behavior change. It was important to inform the parents and the family at the outset of the program intervention that this was expected. It was, however, not typical for the parents and the family to so easily follow through with the plan of treatment. They would, for example, know effective skills but have difficulty in implementing them for various reasons. Parent and family resistance to treatment was, perhaps, the most difficult aspect of program work. This resistance took several forms, depending on the family involved, and often required a major change in the focus of the plan of treatment before an impact on the client's behavior could successfully occur. A few of the major forms of parent and family resistance that we encountered in our work and a brief description of each are presented in the following list:

1. *Marital discord.* Various problems in the parents' relationship emerged that severely impeded or limited their abilities to promote change in the behavior of their son or daughter. Interestingly, problems between parents in some cases emerged *after* significant improvements in client behavior occurred. The HIP dealt with marital issues on a limited basis and made a recommendation for marital therapy if appropriate.

2. *"Burnout."* Parents and family were too tired and frustrated to effectively devote energy to changing the client's behavior. HIP would focus on relieving burnout before concentrating on the parents' responsibility for changing the client's behavior.

3. *Guilt.* Parents felt a recognized or unrecognized sense of self-blame or responsibility for the "problems" of their son or daughter that impeded their abilities to make interactional changes. Setting a limit, for example, was extremely difficult for guilt-ridden parents because they were reluctant to place

their son or daughter in an "uncomfortable situation." This guilt also motivated parents to take on excessive responsibility. There was no simple solution to guilt-based resistance. One effective approach was to focus on parent and family understanding of the manner in which they expressed "love" for their son or daughter: to show love and concern may indeed mean that they need to set that limit or to "push" their son or daughter, despite his or her initial negative responses, so that the son or daughter could develop independent skills and grow as individuals.

4. *Low expectation level.* Parents and family had unrealistic notions of what the son or daughter was capable of. This acted as a form of resistance in that they covertly believed that the behavior of the son or daughter would never improve, an attitude that minimized the extent to which they would follow through on their responsibilities in the treatment plan.

5. *Fear of physical harm.* Parents and family resisted follow-through on the treatment plan for fear of being physically hurt by the son or daughter or for fear of damage to property. This fear was dealt with in several ways: introducing limits gradually, teaching anger control to clients, rehearsing procedures to follow in-home in the event of an outburst, and rearranging the environment to minimize the effects of the outburst.

6. *Unsupportive social-environmental network.* Parents and family resisted follow-through in treatment because of a lack of support from neighbors, close friends, and extended family (e.g., grandparents, aunts, and uncles, who, because they lacked understanding, disagreed with aspects of the treatment plan and convinced the parents to cease their efforts on numerous occasions). To prevent this happening, HIP attempted to include extended family and significant others whenever possible.

13.6.3. Infrequent Severe Behavior Crisis

Another important issue that surfaced early in our program work involved difficulties, from a treatment perspective, in dealing with a client's problem behavior that was great in magnitude but relatively low in its rate of occurrence. Temper outbursts, including very abusive and destructive actions, were characteristic of this category. These low-frequency–high-intensity problems, so easily identified, were the most difficult to treat. From a causal standpoint, numerous possibilities existed for any particular case, ranging from the build-up over time of emotional and psychological stresses, finally aggravated by a seemingly insignificant event, to sexual tension, to possible psychomotor-seizure activity. Neurological evaluations were recommended in some cases to rule in or rule out the latter possibility. HIP interventions for low-frequency–high-intensity outbursts generally focused on teaching parents and family the signals that usually preceded the temper display, on prearranging a plan of action to be followed when the outbursts occurred, on teaching anger control skills to the clients, and on following undesirable behavior with appropriate consequences. Because the problem behaviors occurred with relative infrequency, a particularly useful technique was "fire drilling." This involved repeated practice, during noncrisis or nonproblem times, of the responses and actions of the parents, family, program staff, and so on if the problem actually occurred.

In reviewing case outcomes for evaluation purposes, it appeared that the best results were obtained in those instances where the client was consistently able to "feel" the consequences of his or her behavior. Thus, "one must *feel* consequences to change" became an important "rule of intervention" for us. This feeling of consequences involved the experiences of reinforcement for positive behavior and "aversive" or otherwise appropriate consequences for undesirable behavior. Establishing a program that fostered the use of normal, natural consequences for behavior frequently placed the individual in a situation where, for the first time, she or he was "required" to take responsibility for his or her actions. Replacing items damaged or broken, failing to earn money for a soda, and missing out on lunch because of a refusal to make it were among the many consequences "felt" by the program participants. Although these often were difficult experiences for those who encountered them, they were definite catalysts for positive change.

A final issue pertaining to treatment concerns the fact that the nature and the outcome of the program interventions were necessarily limited by aspects of the situation in which they were implemented. Because the treatment primarily focused on work with significant individuals in the client's natural environment, "success" in treatment greatly depended on the motivations and abilities of these persons to learn and consistently utilize skills. As the capacities for positive change varied, it was important to help each family to become more aware of their individual strengths and limitations and to mutually consider progress, or lack of progress, accordingly. This approach was helpful in determining the extent to which further efforts could be encouraged, and in accepting the fact that the current potential for change had been reached.

13.7. Advantages and Limitations of the HIP Model: A Clinical and Administrative Perspective

13.7.1. The Natural Environment

The most distinct and powerful advantage of the HIP model is that the locus for treatment is based within the context of the client's natural environment. Our presence *in vivo* provided us with unique opportunities to observe problem situations ourselves. We were able to see problems as they typically occurred in the settings where they normally occurred. Initial observations allowed us to understand the nature of the problems more completely and accurately. Frequently, our understanding of a situation as described to us verbally, by phone, or in other "out-of-context" settings was changed quite drastically once we were able to see the events occurring in the home environment. These observations produced valuable assessment data, which then were used in planning the course of the treatment intervention. For example, in a behavioral sense, we were easily able to identify the antecedents and the consequences surrounding particular behaviors by being present; this is vital information for a trained, objective observer and not easily discernible to an overwhelmed parent.

It is appropriate to mention at this point that behavior demonstrated by family members during the early stages of HIP involvement was usually guarded and somewhat tempered in a positive sense as a function of staff presence. Although this "doing what the therapist would want me to" or "halo effect" could be considered a disadvantage of home-based treatment, its effects in each case were relatively short-lived and usually dissipated within one or two weeks' time. Individuals may have "tempered" or "toned down" particular behaviors, but general patterns of behavior, interactions, and coping responses were very obvious and were valuable pieces of information that we used to formulate the course of treatment.

The natural environment was also an excellent setting in which to implement treatment. Just as we learned and understood aspects of client–family problems more completely by being in the home setting, family members were able to benefit from our presence and close contact with them in the places where the problems occurred. We were able to teach skills and alternative coping responses in real, and often quite intense, problem situations. Parents were given the opportunity to observe and learn from us, from our behavior. Conveyed in this process of modeling were not only the basic aspects of a technique, but the more subtle forms of information, such as attitude, intonation, physical movements, and body language, which would be most difficult to describe, and so much more difficult to enact if the situation were not real. Our presence and our attempts to utilize techniques in the context of real problem situations also helped us to understand and respond to the difficulties that the parents had, and would have, in using the same skills themselves. We were able to make the particular treatment more practical or to enhance its potential for continued use and success by modifying a single technique or by uniquely combining techniques for use in particular problem situations.

The effect of therapist's presence in the home setting also seemed to be one that had great utility in helping to "break" firmly established and deeply seated patterns of events and interactions associated with problem situations. We were "there" to encourage and support families in their efforts to change— even in circumstances where emotions were peaked. We had the definite sense that if we weren't present during the initial and crucial stages when the parents would begin to use the treatment techniques, the frustrations that typically accompanied the problems would probably have discouraged their efforts to follow through. (Indeed, some parents were inclined to give up on a new technique even in our presence!)

One example, easily related, was when we were working with parents on breaking their pattern of "rewarding" the undesirable and disruptive behavior of their son. The usual pattern of responding was to give the son excessive amounts of attention (stopping what they were doing, chasing him, calming him down, spending much time with him) whenever the problem behavior occurred. The treatment plan called for a "simple" change in this routine: the entire family was to ignore his behavior. A tremendous effort was needed to persuade the family members, especially the father, to follow through on this changed response. Our therapist team was present in the family's home on the first day of treatment plan implementation when the son began to act out his problem behavior in the usual manner. After a short period of ignoring, tension between the parents increased as the problem behaviors continued and escalated. We gathered the family members together in an isolated part of their house and discussed with them their intense feelings: embarrassment because of the neighbors, guilt about how "bad" their son was acting, and their desire to take responsibility for his behavior. Still, the tension mounted and the "need" to slip into the old pattern of responding increased. Finally, as the father started out of the room in pursuit of his son, the male member of our therapist team took his arm (gently but firmly) and, in a final effort, verbally convinced him to stay. After what seemed to be hours (45–60 minutes), the son returned to the house and calmed down on his own. A family meeting was then called, and the son was verbally reinforced for calming down on his own.

In the above example, we had the advantage of being present at a crucial time, and our intensive involvement with this family up to that point in treatment gave us the rapport necessary to encourage and support them in their efforts to change because of the family's trust in us, an in-depth understanding of the problem, and an understanding of what they had been through in the past. These factors, in combination with the fact that we able to be in the home, enabled us to help them overcome an initial hurdle and begin the process of change. HIP involvement in other aspects of the client's natural environment also had definite advantages. This broad and more inclusive focus enabled treatment to span settings, and it provided consistency and continuity in treatment planning and implementation. In one case, for example, the involvement of vocational services staff who worked with a male client during weekdays was essential in increasing his attendance in that program and in helping to reduce his violent temper outbursts. Similarly, in efforts to span treatment across environments, the HIP became involved with numerous other programs and services, both inside and outside (i.e., school system and social services agency) our mental-health and mental-retardation services agency. These interprogram efforts clearly helped to facilitate the treatment process.

Although the advantages of *in vivo* interventions have been apparent to us, there were some disadvantages worth mentioning. One unavoidable limitation involved the issue of travel time. Although this factor would appear to reduce the overall availability and utilization of "productive" staff time, as we could not "see" clients while driving to their homes, we did attempt to make efficient use of the time spent in transit. For example, travel time provided opportunities for us to prepare and plan for visits while on the way to them and to "process" visits as a team on the trip back. Also, the use of a portable tape-recording device while traveling enabled us to make dictations of case-related information, thereby facilitating the completion of necessary paperwork while maximizing the use of travel time.

Another "disadvantage" of working in the natural environment involved a more clinically related issue. In the majority of cases, the plan of treatment called for the setting of clear and consistent limits regarding problem behaviors. Some clients responded violently to this limit setting, particularly those individuals whose presenting problems involved abusive or destructive behavior. The fact that we were establishing limits *in vivo* meant that violent responses occurred in the homes of some families we worked with. Although abusive or destructive behavior often occurred in these homes anyway, we as staff were "instrumental" in setting the stage for more. By introducing limits, *we* were providing stimuli to which the clients responded violently. In a sense, we felt "responsible" for the damage done—despite our forewarning of family members that such responses might occur, and despite the "necessity" of our actions in producing positive change. This feeling of responsibility, "irrational" as it may have been, was frequently an issue for us in working with families on their "turf" and therefore was a limitation on our work in the natural environment. In the case of one particularly violent individual, we resolved our concerns through the use of visits in our office. These provided an opportunity for us to encourage confrontation and major limit-setting on our own turf. The client, interestingly, did not exhibit violent acting-out responses during these times, as he did at home.

A final disadvantage of services offered *in vivo* was the idea that staff presence in the home was too overwhelming, threatening, or distasteful for some families. These included several identifiable cases where services were made available but were refused by the family. In these instances, the family members expressed concern about having "outsiders" in their home. Some stated that their schedule was not conducive to people coming in. One skeptical foster father stated that he did not want his personal life or the personal life of his family scrutinized by strangers. It is interesting to note that in a majority of these cases, client problems were enmeshed in other, serious family problems, such as alcoholism and abuse. Although in-home intervention was welcomed by and helpful to some families, it did have its limits of acceptability for others.

13.7.2. Team Approach

A "combination of efforts" on the part of staff in the Home Intervention Program, who worked as a therapist team, had many advantages. At the simplest level, working as a team enabled us to share the work load. Thus, individual case assessments, the compilation of data bases, treatment plans, and so on were joint efforts. In addition, the team approach to work with families created a climate within which we could support and reinforce each other. This circumstance was particularly advantageous in working with families' resistance to change, where a combined effort was useful for confronting, understanding, and working through issues that might block progress. At times, we were able to take on specified roles in a joint effort to facilitate treatment. Thus, for example, one of us would be the "heavy" (i.e., the confronter, the limit setter, the identifier of unpopular issues), and the other would assume the role of the "understander" (i.e., the empathetic listener). The fact that there were two of us also provided numerous opportunities to "role-play" together and to model the desired behavior. Finally, as members of a team, we were able to process feelings with each other regarding difficult cases and to maintain a high degree of enthusiasm for our client work.

In addition to these benefits, which would seemingly be present or possible with any team approach to treatment, there were other advantages that appeared to be a function of the fact that the team members (1) were male and female and (2) were married to each other. Although a male–female, unmarried team involved in home intervention would, in our opinion, foster strengths similar in nature to those provided via our husband–wife team approach, we had a definite sense that our married relationship carried with it deeper benefits in our work with families. Central to the utility of this method is the notion that one family unit or system has entered another to effect treatment.

One apparent effect of the male–female team approach was that it fostered relationship building. There were times when, quite simply, the females with whom we were working related best to the female therapist, and the males, to the male team member. At times, however, the opposite was true. It was also quite common that during the initial visits in a two-parent home, the female member of the HIP team would find herself conversing with the mother, and the male team member with the father. This typically would occur after we had discussed "program business" as a group, and it seemed to happen quite naturally. In many instances, the topics discussed during these times seemed "unrelated" to treating the presenting problems: gardening, automobile engines, photography, sewing, and music were among the subjects most frequently discussed. These and future conversations, however, proved to be extremely valuable during the phase of treatment plan implemetation, when the benefits of this relationship building became obvious. One overwhelmed father, for example, related important information to the male member of the therapist team after they had worked together plowing the family's garden for spring planting. The father had previously been uninvolved in the program and reluctant to share his feelings.

Another important benefit of the relationships built between the male or female team member and the same-sexed parent was the establishment of identification bonds. In several instances, it seemed that mothers or fathers would "identify" with the female or male therapist. This identification was manifested most explicitly in instances when the "desired behavior" was modeled by staff. It seemed as if mothers could more easily or willingly model their behavior after that of the female team member. Similarly, fathers appeared to exhibit the behaviors that they had seen demonstrated by the male therapist.

Throughout our work, we have received many inquiries regarding the effects of our working relationship on our marriage relationship and vice versa. Indeed, at this point, the reader must have had a similar curiosity. It is with great honesty (certainly, with somewhat less "pride") that we must state that the husband–wife team approach has, at times, been a hardship in terms of our personal lives. One major factor is "carryovers," which involve some difficulty in leaving "work" at work and, at times (quite honestly), "home" at home. Issues related to work with a case can easily come up at home. This is acceptable at times, if mutually agreed on. "Processing" at home is helpful, but limits were quickly established. Similarly, issues concerning our personal lives have the potential to carry over to our work. Again, limits were mutually set in this area (to get the job done at work).

An important point is that our relationship is such that we have been able to establish a balance that has permitted us to live and work together. A second point is that this is an ongoing effort. Another difficulty that has resulted from working together as a husband–wife therapist team is our increased "need" for time alone. Because we live and work together, we spend a tremendous amount of time "together." Arranging our free time to include "alone time" has been extremely helpful in this regard. The physical and psychological "space" encountered during these times help us to maintain positive and mutually comfortable relationships at home and work. Finally, as there is increased need for individual time alone, there also seems to be a need to spend time alone as a married couple. This time is different from time spent together at home that involves activities aimed at maintaining a household. Experientially, it has been beneficial for us to regularly spend "fun time" together that is unrelated to work or to routines of the household.

13.8. Conclusion

The Home Intervention Program has represented the unique combination of several distinct components: services provided in the natural environment, a husband–wife therapist team, an eclectic approach to treatment, and flexible time scheduling. The present project explored the effects of this particular model with mentally retarded–emotionally disturbed individuals and their families. The project was designed to help fulfill a tremendous need for services and, through a detailed evaluation, to provide useful information to others in the field and to serve as a stimulus for the development of similar programs in other service systems.

In conducting the research, it was generally hypothesized that the HIP model would promote the attainment of specific objectives that were directly related to changes in the behavior of the client and his or her family. The results, as presented on group and individual case bases, indicate that the hypothesis has withstood disconfirmation.

In regard to the client, the program was highly successful in eliminating or decreasing presenting problem behaviors, the majority of which involved abusive-destructive temper outbursts, and in increasing skills focused on personal responsibility and independence. Increased self-control and self-esteem were also noted, especially among the higher functioning individuals in this group.

In regard to the family, parents who participated in the program clearly demonstrated, as a group, increased abilities to consciously, constructively, and effectively utilize behavioral skills with their son or daughter. It was interesting that these parents were able to apply behavioral skills and to implement successful behavior-change programs without significant increases in their tested understanding of theoretical behavioral principles. The program was also successful in reducing parents' overwhelmed feelings and tendencies to "overprotect." Parents also demonstrated positive changes in the area of sensitivity to others, indicative of increased abilities to communicate more effectively with their offspring.

Although the program's focus was primarily on work with the parents or the family to effect changes in problem behavior, there were situations where the families' capacities to make necessary changes were limited. In this regard, the program's ability to focus on parental feelings and attitudes, to be flexible in time and approach, and to involve the total environment in the treatment effort was instrumental in maximizing the potential for positive change. It is clear that these are fundamental requirements for any program intending to meet the needs of this particular population.

Throughout program implementation, the present writers have had the privilege of working closely with families. We have been exposed to portions of their lives, have witnessed their frustration and despair, joy and love. Although the program has offered skills and techniques, it has also provided opportunities for a powerful humanistic exchange that has fostered understanding, trust, and a mutual sharing of thoughts, feelings, and effort. It is felt that the model of service designed and evaluated here would be of benefit to more than the 12 families studied. Although not a panacea, it does offer a way of alleviating frustration and hopelessness, and it enhances the potential for continued community living.

References

1. Berger M, Foster M: Family-level interventions for retarded children: A multivariate approach to issues and strategies. *Multivar Exper Clin Res* 2;2–21, 1976.
2. Tymchuk A: Training parent therapist. *Ment Retard* 13(5);19–22, 1975.
3. Baum MH: Some dynamic factors affecting family adjustment to the handicapped child. *Except Child* 28;387–392, 1962.
4. Evans EC: The grief reaction of parents of the retarded and the counselor's role. *Austr Ment Retard* 4;8–12, 1976.
5. Olshunsky S: Chronic sorrow: A response to having a mentally defective child. *Social Casework* 43;190–193, 1962.
6. Roos P: Parents and families of the mentally retarded, in Kauffmann JM, Payne JS (eds): *Mental Retardation: Introduction and Personal Perspectives*. Columbus, Charles E. Merrill, 1975.
7. Wolfensberger W: Counseling the parents of retarded children, in Baumeister AA (ed): *Mental Retardation: Appraisal, Education and Rehabilitation*. Chicago, Aldine, 1967.
8. Heifetz LJ: Professional preciousness and the evaluation of parent training strategies, in Mittler P (ed): *Research to Practice in Mental Retardation*, vol. 1. Baltimore, University Press, 1977.

9. Matheny AP, Vernick J: Parents of the mentally retarded child: Emotionally overwhelmed or informationally deprived? *J Pediatr* 74;953–959, 1969.

10. Berkowitz BP, Graziano AM: Training parents as behavior therapists: A review. *Behav Res Ther* 10;297–317, 1972.

11. O'Dell S: Training parents in behavior modification: A review. *Psychol Bull* 81;418–433, 1974.

12. Tavormina JB: Relative effectiveness of behavioral and reflective group counseling with parents of mentally retarded children. *Consul Clin Psychol* 43;22–31, 1975.

13. Hawkins RP: It's time we taught the young how to be good parents (and don't we wish we'd started a long time age?). *Psychol Today* 6;28–38, 1972.

14. Guerney BB: *Psychotherapeutic Agents: New Roles for Non-professionals, Parents and Teachers*. New York, Holt, Rinehart and Winston, 1969.

15. Watson LS, Bassinger JF: Parent training technology: A potential service delivery system. *Ment Retard* 12;3–10, 1974.

16. Menolascino FJ: Parents of the mentally retarded: An operational approach to diagnosis and management. *J Am Acad Child Psychol* 7;509–602, 1968.

17. McKibbin, EH: An interdisciplinary program for retarded children and their families. *Am J Occup Ther* 26;125–129, 1972.

18. Garner HG: A truce in the "war for the child." *Excep Child* 42;315–320, 1976.

19. Cianci V: Home supervision of mental deficiants in New Jersey. *Am J Ment Defic* 51;519–524, 1947.

20. Hansen CC: An extended home visit with conjoint family therapy. *Fam Process* 7;67–87, 1968.

21. Kinney JM, Madsen B, Fleming T, et al: Homebuilders: Keeping families together. *J Consult Clin Psychol* 45;667–673, 1977.

22. Cianci V: Home training for retarded children in New Jersey. *The Training School Bulletin* 48;131–139, 1951.

23. O'Leary KD, O'Leary SO, Becker WC: Modification of a deviant sibling interaction pattern in the home. *Behav Res Ther* 5;113–120, 1967.

24. Gray SW: Home-based programs for mothers of young children, in Mittler P (ed): *Research to practice in Mental Retardation*, vol. 1. Baltimore, University Press, 1977.

25. Ramsden M: Shaping the future: Home management: The past six years. *Ontario Psychologist* 6;14–77, 1974.

26. Kiresuk TJ, Lund SH: Goal attainment scaling, in Atkinson CC, Hargreaves W, Horowitz MJ (eds): *Evaluations of Human Service Programs*. New York, Academic Press, 1977.

27. Gordon T: *P.E.T.: Parent Effectiveness Training*. New York, Peter H. Wyden, 1970.

IV

Training Challenges

Introduction

Research, national and state agency surveys, and site visitations in this country confirm that the major service problems in treating and training the mentally retarded-mentally ill individual are a result of improper staff training. Most state and local communities have organized their human delivery-service systems under separate major agencies of mental health and mental retardation. There is very little interaction or communication between staff. As a result, the mental health system is unwilling to work with mentally retarded persons and vice versa.

In order to analyze the training problems and to provide some recommendations, Part IV focuses on the issue of training. Three chapters are presented that focus on, first, an overview of the training needs of mental health personnel in the area of mental retardation; second, the training of paraprofessionals; and third, the practice of social work as a representative model for specific professional training of those individuals who work with this particular population.

Chapter 14 provides a basic analysis of the problem of training mental health personnel in mental retardation and points out specific recommendations both in process and in content in training individuals who specialize in this area. In this chapter, two psychiatrists make specific recommendations for mental health trainees in terms of curriculum knowledge. They point out the need for the trainee to know the basic facts about retardation, definitions, levels of retardation, the diagnostic processes, the social-political forces that operate, and the issues in providing treatment approaches. In addition, the mental health trainee has to understand some of the basic ideological principles and the importance of implementing these principles via a team approach in working with the family. Finally, this chapter makes a number of excellent recommendations about what mental health personnel need to consider for current and future treatment at the undergraduate and graduate, in-service, and continuing-education levels. Such recommendations are for those considering working with the education and training of the mental health professional.

Regardless of how well designed a human-service delivery system is, success or failure often depends on the competence of the staff that provides these services. Because of historical practices, personnel shortages, and financial constraints, a cadre of paraprofessional staff are almost always given the day-to-day responsibility for determining the success of a program. As pointed out in Chapter 15, the success of such programs is often contingent on the type of in-service training such staff have received. Dr. Watson points out that paraprofessional staff in particular need the proper in-service training, as they constitute the majority of work forces in programs for mentally retarded individuals with behavioral disorders. Dr. Watson presents three different programs that are designed to train paraprofessional staff to teach independent-living skills and techniques so as to manage disruptive behavior without violating the client's rights and to comply at the same time with the principles of normalization. The first two staff training programs are based on backward chaining and forward chaining in teaching independent skills. In addition, they are evaluated and data are presented for their efficacy. The third in-service program is designed to teach staff how to manage disruptive behavior based on three different alternatives. Curriculum materials and training techniques are presented and should serve as a valuable resource for paraprofessionals working in this area. In addition, those individuals who are engaged in in-service training will find useful the evaluation techniques in examining the success and the failure of such training programs.

Psychiatrists, psychologists, special educators, rehabilitation specialists, and social workers often represent the bulk of professionals providing services to both mentally retarded and mentally ill individuals. Chapter 16 was selected because it serves as an excellent model that any of these professions can follow in acquiring or upgrading their skills to meet the challenges of working with this complex population. As an experienced social worker engaged in the treatment of this population, Monfils points out skills that should serve as a foundation for social workers, or any other professional, in addressing the needs of the dually diagnosed group. Monfils goes on to describe and examine some of the new challenges that professionals will face in meeting the mental health needs of retarded citizens in both institutional and community settings. Specifically, he points out the challenges that need to be met in institutional settings such as social group work, dealing with sexuality and psychosexual development, and the role that professionals play in preparing clients for placement in a community setting. The challenges that professionals will meet in the community involve extensive work with the family, and a consultation model for this process is presented. In addition, Monfils points out the role, function, and skills necessary for professionals—or more specifically, social workers—in working in community mental-health centers. In short, this chapter presents an overview of some of the new and emerging roles that professionals—more specifically, social workers—may want to adopt in addressing the psychosocial needs of the dually diagnosed population and in accomplishing their treatment, prevention, and outreach efforts.

Training Mental Health Personnel in Mental Retardation

Frank J. Menolascino and Bruce Gutnik

14.1. Introduction

During the last decade, there has been an enhanced interest in providing both general and specialized training experiences in mental retardation for mental health personnel. Increasingly, one notes a variety of course offerings in mental retardation in the mental-health undergraduate, graduate, postgraduate, and continuing education programs. This interest has been spurred by the rapidly increased services provided for retarded citizens, especially in community-based mental-retardation service systems. These systems, usually organized on a regional or statewide basis, have begun to "discover" the high incidence of coexisting mental illness in their clientele. When such systems search for mental health resources to meet these rapidly emerging needs or attempt to develop their own specialized mental-health services, it has become abundantly clear that the traditional mental-health personnel pools and allied resources need reevaluation as to their awareness or knowledge of modern concepts and trends in mental retardation. Concomitantly, a strong interest has been shown in similar educational offerings and efforts that extend the knowledge base of current mental retardation professionals by means of modern information on mental health principles, methods, and techniques.

In this chapter, a brief attempt is made to survey the current components of training approaches that can effectively accomplish the task of training mental health personnel in mental retardation.

14.2. The Current Scene

A current national review of the need for enhanced training efforts, especially as they apply to the current and future delivery of mental health services to retarded citizens, was given in the Report of the Liaison Task Panel

Frank J. Menolascino • Departments of Psychiatry and Pediatrics, Nebraska Psychiatric Institute, University of Nebraska Medical Center, Omaha, Nebraska 68105. *Bruce Gutnik* • Department of Psychiatry, Nebraska Psychiatric Institute, University of Nebraska Medical Center, Omaha, Nebraska 68105.

on Mental Retardation of the President's Commission on Mental Health
(PCMH).[1] The panel noted,

> Information gathered from many of the State Mental Health coordinators indicates
> that the mental health field still responds to the myth that mentally retarded persons
> cannot and do not profit from psychotherapeutic intervention. Others report that
> mental health professionals are generally unfamiliar with the fact and fiction of mental
> retardation. In many cases, their unwillingness to treat mentally retarded persons is
> attributed to their lack of knowledge and training. Mental health delivery systems for
> mentally retarded persons are described as unresponsive, woefully inadequate, and
> often nonexisting. There appears to be a tendency for the mentally retarded client to
> be bounced back and forth between mental health and mental retardation profes-
> sionals, with neither agency offering an adequate service delivery plan to meet the
> client's needs. Often the individual is shuffled among mental health, mental retar-
> dation, and correctional institutions. Some States report that limited services are
> available for mentally retarded persons in local community mental health clinics.
> Others speak of the low priority given mentally retarded persons in local clinics and
> the frequent referrals to State hospitals. (p. 7)

The PCMH, in its recommendations for resolving the above-noted crisis
of nonservice for retarded citizens who are mentally ill, stressed the importance
of providing specific training inputs: initial exposure of the mental health trainee
to basic information and modern treatment approaches in mental retardation,
as well as in-service and other continuing-educational formats.

Thus, the challenges of providing special training in mental retardation for
mental health personnel is well recognized, and there is a national focus on
addressing the delivery of special training in mental retardation for all mental-
health personnel—wherever they practice. Accordingly, a brief overview of
basic and advanced training challenges for all mental-health personnel is presented here.

14.3. Basic Training Components

Although the current mental-health diagnostic and treatment approaches
owe much to their late-nineteenth-century history, where they were entwined
with very similar efforts in mental retardation, this "shared early history" has
not often been presented to mental health colleagues in their past and current
training programs. Accordingly, a historical perspective is a very helpful first
step for the mental health worker—whether a student currently in training or
a graduate of training programs in social work, psychology, psychiatry, nursing,
and so on during the last two decades. Historical overviews have been provided
by Kanner,[2] Kugel and Wolfensberger,[3] Menolascino,[4] and Strider and Menolascino.[5] The study and elaboration of the mutual historical context of mental
retardation and psychiatry (especially clinical psychiatry) clearly show the historical unity of some of the persisting challenges (in both mental retardation
and mental health) that the mental health needs of the retarded still present in
the 1980s. The early studies of the childhood psychoses and their intimate
differential diagnostic relationships to Kanner's later syndrome of infantile autism, the persisting clinical confusion between distinct delays in personality

growth versus personality regression, the realization that the behavioral aspects of phenylketonuria were earlier viewed as symptoms of a functional psychosis, the interrelationships between poorly controlled seizure phenomenon and later personality development, and the benchmark psychiatric-educational efforts of Itard of the Wild Boy of Aveyron—all have a hauntingly modern ring to them.

Thus the trainee should be provided with an overview of basic facts in mental retardation. Key general references, which can provide the trainee a succinct overview of the field of mental retardation, have been provided by Robinson and Robinson,[6] Balthazar and Stevens,[7] and Menolascino and Egger.[8] Through these overviews the trainee has an opportunity to view the differing challenges as to chronological and developmental age-specific problems, the variety of diagnostic–treatment–management modalities that are available, and a knowledge of what mental retardation is (and is not), what can be done, by whom, where, and so on. This training component will put to rest the traditional mental-health professional's repeated faulty impression that the field of mental retardation is narrow or prosaic. For example, the modern approaches of viewing the formal diagnosis of mental retardation as a relative (not a fixed) phenomenon,[9,10] of formulating educational treatment prescriptions based on the level of retardation currently present (without undue focus on its causative factors),[11] and of recognizing the dynamic role of parent advocacy groups in spurring change[4] are still seemingly quite remote to current health personnel.

In addition, the trainee can be introduced to the conceptual issues involved in the formal definition of mental retardation that was initially adopted in 1961 by the American Association on Mental Deficiency, was reaffirmed in 1983,[9] and is also utilized in the recently published DSM-III of the American Psychiatric Association.[10] This definition (i.e., "Mental retardation refers to significantly sub-average general intellectual functioning existing concurrently with deficits in adaptive behavior, and is manifested during the developmental period"—Grossman[9]), stressing as it does the *dual* concept of lowered global intelligence and delayed social-adaptive functioning, will help the trainee to appreciate and understand the "label" of mental retardation versus its distinct impact on the adjustment potentials of a fellow citizen. Therefore, the mental age myth (e.g., "He has the mind of a 12-year old and the body and wants of a 25-year old person") or the "magical IQ 70" figure (e.g., "If your IQ is below 70, you are retarded and incompetent, period!") will hopefully not be utilized by the trainee in his or her future professional work.

14.3.1. Diagnosis and Levels of Retardation

As to diagnosis, the trainee should be introduced to the syndromes with which the symptom of mental retardation is most frequently associated—as described in the classification system of the American Association on Mental Deficiency (AAMD). This diagnostic standard organizes the more than 350 causes of mental retardation into eight distinct groupings on the basis of the

known (or suspected) causative factors and the associated clinical manifestations. In reviewing the different *major* syndromes (not the rare or exotic ones),
the trainee should be counseled as to whom to turn to for further consultation
in these challenges: geneticists, pediatricians with a special interest in genetics,
and so on. The mental health trainee may be surprised to learn that much more
is known about the causes of mental retardation than about the causes of mental
illness.[8] Similarly, the impact of secondary handicaps on the retarded (e.g.,
seizures and special sensory impairments) and their specific impacts on personality development can make the trainee both knowledgeable about and more
understanding of retarded individuals' transactions with a reality that they
poorly perceive or integrate into consciousness. Clear-cut syndromes such as
hydrocephaly or Down's syndrome are very helpful in illustrating signs, symptoms, cognitive levels, and modes of impaired personality growth for the student. Concomitantly, these diagnostic experiences—beyond the mere listing
of somatic symptoms—can give the trainee a poignant insight into how parents
view their child as "different" and how the perceived "stigmata" can be cos-
metically mitigated (e.g., longer hair for the youth with arrested hydrocephaly
and tinted glasses to obscure the eye signs for the Down's syndrome lad). The
trainee can thus focus on a wide variety of interventions, rather than the traditional professional approach of an exclusive focus on diagnostic categorizing
and a resultant shrugging of the shoulders in resignation about possible treatment approaches. The wide range of treatment and management approaches
to the known genetic disorders (e.g., active informant inborn errors of retardation, such as galactosemia and homocystinuria) and the correctible metabolic
(hypothyroidism), toxic (e.g., lead intoxication), cranial malformations (e.g.,
neurosurigcal intervention for craniostenosis), and allied challenges should be
shared with the trainee to underscore the great progress that has been accomplished in this field, in which hopeless prognoses were the automatic answers
of the recent past.

Next, the different *levels* of mental retardation and their manifestations at
differing chronological ages are reviewed, and the trainee can be directly shown
how to translate these levels into the three types of diagnostic approaches by
which the mentally retarded are usually identified:

1. Multidisciplinary diagnostic-team assessments usually confirm the diagnosis of profound, severe, or moderate mental retardation in infancy and the
preschool years. These infants and children tend to have early histories of high
"at-risk" factors and allied distinct indices of slow developmental progress.

2. Poor performance on school and achievement tests and general under-
achievement are usually the cardinal signs that prompt the identification and
the subsequent diagnostic evaluation of the mildly retarded. Mental retardation
is rarely suspected in these youngsters before their initial school attendance
and subsequent academic performance difficulties. Interestingly, mental health
professionals often tend to obscure the coexistence of the symptoms of mental
retardation in syndromes such as the hyperactive child—viewing delayed cognitive functioning as secondary to the presenting behavioral problems. Con-

versely, the indices of retardation may be ignored for the time being because retardation is viewed as "untreatable" as long as the remainder of the child's problems have not been as "fixed." In either of the two above viewpoints, the child's *total* clinical picture becomes blurred, the relative nature of the AAMD definition of the symptom of mental retardation is overlooked, and the child and his or her parents remain perplexed.

3. At all chronological ages, the recognition of some degrees of social maladaptability and vocational inadequacy becomes a major reason for diagnostic referral. If this social maladjustability or vocational inadequacy is erroneously viewed as primitive or regressed behavior, then a misdiagnoses of schizophrenia can mislead or blur appropriate treatment potentials. To paraphrase Gertrude Stein, the retarded are not just the retarded—the level of this symptom is of major diagnostic, treatment, and prognosis significance.

Lastly, as to the levels concept, the trainee learns that the President's Committee on Mental Retardation[12] noted that 86% of all mentally retarded persons are mildly retarded, 6% are moderately retarded, 3.5% are severely retarded, and 1.5% are profoundly retarded. These levels of retardation provide the following general predictions of future attainments by the retarded if modern treatment and management approaches are utilized:

Mildly retarded persons are almost always capable of learning to do productive work, of learning academic school subjects to varying degrees, and, as adults, of living independently and becoming self-supporting if they have received appropriate services during childhood, adolescence, and early adulthood.

Moderately retarded persons can almost always learn to care for themselves, can profit in varying degrees from classroom instruction, and can be trained for semicomplex vocational tasks. With an appropriate background of stimulation and training from early childhood, most are able to become at least partially self-supporting and are able to live in the community with some degree of supervision.

Severely retarded persons generally require specialized services at all stages of their lives. They are capable of learning to care for themselves, and many can become marginally productive, as adults, under supervision in sheltered work settings. Recent studies, both in America and abroad, certainly demonstrate that the severely retarded are capable of performing many tasks that were previously thought to be beyond their capability.

Profoundly retarded persons nearly always require major inputs of medical and/or nursing supervision in order to remediate physical and medical disabilities and maintain life. Yet, many can be taught some degree of self-care skill such as feeding, dressing, and ambulation. Issues related to the humanistic care of these very handicapped individuals can become an introduction to the ethics of human services provision and quality-of-life issues and can provide trainees with a close look at their own interdependence.

The trainee can then be presented with an overview of the many outstanding developments in refined diagnostic approaches that have recently been attained. Genetic counseling of prospective parents has enlarged the vista of prevention. For example, evaluation of the fetus *in utero* (via amniocentesis) has now evolved into a safe technique by which 35 different causes of mental retardation can be detected *in utero*. This crucial information permits the parents to make scientifically based decisions about their child. Although this topic is fraught with much controversy today, the trainee should be exposed to the valid professional viewpoint that amniocentesis is very often a life-giving procedure—especially for couples who are afraid to intitiate pregnancy because of a known high risk. Similarly, new assessment techniques in the newborn period have evolved to the point where a new branch of pediatrics (neonatology) stands ready to evaluate, in the early hours and days of life, a wide number of conditions that can be ameliorated. The nationwide expansion of mandatory metabolic screening early in life for the inborn errors of metabolism (e.g., PKU and hypothyroidism), for the debilitating infections noted in the newborn period (e.g., syphillis and cytomegalic virus), and for toxic substances in early childhood (e.g., lead and abused pharmaceuticals) underscores for the trainee the need for very early diagnosis and rapid intervention.

The trainee should be also exposed to the social-political forces at work in the area of mental retardation. For example, the advocacy–public-health–political thrusts that have combined their efforts to obtain mandatory immunizations in childhood have had a magnificient payoff in the sharp drop noted in the incidence of rubella and its past handicapping residue in many children. Also, in spite of the recent giant strides in early diagnostic evaluation, a rapid expansion of the federally funded Early and Periodic Screening, Diagnosis, and Treatment Program is desperately needed. First initiated in 1967, this program has had more than its share of implementation problems. As of June 1979, only 3.5 million children (out of a possible 13 million eligible) had received their first screening evaluation. Yet, the trainee can be shown that the positive impact of early diagnosis, which is rapidly followed by prescriptive and treatment approaches, cannot readily be questioned for any handicapped child.

14.3.2. Treatment Considerations

As to treatment considerations, the previously noted historical review should remind the trainee of the "hopelessness" regarding the treatment of mental retardation that prevailed 25 years ago. This hopelessness has been dispelled by the encouraging results of numerous basic and applied studies, which have documented what can be done. Thus, the mental health trainee should be exposed to the modern concept(s) of prevention (as in Rh, rubella, and so on), cure for a few (secondary prevention—surgical intervention in premature closure of the skull sutures), and treatment and habilitation (tertiary prevention—modern educational and habilitation approaches) for *all* of our retarded citizens.

Primary prevention removes the causes of the initial occurrence of a disorder. Application of the fruits of basic research, coupled with public health and public education, has provided dramatic eradication of some potential causes of mental retardation. Phenylketonuria, hypothyroidism, rubella, lead poisoning, Tay–Sachs disease, and Rh-factor incompatability are sterling examples. Amniocentesis has permitted early active treatment intervention (*in utero*) in a number of inborn errors of metabolism (e.g., Murphy's disease). Unfortunately, there is still a wide gap between current knowledge and the application of known prevention technology to eradicate known causes.

The major challenges in actively using this increasing body of knowledge lie in the area of public education—and then the mental health trainee can review data that clearly document the presence of primary prevention in mental retardation; this is almost unheard of in mental health or, at best, is viewed as a speculative matter. For example, the causative mechanisms of both rubella and Rh-disease are well understood. Yet, the direct application of this knowledge depends on whether the prospective parent is immunized or desensitized. The trainee is introduced to the immediate steps that can accomplish protection (i.e., dissemination of health information to grade- and high-school students, professionals, and the general public). Areas of primary-prevention concern that could become key training ingredients include the following: (1) at preconception, genetic assessment to determine potential chromosomal genetic risks in pregnancy, timing and spacing of pregnancies through family-planning strategies, adequate nutrition for women of childbearing age, and immunization; (2) during pregnancy, protection of mother and fetus against disease, proper nutrition, monitoring pregnancy through medical supervision, use of amniocentesis to determine the condition of the fetus in high-risk mothers, and parental choice about termination of pregnancy when amniocentesis confirms that the fetus is defective; (3) at delivery, medical supervision of delivery in a hospital, including screening for conditions causing mental retardation to identify newborn children at risk and taking indicated remedial action; protection of Rh-mothers with Rho-Gam within 72 hours after delivery; and the intensive care of children who are born ill or prematurely; and (4) in early childhood, proper nutrition for nursing mothers, infants, and very young children; dietary management of metabolic conditions leading to mental retardation; removal of environmental hazards such as lead-based paint; and very early social-educational stimulation for infants and young children who are "at risk" for developing mental retardation. As noted by many mental-health workers,[13] these "organic" considerations in mental retardation are closely akin to the spectrum of causes for many of the psychiatric disorders of childhood.

Secondary prevention and treatment measures attempt to roll back (i.e., cure) or substantially ameliorate the degree of mental retardation present in the past. The prototypical examples of secondary prevention in mental retardation were the energetic treatment of hypothyroidism, PKU, and galactosemia in the early months of life, as well as surgical treatment of secondary handicaps (e.g., motor, sensory, emotional, and seizure phenomena). Prompt alleviation and/or control of these secondary handicaps can often sufficiently enhance the individual's social-adaptive skills to permit functioning at near-normal levels. The treatment of some of these secondary handicaps could be advanced by the application of new technology such as telemetry, direct brain stimulation, and sensory and motor prosthesis.

Developmental enrichment programs for both the parents and the at-risk child are showing great promise for altering the early manifestations of retardation in culturally, familially, and psychosocially deprived youngsters. Here again, the interchangeability of these factors and the training opportunities for obtaining a fuller understanding of both mental-retardation and mental-health repercussions in an individual are remarkable. These programs, which are still preciously few in number, have great potential for both primary and secondary prevention in the largest grouping of the retarded: the mildly retarded. Advances in emergency care procedures and rehabilitative medicine have lessened the intellectual impairment of victims of trauma. Similar medical treatment advances in the management of toxemia (i.e., treatment of the mother's borderline hypertension status) and pretesting of immunization substances before routine administration have reduced the frequency of residuals of intoxication as a cause of retardation. Early and definitive treatment of the infectious causes of mental retardation, such as meningitis, is also now possible. Lastly, treatment programs that focus on infant stimulation and behavior modification technology show promising secondary prevention potential.

Until recently, the challenge of *tertiary prevention* was typically met by a shrug of the professional's shoulders or "helpful" advice to keep the child happy or to send him or her away "to be with his or her own kind" (institutionalization). Today, the trainee will note that it is generally recognized that the overwhelming number of retarded citizens can be nurtured and trained to lead personally fulfilling lives within the structure of their families, homes, and communities. Effective amelioration of mental retardation is predicated on accepting retarded persons as entitled to the same legal rights and privileges as other citizens. Continued infringement of these rights has led to some major legal confrontations during the last decade. The courts have upheld, in a number of benchmark class-action suits, the retarded citizen's legal rights to public education, treatment, compensation, freedom from harm, and valid calssification assessments. Court mandates have ushered in a new era of accountability for professionals and public agencies. Legal decisions have also required that the retarded citizen (and his or her parents) be given the opportunity to actively participate in the development and implementation of treatment and habilitation plans. This entire topic can provide the trainee with a foundation for more fully understanding the veritable revolution in patients' rights—in both mental retardation and mental health—that is currently occurring in our society.

14.3.3. Unique Family Issues

Family issues of the mentally retarded present an opportunity to further clarify a basic training need for all mental-health personnel in the area of mental retardation. Contrary to the frequent clinical occurrence, where a mentally ill child represents the emotional precipitate of parental problems, parents of the retarded typically face the challenge of a developmentally delayed child who is literally dropped into their family and henceforth disrupts family functioning. This atypical precipitation of emotional stress in the family unit, which is experienced by a majority of parents of the retarded, has been succinctly discussed by Roos.[30] Yet, the parents of mentally retarded individuals have a long history of being literally mishandled by mental health professionals. They have, for example, sometimes been miscast as emotionally disturbed people in desperate need of psychiatric care, and their realistic "sorrow" for their child's developmental delay has been inappropriately interpreted as psychopathology. Similarly, their militant demands for improved services have been viewed as manifestations of displaced hostility.

A recent conceptualization of the unique crises faced by the families of the retarded are described (replete with specific treatment recommendations) by Menolascino.[29] Only in recent years have mental health professionals begun to recognize and appreciate the fortitude and dedication of the parents of the retarded in their ongoing efforts to foster the development of appropriate services for their children and/or similarly affected adults. Utilizing supervised clinical experiences (e.g., multidisciplinary diagnostic interviews and family counseling services), the trainee will clearly understand that the emotional impact for parents of having a mentally retarded child can be minimized by specialized counseling procedures and by the professional posture of the family helper. For example, such an experience may exacerbate basic existential anxieties in parents and may represent a mental health problem that warrants help. Their needs require a special sensitivity and understanding of their retarded family member within their total life experience. Other parents need help in coping with the realistic problems of raising a retarded child. Yet, despite these burdens, greater numbers of mentally retarded persons are living with their families or are being supported in private living situations close to home. The family has been, and continues to be, a vital resource and, as such, has prevented or delayed costly institutionalization for many retarded citizens. If these families are to continue to maintain the primary responsibility for their mentally retarded member, then the mental health professional must help sustain them.

14.3.4. Interpretation of Diagnoses and Family Counseling

Trainees can develop specific skills in interpreting findings and in providing family counseling to parents of the retarded—a set of skills that has remarkable carry-over to parents of *all* developmentally disabled children or adults (i.e., the learning disabilities, autism, epilepsy, and cerebral palsy). Initially, the trainee needs aid and experience in the adequate interpretation and transmission of the diagnostic findings to the parents, as this is the first step in inaugurating a specific treatment-habilitative program for both the child and his or her parents. Knowledge of the clinical disorders that frequently produce mental retardation allows the trainee to share his or her conclusions with the parents without feeling uneasy with terms, findings, and parental questions about specific facts and prognostic implications. The practice of interpretation and parental counseling is a most demanding one, and the trainee will need certain skills in order to be effective (i.e., to know when and how much to interpret demands on an intimate understanding of the family dynamics—a traditional forte of mental health personnel). Here, the trainee needs help not only in attempting to delineate the role that family psychopathology may have had in the origin of the child's presenting problems, but also in assessing possible reactive components secondary to the child's impairments and behavioral characteristics.

Counseling parents of the mentally retarded can be both therapeutically gratifying and self-educative for the trainee. A host of specific parental counseling questions arise here: Are the parents perplexed by the child's slow development and behavioral characteristics, but not necessarily a negative influence on his personality growth? How much does family crisis contribute to the presenting problem? Has the family's interpersonal milieu produced the presenting clinical picture or otherwise contributed to the child's adaptive problems (for example, an adjustment reaction with or without associated primary mental retardation)? How much do the parental responses stem from disillusionment about the developmental course of their child (e.g., this factor may have literally demolished their expectations for and from their child)? Such considerations underscore the relatively normal reactions to chronic stress that one so commonly sees in parents of the retarded. Counseling and/or guidance of parents of the mentally retarded seemingly needs more focus on the "here and now," rather than the "past" historical focus of most mental-health psychotherapeutic approaches. Similar reorientation to family counseling will remind the trainee rather forcibly that not all family psychopathology reflects earlier stages of conflict-induced fixation in the respective parents' development. As previously noted, such considerations are unique to the field of mental retardation, and it appears that attempts to employ models from other clinical fields (for example, the traditional child-psychiatry approach to families of disturbed children) may be both misleading and harmful to the retarded citizen and/or his or her parents. A trainee can appreciate these particular family counseling constellations as being unique *only* if he or she has had the opportunity to fully evaluate the parental-family problems in adaptation and has directly observed therapeutic approaches that are specifically tailored for such families and their retarded son or daughter.[6]

Mental retardation places many stresses on the family in the problems of care and management over the lifetime of the afflicted members: educational needs, vocational training, and long-range planning for future care. Here, the trainee will quickly realize that his or her expertise does not extend to these other areas of professional endeavor. Reviews of these topical areas should be presented to the trainee in conjunction with visits to preschool programs, special-education classrooms, sheltered workshops, group homes, and so on. Parenthetically, this acquired knowledge base in the multiple service needs of lifelong planning for the retarded is an excellent introduction to *similar* issues that the mental health trainee will encounter in the care of the chronically mentally ill. As noted in the recent book by Lamb,[14] the long-term care of the chronically mentally ill presents treatment–management issues that are remarkably similar to those noted for any chronically handicapped individual.

14.3.5. Ideological Principles

Much of the current wave of change in the field of mental retardation has been due to groundswells around new principles of care and management of the individual retarded citizen. The recently formulated principle of normalization,[15,16] the developmental model,[4] the least restrictive alternative, and citizen advocacy have eventuated in the rapid rise of community-based systems of service for the mentally retarded. The trainee will note that the normalization principle has transformed both the nature and the physical location of service delivery for the mentally retarded. This principle and the concept of the least restrictive setting have provided the ideological underpinnings for the currently vibrant deinstitutionalization movement in the field of mental retardation. In contrast, in the field of mental health, there was precious little ideological rationale for the exodus from the state mental hospitals in the 1960s, without the presence of community-based alternative systems of service or a vocal and active group of advocates who could monitor these less restrictive community settings. Yet, many of these concepts have directly evolved from major contributions of mental health professionals to our knowledge of early personality development and child-care principles. Indeed, the recent changes in the care of the mentally retarded, to a great extent, have had their roots in the advances made in child psychiatry over the last 30 years. These changes fall into three main areas: (1) improved understanding of early personality development and the process of attachment; (2) an enhanced scope of treatment modalities for emotional illness early in life; and (3) movement toward community placement and treatment of mentally and emotionally handicapped persons.[17] Each of these three "crossover" areas between mental retardation and mental health can be presented to the trainee in the following three training formats: developmental issues, enhanced medical management, and the national move toward community-based programs.

14.3.6. Community-Based Programs

It is significant that the great strides in improved understanding of the importance of early close relationships to normal development occurred within the last three decades; that the striking gains in the medical control of epilepsy, motoric impulse disorders, emotional disturbances, and the allied handicaps in the retarded have also come within the last 30 years*; and that the major movement toward community-based programs for the mentally ill and the retarded has occurred in the past 15 years. Although the work on normal human development and the problems of detachment pointed to the need for greater family and community care of retarded persons, these changes would have

---

* Truly, the application of behavioral analysis, via specific behavioral-modification treatment paradigms, must be listed in these dramatic and significant treatment advances of the last 20 years. They are not stressed herein because Drs. Gardner and Cole have clearly documented their efficacy (and training challenges) in Chapter 4.

been greatly delayed without the improvements in medical management that have made community care a practical reality for many retarded individuals.

With the advent of community-based programs for both the mentally ill and the mentally retarded, a series of mutually reinforcing events has unfolded. Many of the symptoms of institutionalization have been prevented in the group of younger retarded persons, and the incidence of many types of psychiatric complications has been significantly reduced. The improved medical management of emotional and behavioral problems in the retarded has significantly increased the morale and the confidence of persons who work with the retarded on a daily basis. They can now treat the retarded person in more humane and less restrictive ways. Greater confidence and flexibility in dealing with the retarded and the disturbed have given caretakers a positive message regarding their potential for acceptable behavior. The decreased need for minute-to-minute staff control has made it possible to develop more comprehensive training programs for the retarded. All of these events have led to significantly increased independent and semi-independent functioning for many retarded persons and has greatly improved the quality of community-based programs for the retarded. In addition to the advantages of avoiding the institutional syndromes of detachment, the community-based programs can provide a normalizing set of life experiences in the community with regard to school, recreational, work, and home environments. They allow the mentally retarded citizen to be close to their families, to maintain close relationships with other caretakers, to live in an actual neighborhood and a homelike setting, and to be close to sources of sophisticated medical support.

The previous overemphasis on severe mental retardation and severe behavioral problems not only produced a distorted view of the mental health dimensions of the mentally retarded but also failed to focus psychiatric effort where it was quantitatively, socially, and programmatically more desperately needed: on the mildly retarded. The large group of mildly retarded citizens are those whom the majority of mental health trainees will see and try to help during their professional careers. Thus, the trainee should have an opportunity to understand the linchpins of modern community-based programs for the retarded, from their ideological underpinnings and the closely allied progress in mental health advances, to the actual systems of service that are currently operative.

14.4. Advanced Training Components

The above-noted training components, if not embellished by actual clinical training experiences, may be integrated by the trainee at only an intellectual (i.e., knowledge base) level of acceptance of the challenges presented by retarded citizens with associated mental illness. Some key sets of training expertise and a positive attitudinal set for the trainee are now reviewed.

14.4.1. Multidisciplinary Team Approach

By its very nature, the evaluation, treatment, and habilitation of the mentally retarded individual presenting with associated mental health problems require the skills of a number of disciplines. To be effective in evaluation and treatment, a truly integrated interdisciplinary approach must be flexible enough to change, as required, from a medical to a mental focus, or to an educational or vocational one, without threatening the competency and/or the security of the trainee. With the increasing emphasis on family and community psychiatry, mental health workers of the future will undoubtedly find themselves thrust more and more into positions in which they not only give direct services to the mentally retarded individual but also activate and coordinate those resources and agencies that concern themselves with the problem of mental retardation on a broad front.

Gone is the day when the psychiatrist, after interviewing a youngster who was referred as possibly being mentally retarded, would share the diagnosis with the parents and refer them for "schooling." Instead, the trainee would profit greatly from extended experiences in a local university-affiliated program that specifically utilizes a multidisciplinary approach to the diagnosis and management of the symptom of mental retardation. Directly viewing the retarded citizen's current level of functioning—in the family, at school, or at the training center, during a specific pediatric examination, a psychiatric consultation, speech and hearing assessments, vocational rehabilitation assessments, and so on—provides a composite picture of what he or she can or cannot accomplish at the present time. For example, direct observation of the actual assessment of both the quantitative and the qualitative aspects of a retarded individual's intellectual functioning provides the trainee with a firsthand appreciation of the methods available, the limitations of those methods at various ages, and their application when special handicapping conditions (e.g., motor impairments, deafness, and specific language disabilities) are present. Evaluating the intellectual potential of a retarded citizen thus becomes much more than simply assessing the global level of intellectual functioning. The presence and role of a host of multiple handicaps and other specific cognitive and conceptual deficits need to be determined and appreciated by the trainee. Furthermore, these deficits must be differentiated from the disorganizing effect of anxiety that accompanies an emotional disorder. Partaking in the synthesis of these findings, at case conferences with all of the interdisciplinary team members interacting, is an excellent prelude to sitting in on the interpretation and follow-up treatment sessions with the parents. Though this training ingredient does not sound very "modern" in the 1980s, the writers did not experience it in their own training in mental health and are suspicious that it is still not readily available even today! It is a vital set of clinical training experiences wherein the complexity of the diagnostic and treatment challenges—and their appropriate management—can be viewed at close quarters, compared to past and current approaches in mental health, and then integrated into the trainee's professional armamentarium.

If the trainee shows further interest in specific diagnostic techniques, then formal or informal training (and experiences) in the cytogenetic, biochemical, metabolic, and neurological aspects of mental retardation can broaden the trainee's understanding of the complex interrelated factors that are often involved in the genesis of even the most easily recognizable conditions associated with mental retardation, such as Down's syndrome or phenylketonuria. Such training experiences will underscore the necessity of thinking in terms of multifactorial etiological models for basic causes, as well as the resultant interaction of dynamic processes that eventuates in the syndrome of mental retardation. Thus, retarded intellectual functioning, psychiatric disturbance, and the neurological manifestations of brain damage and/or dysfunction can all be viewed in terms of their respective contributions to a particular child's problems. These considerations can help the mental health worker avoid far-too-common unitary viewpoints on etiology such as "Something is wrong with his brain" or "she's just mentally retarded."

14.4.2. Personality Assessment

A purely descriptive or psychoanalytic approach is often not adequate in assessing the concrete (and often reality-based) problems and needs of the retarded individual. Thus, the mental health trainee should have an extended opportunity to view the personality development of retarded children (or adults) in the context of the often varied and kaleidoscopic manifestations of the various physical, neurological, and psychiatric disorders occurring during early infancy and childhood—factors that often significantly alter the normal sequences of personality differentiation and maturation. The comprehensive evaluation of the mentally retarded child confronts the trainee with the necessity of viewing developments from a truly psychobiological point of view.

The mental health trainee will quickly note, when relating with retarded citizens whose level of retardation is below the mild range, that characteristic thinking (i.e., concrete), language (i.e., delayed and/or with associated articulation disorders), and overall personality immaturity dimensions are frequently observed in the interview setting.[18,19] With guidance and experience, the trainee will learn to "get with" these atypical developmental handicaps and thus truly listen beyond the noted handicaps. Similarly, the trainee will note that one has to be far more active in the diagnostic interview setting, in sharp contrast to the more passive mode of interviewing a psychiatric patient, lest the retarded citizen's pervasive fear of failure[20] be viewed as volitional in origin, and the retarded citizen retreat to the "benign autism" that Webster[21] so aptly described. Helping the trainee to feel more comfortable with the atypicality of general personality immaturity (and delayed language) of the retarded will permit further exploration of the usually rich emotional life of the retarded citizen. A tactic that we frequently utilize to underscore this point is to have the trainee read The World of Nigel Hunt,[28] one of three available autobiographies written by Down's syndrome individuals. Invariably, trainees are amazed at Mr. Hunt's breadth of reflection on his life, his parents, his travels, and so on. As one trainee commented, "I always thought those mongoloids(!) were drooling idiots who belonged in Endsville. Who would have thought that they were as observant, sensitive, and involved with the people all around them as Nigel obviously is?"

Thus, the acquisition of new techniques, flowing from actual clinical transactions buttressed by specific reading assignments, can have many influences on professional attitudinal changes. Such experiences help trainees to learn to fully appreciate the diagnostic considerations that lead to realistic treatment guidelines. When they can appreciate and empathize with the retarded citizen's multiple handicaps and limitations, his or her strong suits as to life attainments, and the realistic problems of his or her family, then these diagnostic challenges can be realistically translated into treatment targets and can be actively worked with in a positive fashion. This attitudinal change leaves little room for the currently too common mental-health professional's rationalizations that lead to nihilistic treatment and prognostic postures toward chronically handicapped individuals.

14.4.3. Programming Treatment and Habilitative Services

The comprehensive approach to the problems of the mentally retarded individual noted here can provide the trainee with a more realistic assessment of the child's assets and deficits. Consequently, it leads to more appropriate and specific treatment and habilitative planning for the child and his or her parents. Aspects of this total treatment approach underscore the need to introduce the trainee to the broad range of community services and educational-vocational facilities available for mentally retarded individuals, and to the selective utilization of these resources. The trainee can also be introduced to such areas as recent social-security and tax rulings that can aid the retarded individual and his or her family, to the question of estate planning and legal protection, and to a multitude of other factors that can enrich the trainee's knowledge base of treatment and management adjuncts. Concomitantly, these experiences will increase his or her scope and understanding of the broad personal, social, and cultural issues that are present here. Such an awareness can be extended to practical exercises, such as working with local associations for retarded citizens, and to community leadership roles in expanding the available continuum.

14.4.4. Flexible View of Psychotherapy Needs

The necessity for high intellectual endowment has been overemphasized as a prerequisite for psychotherapy.

For example, psychotherapeutic efforts with emotionally disturbed–mentally retarded children can focus heavily on play therapy, with an emphasis on nonverbal techniques. Accordingly, both the attitudinal and the methodological treatment issues in the psychotherapy of the retarded must be understood by the trainee. Appreciation of the retarded child's problems in interpersonal adjustments, which are so often associated with his or her intellectual deficits, can lead to more empathic and realistic psychotherapeutic relationships with the child and a greater use of his or her personality assets. With guided experience, the trainee can also more fully appreciate the difference between psychotherapeutic approaches based on uncovering techniques (with the possible aftermath of heightened management difficulties) and therapeutic-educational approaches that place a premium on behavioral control and acquisition by training of socially acceptable modes of behavior.

14.4.5. Psychopharmacological Challenges

A wide spectrum of pharmacological agents may be necessary in an effort to increase, decrease, or alter the level of arousal and of motor overactivity, convulsive threshold, and general emotional status. For example, the recognition of the hyperkinetic behavioral syndrome so commonly seen after postnatal infections can induce the trainee to become more familiar with a wide range of drugs that may very well control the behavior of affected children. Experience with the pharmacological adjuncts to treatment will also make the trainee aware of our pressing need for more selective agents for the management of psychomotor overactivity without jeopardizing the child's profitable participation in educational programs. The specific beneficial effects of haloperiodol in dampening ticlike movements, as well as the rapid diminution of autistic and bizarre features in psychotic phenylketonuric individuals placed on the Lofenolac diet, serves to remind the mental health trainee rather forcibly of some of the organic determinants of human behavioral derangement and their treatment by pharmacological agents. Lastly, the trainee can be introduced to the exciting pharmacological research into the purported memory and/or learning enhancers (e.g., choline) that may hold great promise of "cure" for the primary symptom of mental retardation.

14.4.6. Preventive Psychiatric Dimensions

Preventive mental-health aspects of mental retardation[22] can also be rewarding educational experiences for the trainee, because of his or her possible future professional roles in both prevention and intervention. The concept of the at-risk child, which is so central to recent mental-health research studies, has its corollary in the at-risk physical and emotional status of the pregnant mother and the quality of the resultant early mother–child interaction. Supportive psychotherapeutic aids in the clinical management of the mother who is having periodic bleeding during pregnancy, or mixed feelings toward being pregnant, or fears of the possibly retarded child as a carry-over from past pregnancies, can be crucial in ensuring that the mother's engagement and investment in her child will be a positive one. Emotional support of mothers with an atypical or retarded newborn child can also maximize the initial and ongoing mother–child interaction. These preventive psychiatric concepts are important therapeutic attempts to prevent maternal perplexities and/or relationship disengagements that can produce such disastrous emotional, developmental, and intellectual residues in children. Such considerations allow trainees to enlarge their view of current research projects in child psychiatry as to early mother–child relationships and their influence on future developmental and personality growth.

14.4.7. Future Service Delivery

Experience in meeting the broad treatment and habilitative needs of the retarded citizen can serve as a model of providing similarly comprehensive services to *any* citizen with complex problems. These experiences can help to prevent the all-too-common "checkerboard" treatment approaches to children or adults who need complex services. The traditional mental-health treatment approach can thus be extended so as to capitalize on the treatment and rehabilitative resources of the retarded individual, his or her family, and the community. Recent trends in the management of mentally retarded children may contribute to the further development of comprehensive treatment and habilitative programming for emotionally disturbed children who may or may not be mentally retarded. Although service patterns in mental retardation and mental health tend to go hand-in-hand, currently there appears to be a relatively greater revolution in the field of mental retardation than in the mental health field. Manifestations of this revolution are the present proliferation of research and the rapid move toward new community-service patterns for the mentally retarded. The mental health worker can profit from both of these trends. An example is the recently stressed emphasis on behavioral analysis as a basic tool for training the mentally retarded, in contrast to the traditional psychodynamically oriented teaching approach with the mentally ill. Conversely, current research in many aspects of the use of behavior modification in mental retardation is directly applicable to psychiatric service patterns, especially for children, and even more specifically for children whose intellectual development is being distorted by emotional conflicts.

Comparative international perspectives can be reviewed for the trainee by noting that current treatment–management approaches to mental retardation in our country may well benefit from the adoption of some European service patterns. In our country, a diagnosis of mental retardation often tends to exclude the child from care and educational services. By contrast, current European approaches to the same diagnostic grouping serve as an impetus to stimulate treatment avenues that strongly focus on educational placement and active case work with the family. Education is stressed as an integral part of the treatment approaches to these children—rather than the far too frequently separated part (despite PL 94-142!) it plays in the United States.[23] These considerations can open the trainee's vista to future changes in the field of mental health, can stimulate a literally global view of treatment approaches, and can develop an appreciation of the dynamic continuity of ongoing international professional efforts to help the mentally retarded—past and present.

14.4.8. Trainee Exposure to Current and Futuristic Research

Because an ultimate goal is the primary prevention of the disorders that produce the sympton of mental retardation, the trainee should be given an overview of current research in this area. Prevention could also be fostered as a result of a better understanding of basic neurological and perceptual processes. Relatively little is known about the working of the brain and its 10 billion nuerons and billions of synaptic junctions. Likewise, research is desperately needed on attention, perception, and memory. An important current research focus relates to the influences of abnormal genes. For example, current research in genetics is directed at altering a missing or low level of essential body substances and a supplementing of enzymes (e.g., via replacement, induction, and coenzyme functions). Current research into the mechanisms by which social, environmental, infectious, immunological, nutritional, and traumatic and psychogenic factors impair intellectual performance is a fascinating area of training challenges. Special emphasis should be directed at unraveling the variable responsible for the well-known overrepresentation of mildly retarded persons in the most disadvantaged segments of our society. One can explain to the trainee that to develop massive intervention programs that remedy all of the known environmental deficits for millions of impoverished citizens may be beyond the scope of what can be done in the near future. A more feasible goal involves the determination of which factors are most critical, when and how long-term intervention strategies should be applied, and what aspects of an at-risk child's specific daily living experiences must be modified to prevent intellectual and behavioral deficit.

Lastly, the trainee should be exposed to the futurist-oriented research that holds great promise in finding improved approaches to the amelioration of mental retardation. Special attention should be directed to work concerning the refinement of behavior modification techniques, the application of telemetry, sensory and motor prostheses, direct stimulation of the brain, the use of space technology, and the design of total prosthetic environments. Similarly, in the field of education, the trainee can be exposed to the research in progress concerning such diverse areas as engineered classrooms, self-contained audiovisual training devices, computer-assisted programmed instruction, career-recycling approaches to adult education, and "analogue education" that capitalizes on right-cerebral-hemisphere functions. Beyond mental retardation, the trainee tends to quickly grasp that current biomedical research issues and techniques strike at key components of the personality, such as the possible enhancement of memory and learning capabilities.[24] The interrelationships of these research thrusts with the maximizing of personality function are quickly understood, as are the clear implications for significant future help for elderly citizens with Alzheimer's disease.

14.5. General Training Ingredients

Beyond the reviewed basic and advanced training components that can greatly aid in the current and future training of mental health personnel in helping mentally retarded citizens with allied mental illness are a number of training ingredients that can be interwoven into their ongoing professional training experiences:

- Senior staff members should be used to train personnel from an allied field. The message transmitted to the trainee—especially as to professional modeling—is clear: the boss believes in this work and practices it daily. For example, it is not sufficient to present lectures concerning the specific indications associated with psychopharmacological agents for mentally ill–mentally retarded individuals. More effective are clinical rounds with a practicing, teaching clinical psychiatrist who has a major interest in psychopharmacology, and then seminars to expand on what has been seen and done.

- Audiovisual materials—especially videotaped segments of diagnostic, treatment, and management challenges—should be heavily used. One videotape of a concrete "show-and-tell" nature is more effective than a number of lecture presentations on "what happened," especially when the relative merits of differing treatment approaches are being discussed.

- The trainee should be exposed as much as possible to a large sample of nondisturbed mentally retarded citizens and their parents. For example, periodic invited dinners at a group home for the retarded or regular attendance at meetings of associations for retarded citizens underscore the real world—rather than the selectivity of the clinic- or hospital-based populations.

- Excellent films are available in the field of mental retardation. For example, the recent film *Harry*[25] is a superb illustration of the effective use of behavioral analysis techniques in a mentally retarded citizen who has severe behavioral problems. Similarly, the film *Cry Sorrow, Cry Hope*, by the Pennsylvania Association for Retarded Citizens,[26] is, in our opinion, the best one-hour training–learning package available concerning the personal and family crises that the parents of the retarded experience. These and other films should never be seen alone by the trainees. Rather, they should be presented to very small groups and then immediately become the focus for extended interpretation, discussion, and synopsis of the large informational blocks of knowledge that they so excellently transmit.

- Special presentations, by local or visiting experts in the field of mental retardation, can greatly help mental health trainees to expand their views beyond the primary training setting. For example, our training program had a presentation by a Dybwad Award winner concerning innovative parent-to-parent (of the retarded) training programs in Europe. Viewing the parent as a trainer—and not as a "patient" or a "consumer of services"—was an unsettling experience for some of our mental-health trainees, who were molded a bit too heavily in the "medical model." Having the pilot parents actually present to discuss their own work (and results) was a tremendous desensitizing experience for these mental-health trainees, and the distribution of a recent professional journal reprint on the topic[27] provided further memory-trace enhancement for them.

- Structured experiences in direct and indirect consultation* and education programs in schools, local group homes, vocational training centers, and so on permit the trainee to directly view these community psychiatry consultative models of service (and public information) in mental retardation.

- Trainees should directly observe and participate in meetings of professionals and parents concerning expressed and specific parental disapproval of their child's current program. Such experiences show the trainee the multiple hazards and opportunities of advocacy "out in the real world."

Lastly, the trainee should continually be challenged with the best of the current professional literature via a regularly scheduled journal club. This activity will provide trainees with an excellent vehicle for continuing to deepen their professional expertise in this exciting field.

14.6. Summary

The topical area of training current and future mental-health workers so that they can be more attuned to the mental health needs of the mentally retarded has been reviewed. Specific recommendations have been provided as to basic and advanced knowledge bases and "in-the-field" sets of clinically oriented training experiences that will provide multilevel experiences for the trainee. The unique aspects of mental retardation, when amalgamated with both the traditional and the modern intrapersonal-interpersonal training curriculum of mental health workers, show great promise for spurring their professional competency to become excellent helpers for retarded citizens who have allied signs and symptoms of mental illness.

References

1. President's Commission on Mental Health: *Task Force IV Report*, vol 3. Washington, D.C., Government Printing Office, 1978.
2. Kanner L: *History of the Care and Study of the Mentally Retarded*. Springfield, IL, C Thomas, 1959.
3. Kugel RG, Wolfensberger W (eds): *Changing Patterns in Residential Services for the Mentally Retarded*. Washington, D.C., Government Printing Office, 1969.

---

* An excellent recent reference on this topic is *Psychiatric Consultation in Mental Retardation*, by the Group for the Advancement of Psychiatry (New York, Author, 1979).

4. Menolascino FJ: *Challenges in Mental Retardation: Progressive Ideologies and Services.* New York, Human Sciences Press, 1977.
5. Strider F, Menolascino FJ: Resources for the mentally retarded: A bibliographic essay, in Menolascino F, McCann BB (eds): *Bridging the Gap: Mental Health Needs of the Mentally Retarded Person.* New York, University Park Press, 1983.
6. Robinson HB, Robinson NM: *The Mentally Retarded Child: A Psychological Approach,* ed 2. New York, McGraw-Hill, 1980.
7. Balthazar EE, Stevens HA: *The Emotionally Disturbed Mentally Retarded: A Historical and Contemporary Perspective.* Englewood Cliffs, NJ, Prentice-Hall, 1975.
8. Menolascino FJ, Egger ML: *Medical Dimensions of Mental Retardation.* Lincoln, Nebraska, University Press, 1978.
9. Grossman HJ: *Manual of Terminology and Classification on Mental Retardation.* Washington, D.C., American Association on Mental Deficiency, 1983.
10. American Psychiatric Association: *Diagnostic and Statistical Manual of Mental Disorders,* ed 3. Washington, D.C., Author, 1980.
11. Tizard J: Mental retardation and child psychiatry, in Menolascino F (ed): *Psychiatric Approaches to Mental Retardation.* New York, Basic Books, 1970.
12. President's Committee on Mental Retardation: *Mental Retardation: Century of Decision.* Washington, D.C., Government Printing Office, 1976.
13. Eisenberg L: Caster, class and intelligence, in Murray R. Rossner P (eds): *The Genetic, Metabolic, and Developmental Aspects of Mental Retardation.* Springfield, IL, CC Thomas, 1972.
14. Lamb HR (ed): *Alternatives to Acute Hospitalization—New Directions for Mental Health Services.* San Francisco, Jossey-Bass, 1979.
15. Nirje B: The normalization principle and its human management implications, in Kugel R, Wolfensberger W (eds): *Changing Patterns in Residential Services for the Mentally Retarded.* Washington, D.C., Government Printing Office, 1969.
16. Wolfensberger W: *The Principle of Normalization in Human Services.* Toronto, National Institute for Mental Retardation, 1972.
17. Menolascino FJ, Donaldson JY: Therapeutic and preventive interventions in mental retardation, in Sholevar GP, Benson RM, Blinder BJ (eds): *Treatment of Emotional Disorders in Children and Adolescents.* Holliswood, NY, Spectrum Publications, 1980.
18. Menolascino FJ, Bernstein NR: Psychiatric assessment of the mentally retarded child, in Bernstein NR (ed): *Diminished People.* Boston, Little, Brown, 1970.
19. Szymanski L: Psychiatric diagnostic evaluation of mentally retarded individuals. *J Acad Child Psychiatr* 16;67–87, 1978.
20. Zigler E, Abelson A, Seitz V: Motivational factors in the performance of economically disadvantaged children on the Peabody Picture Vocabulary Test. *Child Dev* 44;294–303, 1973.
21. Webster TG: Unique aspects of emotional development in mentally retarded children, in Menolascino FJ (ed): *Psychiatric Approaches to Mental Retardation.* New York, Basic Books, 1970.
22. Menolascino FJ, Strider FD: Advances in the prevention and treatment of mental retardation, in Arieti S (ed): *American Handbook of Psychiatry,* ed 7. New York, Basic Books, 1981.
23. Menolascino FJ: Handicapped children and youth: Current-future international perspectives and challenges. *Except Child* 46(3);168–176, 1979.
24. National Association for Retarded Citizens Research and Demonstration Institute: *Bridges: A Rationales for Residential Services,* vol 1. Arlington, TX, National Association for Retarded Citizens, 1980.
25. Fox RM: *Harry* (film). Champaign, IL, Research Press, 1980.
26. Pennsylvania Association for Retarded Citizens: *Cry Sorrow, Cry Hope* (film). Philadelphia, 1977.
27. Menolascino FJ, Coleman R: The pilot parent program: Helping developmentally disabled children through their parents. *Child Psychiatr Hum Dev* 11(1), Fall 1980.
28. Hunt N: *The World of Nigel Hunt.* New York, Taplinger, 1967.

29. Wolfensberger W, Menolascino FJ: A theoretical framework for the management of parents of the mentally retarded. In Menolascino FJ (ed): *Psychiatric Approaches to Mental Retardation*. New York, Basic Books, 1970.
30. Roos P: The handling and mishandling of parents of mentally retarded persons. In Menolascino FJ, McCann BM (eds.): *Mental Health and Mental Retardation: Bridging the Gap*. Baltimore, University Park Press, 1983.

15

Teaching Behavior Modification Skills to Paraprofessionals

Luke S. Watson, Jr.

The success of behavior modification programs depends, to a great extent, on the type of in-service training staff receive.[1-5] Programs designed to teach mentally retarded persons independent living skills and to manage their disruptive behavior often fail because staff have not received the necessary training.[6] Paraprofessional staff, in particular, need the appropriate training because they constitute the major work force in residential facilities, including group homes, special-educational, and/or day-care programs.

Three different staff training programs are described and evaluated in this chapter.[7-9] Two were designed to train paraprofessional staff to teach independent-living skills to mentally retarded clients, and the purpose of the third is to teach staff to manage disruptive behavior without violating a client's human and legal rights,[10,11] while complying with principles of normalization.[12]

15.1. Teaching Independent-Living Skills

15.1.1. Backward Chaining

The first staff training program to be described teaches paraprofessional staff how to teach clients independent-living skills by means of the backward chaining approach.[13] In backward chaining, clients are taught the last step in a training sequence first, and the first step is taught last. For example, if a client is being taught to take off his pants (assuming this hypothetical child is male), the steps in the sequence would be taught in the following order: (1) removes pants from one foot; (2) removes pants from both feet; (3) pushes pants down from calves; (4) pushes pants down from thighs; (5) pushes pants down from groin; and (6) pushes pants down from waist.

The client is taught Step 1 first, removing his pants from one foot. Once he completes Step 1, he gets to practice Step 2, followed by Step 1. He takes his pants off one ankle and foot and then off the other ankle and foot. After the client passes Step 2, he begins to train on Step 3. He pushes the pants down

---

Luke S. Watson, Jr. • Therapeutic Homes, Inc., 6214 Presidential Court, S.W., Suite C, Fort Myers, Florida 33907.

from his calves, takes them off one ankle and foot, and removes them from the other ankle and foot. And so on.

Three types of prompts are used with this technique: verbal, gestural, and physical. The trainer begins with a verbal prompt: "Billy, take off your pants." If the client does not respond to a verbal prompt or responds incorrectly, the trainer goes to a verbal prompt paired with a gestural prompt, for example, "Billy, take off your pants," paired with a gestural prompt. If the client fails to respond to the gestural prompt or responds incorrectly, the trainer goes to a verbal prompt paired with a physical prompt. The client is given three types of reinforcement as he completes the steps in the program: verbal, social, and tokens or food-type reinforcement. Verbal and social reinforcement may be given as the client goes through a series of steps. Tokens or primary reinforcements are usually given at the end of a trial.

This method appears to work especially well with the severely and the profoundly mentally retarded,[14] and it was one of the first practical living-skill training techniques developed for the mentally retarded.[15,16]

Students who enroll in this program are taught the principles of reinforcement and stimulus control, shaping procedures, the management of disruptive behavior, and data collection. The program consists of an academic phase and a practicum phase. Academic training requires approximately 20 hours to complete, and the practicum training requires 4–6 hours. Classes typically run for about 2 hours each, so it takes about three weeks to complete the staff training program. The materials used in teaching the course are three manuals: an instructor's manual,[7] a student's manual,[13] and a manual of client training programs.[17] In addition, approximately 350 35-mm slides are used. The instructor's manual provides a guide to teaching both phases of the course. The student's manual is a programmed text modeled after the procedure developed by Keller.[18] It uses very little jargon and can be read by anyone who can read newspapers. Topics are presented in layman's language. For example, *reinforcement* is defined as something a client likes and is willing to work to get. The manual of programs contains a series of self-help skills and language and recreational programs. They are set up in a task analysis format and contain detailed instructions for teaching each step in each program. The slides are designed to be used as audiovisual aids during the lecture. They illustrate and supplement the principles and procedures presented in the lecture.

When the trainees come to class on the first day, they are given a student's manual and are told how the class will function. They are told that a reading-assignment–lecture–discussion format is used and that tests are given to evaluate how well the students understand the reading assignment and the lecture. They also are told that they will have the opportunity to discuss the contents of the tests each day when they first come to class. The trainees are assigned the first chapter in the student's manual to read, and the class is dismissed.

When they come to class the second day, they begin with a preexamination discussion. All true–false, fill-in, and essay examination items that will be given that day are reviewed. Students take turns answering the test items and are given the opportunity to ask questions about them or to discuss them to their satisfaction. The preexamination discussion is intended to serve as a review to provide the trainees with an additional opportunity to go over the major points or principles prior to the examination or lecture.

Then trainees are given a true–false and a fill-in examination. They complete the true–false exam, hand it into the instructor, and are given the fill-in exam. The true–false examination is handed in before the fill-in exam is given out because answers to the fill-in exam can be obtained from the true–false examination. The criterion for passing each exam is 90% correct. If anyone fails to pass a test, that student is given the opportunity to briefly review the missed test items and is retested—but only on the missed items.

When all students have completed the true–false and fill-in examinations, they receive the lecture. As the instructor gives the lecture, he or she uses the 35-mm slides to illustrate the points made or the procedures used. The lecture is designed to supplement and illustrate the material presented in the reading assignment.

When the lecture is completed, the students are given an essay examination. The exam is graded as soon as it is handed in. The criterion for passing this exam also is 90%. Anyone who fails to meet the criterion must retake the missed test items, after he or she first reviews them, either by looking them up in the student's manual or by asking another student. The average number of test retakes per student for the 10 lectures is two.

Notice the progression in requirements for information in the test sequence. At first, the student has to identify only whether a statement is correct or incorrect (true–false). Then, the student must supply certain key words or terms (fill-in). Finally, the student is required to write the entire sentence (essay). The purpose of this test sequence is to *shape* the student's *verbal behavior*.

The last lecture presented during the academic phase of training is on data collection. Once the student has completed the lecture on data collection, he or she is required to keep client training-records daily.

Before beginning the practicum phase of training, the students are given the manual of programs.[17] They then see a movie or a role-playing demonstration that shows how to determine reinforcement preferences, to shape eye contact, to obtain compliance, to do baselines, and to teach self-help skills. After the movie or demonstration is completed, the trainees role-play these techniques in pairs and are rated by the instructor on the Training Proficiency Scale (TPS),[19] a 45-item, 5-point rating scale. They must make a 95% score on the TPS on each of three role-playing evaluations: prerequisite skill training (reinforcement preferences, eye contact, and compliance), baselines, and self-help skill training. The average number of attempts required for students to meet criterion on each of these three role-playing examinations is two.

When students pass their three role-playing examinations, they are assigned to clients and begin teaching them one self-help skill each. At this point, they start a six-month internship. They are supervised daily and must make a 95% score on the TPS every 30 days to complete the internship satisfactorily.

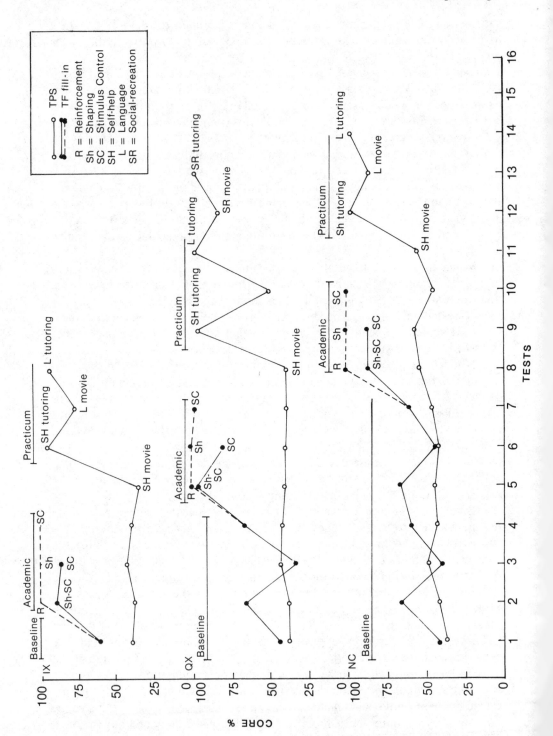

After they train for six to eight weeks, the trainees are usually assigned additional self-help skills to teach to clients.

15.1.2. Evaluation of Backward Chaining

15.1.2.1. Field Test I

The first field test was carried out in Franklin County, Ohio, with a parent training program.[20] The purpose of the field test was to assess the relative effectiveness of the academic and practicum phases of the staff training program with parents. The influence of academic training on clinical behavior-modification skills was compared with the practicum training. With regard to practicum training, the influence of seeing a movie, which was to be modeled by the instructor after it was shown, was compared with tutored-TPS feedback.

Three parents served as subjects. One was the mother of a 3-year-old, mildly retarded, mute girl. The second was the mother of a 6-year-old, profoundly retarded, hydrocephalic, semiambulatory, mute girl. The third was a foster parent of a 6-year-old psychotic male, who also was mentally retarded. The two younger mothers (both in their 20s) were high-school graduates, and the foster parent (in her late 50s) had completed two years of college.

Three principles taught in the academic phase of training were assessed: reinforcement, shaping, and stimulus control. To accomplish this objective, only three lectures were given: one on reinforcement, one on shaping, and one on stimulus control. Three phases of practicum training also were evaluated: self-help skill training, language training, and social-recreational skill training. By evaluating three phases of each type of program, it was possible to obtain some measure of generalization effects. The teaching procedure and materials used were the same ones described earlier.

True–false and fill-in test scores were used to assess written knowledge of principles, and Training Proficiency Scale (TPS) scores were used to evaluate clinical behavior-modification skills. True–false and fill-in test items were sampled from the student's text, *Child Behavior and Modification.*[13]

A multiple-baseline type of design[21] was used to evaluate the program. Prior to beginning academic training, pretraining baselines were obtained on all three parents (see Figure 1). Each time a probe was given, both true–false/fill-in exams and the TPS checklist were administered.

The results of the study are summarized in Figure 1. As the figure indicates, academic training influenced both the particular topic taught (see broken lines in academic phase, i.e., TF/Fill-in) and the academic topics that were not being

Figure 1. Relative performance of three parents in the academic and practicum phases of the parent training program. The solid lines in TF/fill-in indicate tests on academic phases that were not taught at that time, and the broken lines indicate tests on academic phases that were taught during that session. All parents were required to make a 90% correct criterion before moving from one phase of the academic program to the next, and a 95% criterion was required for moving from one phase of the practicum to the next.

taught that day (see solid lines in academic phase, i.e., TF/Fill-in). There appeared to be no effect of academic training on practicum performance (see TPS score plot in academic phase). Practicum performance evidently was effected primarily by practicum training, and training on one topic (e.g., self-help skills) appeared to generalize to other topics (e.g., language skills). Finally, seeing a movie of someone else training did not appear to be as effective as tutored TPS feedback for developing criterion-level practicum performance. An average of 21 hours was required to complete the academic phase of training, and a mean of 3 hours was required to carry out practicum training. An average of two true–false, fill-in, and essay exams was failed during academic training, and an average of two role-playing sessions was required to meet criterion in practicum training.

The parents who completed this program were able to teach self-help and language skills to their children. In addition, the parents maintained these skills over a period of time. Parents who were assessed with the TPS one to three years after they had completed the program made an average score of 90%.

15.1.2.2. Field Test II

The next field test involved a second parent training program.[22] This program was located at the Special Education District of Lake County in Illinois. Six parents were involved in the study. The mothers ranged in age from 24 to 43 and ranged in educational levels from high-school graduates to college graduates. All parents went through the staff training program in the manner described earlier.

The results of the field test were substantially the same as for the first field test. Academic training primarily affected academic performance, and practicum training was the factor that influenced clinical training skills. As in the first field test, an average of 21 hours was required to complete the academic phase of training, and a mean of 3 hours was required to carry out the practicum training. An average of two examinations per student was failed during academic training, and an average of two role-playing sessions was required to complete the practicum training. The parents who went through this program were able to teach dressing and toileting skills to their children.[6]

15.1.2.3. Field Test III

A field test of the same staff training program was carried out with paraprofessional staff in a large residential facility in Alabama.[23] As in the two previous field tests, both academic and practicum training were evaluated. Twenty-four mental health workers participated in this study. They had a mean age of 34.2 years, with a range from 24 to 50. All staff worked on a unit that housed multihandicapped mentally retarded residents.

A multiple-baseline type of design[21] was used to evaluate the treatment efects. The subjects were divided into two groups. As Figure 2 indicates, both groups received a true–false and a fill-in test, as well as a TPS evaluation prior

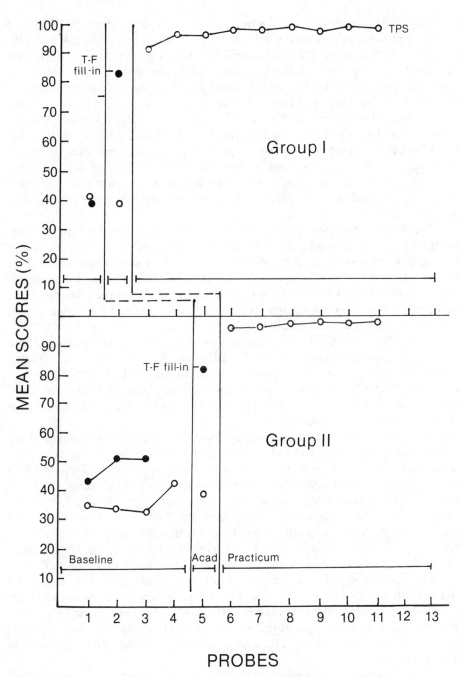

Figure 2. Relative performance of two groups of paraprofessional staff on academic and practicum phases of a staff training program. True–false and fill-in tests were used to assess academic training, and the Training Proficiency Scale (TPS) was used to evaluate practicum training.

to any training (pretest). Then, the first group received academic training, and both groups were tested with the true–false/fill-in examinations and the TPS checklist. At this point, the second group, which had served as a control for the first group, received academic training. When the second group completed academic training, they were assessed with the true–false/fill-in examinations and the TPS checklist, and Group I was evaluated with the TPS. The same methodological procedure was used for practicum training. Follow-up assessment involved administering the TPS checklist periodically for several weeks. Once Group II met criterion in practicum training, both groups were given the TPS every 2 weeks for a 4-week period and every 4 weeks for an additional 12-week period. The same teaching procedure described earlier was used here. The students received 10 lectures in academic training followed by practicum training.

The results of the study are summarized in Figure 2. As the figure shows, Group I received a mean pretest score of 0.397 on the true–false and fill-in tests and a posttest score of 0.830. The mean pretest scores for Group II on the true–false and fill-in tests were 0.426, 0.512, and 0.512 for the three pretest probes. After academic training, Group II scored 0.822 on the true–false and fill-in tests. This score is comparable to the score obtained by Group I after they completed academic training.

TPS scores were used to evaluate clinical skills in practicum training. There was no substantial increase in scores for either group until after they completed practicum training. The initial posttest score for Group I was 0.912, and for Group II, it was 0.989. The scores for both groups increased with time, and the TPS scores for Group I approximated 99% on subsequent probes, and the Group II scores approximated 98%.

The results of this field test suggest that academic training influenced academic performance but had little influence on practicum performance. True–false and fill-in test scores increased markedly after academic training, but TPS scores showed only a minor fluctuation prior to practicum training. Once the two groups had completed practicum training, there was a dramatic increase in the value of the TPS scores. In addition, the TPS scores remained above the 95% criterion for completing the practicum throughout the field test period, an interval of 22 weeks for Group I and 16 weeks for Group II. The maintenance of the TPS scores at a high level probably was due to the fact that staff were monitored and received feedback daily. Staff on another unit, who had received the same in-service training, were monitored and given feedback routinely for two years and were evaluated monthly with the TPS checklist. Their TPS scores were 95% or higher throughout the two-year period. These staff were required to score at least 95% on the TPS every month to maintain their certification as trainers.

A final factor that is of interest is the success that the paraprofessional staff had in teaching self-help skills to the residents once they had completed the staff training program. Approximately 35 staff assigned to this unit taught 560 self-help skills to multihandicapped clients over an 18-month period. Approximately 242 staff on three other units, who had completed the same in-

Table 1. Summary of Time Required and Cost of Teaching Specific Self-Help Skills to Severely Mentally Retarded Adult Residents

Skill	Hours to teach	Cost
Buttoning	37.67	$106.98
Shoelacing	41	$116.44
Showering	33	$ 93.72
Undressing—pants	6	$ 17.04

service training, taught a total of 4,993 self-help skills over a two-year period to severely and profoundly mentally retarded ambulatory clients.

15.1.2.4. Field Test IV

The fourth field test took place in a large residential facility for the mentally retarded in Idaho.[23] This field test also assessed the academic and practicum phases of the backward-chaining staff training program. The same methodological procedure and staff training method used in Field Test III were used here. Ten aides and supervisory paraprofessional staff were involved in this study. They had a mean age of 30.3 years (18–58), and their educational level was 12.2 years (10–16). The results were essentially the same as for the previous field tests. Academic training appeared to be the primary factor influencing academic performance, and practicum training seemed to be the basic factor influencing practicum performance.

After staff completed practicum training, they were assigned 18 adult, ambulatory, severely retarded males to teach self-help skills. The skills taught were undressing, buttoning, shoelacing, and showering. The average time required to teach each skill and the average cost are summarized in Table 1.

15.1.2.5. Field Test V

The final field test to be reported took place in a large residential facility in Ohio. Twelve aides and supervisory paraprofessional staff were involved in this field test. They had an average age of 37.1 years (22–49), and their average educational level was 11.2 years (8–17). Again, the methodological and teaching procedure was the same as it was in the previous two field tests.

The results were essentially the same as in the previous field tests. Academic training appeared to be the major factor influencing academic performance. Academic training apparently had little effect on practicum performance. Finally, practicum training appeared to be the primary factor influencing practicum performance.

15.1.2.6. Conclusions

The results of these five field tests were very consistent. Both parents and aide-level staff in residential facilities can complete the backward-chaining staff training program successfully and can apply the independent-living-skill techniques to both ambulatory and multihandicapped mentally retarded persons. Staff in all five field tests failed an average of two tests during academic training and required a mean of two role-playing attempts to complete practicum training. Ninety-eight percent of the staff who went through this in-service training program completed it successfully. Staff who were monitored by supervisors and were certified as trainers on a monthly basis maintained their training skills over an extended period of time.

15.1.3. Forward Sequencing

When clients are taught independent-living skills using the forward sequencing approach, skills are taught in the natural order in which they are usually performed. If a client is being taught to apply deodorant (assuming again that he is a male), the steps would be taught in the following order: (1) pick up the deodorant; (2) shake the deodorant container; (3) remove the cap; (4) hold the bottle up; (5) rub the deodorant onto the underarm; (6) put the deodorant in the other hand; (7) hold the bottle up; (8) put the deodorant onto the underarm; and (9) put the cap back on the deodorant.

Four different kinds of prompts are used with this training approach: verbal prompts, modeling, gestural prompts, and physical prompts. Training begins with the instructor placing the deodorant in front of the client on a table. If the client fails to pick up the deodorant voluntarily, the trainer uses a verbal prompt, "Billy, use the deodorant." If the client does not respond or responds incorrectly, the trainer uses a verbal prompt and models the first step for the client. If the client still fails to respond or responds incorrectly, the trainer pairs a gesture with a verbal prompt. If he still fails to respond or responds incorrectly, the trainer pairs a verbal prompt with a physical prompt. This prompting sequence is followed for all steps in the deodorant program. The same reinforcement procedure used for backward chaining is employed in this training technique. The client receives verbal reinforcement, pats or hugs, tokens or points, or some type of edible reinforcement.

The forward sequencing approach is ideally suited for clients who have enough receptive language skills to follow verbal instructions, such as mildly and moderately mentally retarded clients and some severely mentally retarded clients. These kinds of clients can be taught independent-living skills primarily with verbal prompts and modeling and are not so dependent on gestural and physical prompts.[14]

Like the backward-chaining staff training program, this in-service training program is divided into an academic phase and a practicum phase. The academic phase requires approximately 22 hours to teach, and the practicum phase lasts for about 6 hours. Classes usually run for 2 hours each, and about three weeks are required to complete the course. The materials used in this program are a student manual[24] and an instructor's manual[8] plus six 8" by 10" transparencies.

The academic phase of training begins with the instructor giving the students their textbooks and describing for them the format that will be used to teach the course. They are told that at the end of class each day, they will be given a reading assignment in their student manual. As they read through their assignment, they should do the true–false, fill-in, and essay test items as they come to them. When they come to class each day, there will be a preexamination discussion. They will be given the opportunity to review all test items that were in their reading assignment, which are also the same items that will be on their test. Then, they will be given a true–false and fill-in exam, and everyone must make a 90% score to pass the exam. After the examination is completed, there will be a lecture, and all material presented in the reading assignment will be covered during the lecture. Then, there will be a discussion of the major principles and procedures presented in the lecture, followed by an essay examination.

The instructor points out that, at the beginning of the practicum phase, a role-playing demonstration will be presented to show how the training technique is used. He or she adds that, following the demonstration, all students will role-play the technique in pairs and will be certified with the TPS checklist. They must make a 95% score to be certified and to complete the first practicum.

The class is told that after the practicum is completed, they will begin a six-month internship. They will be assigned two clients each and will begin by teaching each client one practical living skill. After four to six weeks, they will be assigned additional skills to teach these same clients. After the internship, the students will return to class and receive a lecture that reviews the 11 most common problems that prevent clients from learning independent-living skills and the solutions to these problems. The lecture will be followed by another practicum, during which the trainees will have the opportunity to role-play each of the procedures that are used to overcome the various training problems. All students will be certified in each of the procedures by means of a checklist.

The format used in each lecture is similar to that used for the backward-chaining in-service training program, with the exception that there are no slides to illustrate the procedures. Instead, the instructor utilizes role-playing demonstrations. The 8″ by 10″ transparencies are used to teach students data collection procedures. The instructor models the correct data-collection technique using the 8″ by 10″ transparencies; that is, he or she fills them out as he or she explains each step in data collection, and the students model the instructor using the same data sheets.

15.1.4. Evaluation of Forward Sequencing

This staff training program has been field-tested in two different geographical settings. An earlier version was field-tested at the Kankakee Developmental Center, Kankakee, Illinois, with approximately 20 clients. It was revised, and the present version of the program was field-tested at Partlow State School and Hospital, Tuscaloosa, Alabama, with approximately 115 paraprofessional and professional staff. Staff at Partlow who completed this pro-

Table 2. Summary of Self-Help and Social-Recreational Skills Taught to Moderately and Mildly
Retarded Clients

Clipping nails	Skittles bowling
Taking a coat off a hanger	Horseshoes
Putting a coat on a hanger	Chinese checkers
Clothes folding	Checkers
Vacuuming	Shining shoes
Putting on lipstick	Tablesetting
Applying base makeup	Ironing
Applying blush makeup	Telephoning for help
Applying eye makeup	Handwashing lingerie
Changing clothes regularly	Putting on pantyhose
Carrying on a conversation	Taking off pantyhose
Relating to facility staff	Self-identification
Riding a bicycle	Crossing sidewalks and intersections
Ball darts	Operating a clothes washer
Slapjack	Operating a clothes dryer
War	Matching clothes
Old maid	Ordering meals in restaurants
Go fishing	Taking care of personal possessions
Lotto	Wearing clothes appropriate to situation
Dominoes	Shopping
Darts	

gram were able to teach a variety of independent-living skills to severely, moderately, and mildly mentally retarded clients.[6] Approximately 855 self-help and
social skills were taught to these kinds of clients. A summary of the skills taught
can be found in Table 2.

15.1.5. Managing Disruptive Behavior

The third in-service training program is designed to teach both paraprofessional and professional staff to manage clients who exhibit aggressive, self-
destructive, and bizarre behavior, as well as destroying property. Students are
taught a three-alternative approach to managing disruptive behavior. Alternative I consists of scheduling programs and interesting activities to reduce
disruptiveness. For clients who do not respond to this alternative, Alternative
II is implemented (but Alternative I is continued). It consists of fines and loss
of privileges, required relaxation, interrupting the chain, and the backup trainer
approach. If clients fail to become manageable after Alternative II is introduced, Alternative III is attempted (and Alternative I is still continued). Alternative III includes required relaxation with holding, various forms of time-
out, overcorrection, and positive practice.

This program utilizes the same format as the forward-sequencing staff
training program. Classes consist of lectures followed by role-playing discussions. The course is almost exclusively of a practicum nature, rather than being

divided into academic and practicum phases. The course requires approximately 24 hours to complete. Classes run for approximately 2 hours each.

The materials used in this program are a student manual, an instructor's manual,[9] and various checklists. When the students arrive at class on the first day, the instructor gives them their textbooks and tells them how the class will function. Each day they will be given a reading assignment. When they come to class the following day, they will be presented with a lecture that reviews all of the principles and procedures found in the reading assignment. Then, there will be a discussion of the content of the lecture and the main points that are covered in a true–false and fill-in examination. Then, the students are given the exam, and it is graded immediately. The criterion for passing the exam is 90%.

After all students complete the examination satisfactorily, the practicum is presented. The items in each checklist that are used to certify students on each procedure taught in the practicum are reviewed, and the procedures themselves are demonstrated by the instructor. Following the demonstration, the students role-play each procedure in pairs and are certified by the instructor by means of the checklists. The students must make a 95% score to be certified on a checklist.

15.1.6. Evaluation of the Disruptive-Behavior-Management Program

This program has been field-tested at Partlow State School and Hospital with approximately 100 professional and paraprofessional staff. About 90% of the persons who enrolled in the program completed it successfully. Persons who failed the program were typically extremely overweight or had a health problem such as a coronary condition or hypertension.

15.2. Conclusion

These three staff training programs make it possible to teach a variety of independent-living skills to the mentally retarded and to manage their disruptive behavior. Most paraprofessional staff have no difficulty in completing these programs. The backward chaining and forward sequencing procedures seem to be suited for different populations of mentally retarded persons. Backward chaining evidently works well with the severely and the profoundly mentally retarded, and there are a fairly large number of training programs that can be adapted.[14] This technique is relatively easy to teach to paraprofessional staff.[14] The main disadvantage is that some clients become dependent on physical prompts. The forward sequencing approach appears to work well with severely, moderately, and mildly mentally retarded clients who have receptive language skills and who do not require extensive physical prompting.[14] There are many programs that can be taught by means of this technique. It appears to be the choice for training the moderately and the mildly retarded. This program is also readily learned by most paraprofessional staff. The staff training program for managing disruptive behavior contains a variety of procedures that will work effectively with mentally retarded persons ranging from the profoundly mentally retarded to the mildly mentally retarded. Because a three-alternative sequential approach to managing behavior problems is employed, it should not violate a retarded person's human and legal rights.

References

 1. Kazdin AE: Implementing token programs: The use of staff and patients for maximizing change, in Patterson RE (ed): *Maintaining Effective Token Economies*. Springfield, IL, C. C. Thomas, 1976.
 2. Thompson T, Grabowski J: *Behavior Modification of the Mentally Retarded*. New York, Oxford University Press, 1972.
 3. Watson LS: Behavior modification of residents and personnel in institutions for the mentally retarded, in Baumeister A, Butterfield E (eds): *Residential Facilities for the Mentally Retarded*. Chicago, IL, Aldine Press, 1970.
 4. Watson LS: Shaping and maintaining behavior modification skills in staff using contingent reinforcement techniques, in Patterson R (ed): *Maintaining Effective Token Economies*. Springfield, IL, C. C. Thomas, 1976.
 5. Watson LS, Gardner JM, Sanders C: Shaping and maintaining behavior modification skills in staff members in an MR institution. *Ment Retard* 3;39–42, 1971.
 6. Watson LS: *A Management System Approach to Teaching Independent Living Skills and Managing Disruptive Behavior*. Tuscaloosa, AL, BMT, 1978.
 7. Watson LS: *A Manual for Teaching Behavior Modification Skills to Staff: An Inservice Training Program for Parents, Teachers, Nurses, and Resident Direct Care Staff*. Libertyville, IL, BMT, 1974.
 8. Watson LS: *How to Teaching Independent Living Skills and Manage Disruptive Behavior: Instructor's Edition*. Tuscaloosa, AL, BMT, 1978.
 9. Watson, LS, Uzzell R: *A Positive Approach to Managing Disruptive Behavior: Instructor's Edition*. Tuscaloosa, AL, BMT, 1980.
10. Martin R: *Legal Challenges to Behavior Modification*. Champaign, IL, Research Press, 1975.
11. stolz, SB: *Ethical Issues in Behavior Modification*. Washington, Jossey-Bass, 1978.
12. Roos P: Reconciling behavior modification procedures with the normalization principle, in Wolfensberger W (ed): *Normalization*. Toronto, National Institute on Mental Retardation, 1972.
13. Watson LS: *Child Behavior Modification: A Manual for Teachers, Nurses, and Parents*. New York, Pergamon Press, 1973.
14. Watson LS, Uzzell R: Teaching self-help skills, grooming skills and utensil feeding skills to the mentally retarded, in Matson J, McCartney J (eds): *Handbook of Behavior Modification with the Mentally Retarded*. New York, Plenum Press, 1981.
15. Bensberg GJ (ed): *Teaching the Mentally Retarded: A Handbook for Ward Personnel*. Atlanta, Southern Regional Educational Board, 1965.
16. Bensberg GJ, Colwell CN, Cassell RH: Teaching the profoundly retarded self-help activities by behavior shaping techniques. *Am J Ment Defic* 68;674–679, 1965.
17. Watson LS: *How to Use Behavior Modification with Mentally Retarded and Autistic Children: Programs for Administrators, Teachers, Parents, and Nurses*. Columbus, OH, BMT, 1972.
18. Keller FS: Goodbye teacher. *J Appl Behav Anal* 1;79–90, 1968.
19. Watson LS: *Training Proficiency Scale: An Assessment Instrument for Evaluating Behavior Modification Training Proficiency of Staff*. Libertyville, IL, BMT, 1974.
20. Watson LS, Bassinger JF: Parent training technology: A potential service delivery system. *Ment Retard* 12;3–10, 1974.
21. Baer DM, Wolf MM, Risley TR: Some current dimensions of applied behavior analysis. *J Appl Behav Anal* 1;91–97, 1968.

22. Watson LS: An inservice training program for teaching behavior modification skills to parents of retarded children. Submitted to *Ment Retard*, unpublished.
23. Watson LS, Uzzell R: A program for teaching behavior modification skills to institutional staff. Applied Research in Mental Retardation *1*;41–53, 1980.
24. Watson LS: *How to Teach Independent Living Skills and Manage Disruptive Behavior: Instructor's Edition*. Tuscaloosa, AL, BMT, 1978.

16

New Challenges in Social Work Practice with the Mentally Retarded

Michael J. Monfils

During the past 15 years, dramatic developments have occurred within the fields of mental retardation and mental health. The number of residents in public institutions for the retarded in the United States has shrunk from a high of near 193,000 in 1967[1] to a current figure of around 139,000.[2] Mentally retarded citizens have moved into community-based residential and vocational settings and are participating in a wide variety of community services and programs. The impact of Public Law 94-142 (the Education for All Handicapped Children Act of 1975) has been felt across the country as increasing numbers of mentally retarded children are being served in the public schools. Many of these children, who previously had been educated in self-contained special classes or in institutions, have now been placed in regular classes for part or all of their school program. Because of recent court decisions and advocacy on the part of parent and professional groups such as the Association for Retarded Citizens, the legal and basic human rights of the retarded have been affirmed and promoted. A new diversity in service provision to the retarded has thus arisen, as the mental health needs of these citizens are addressed in an assortment of settings.

16.1. Social Work Response

Unfortunately, social workers have not assumed a position of leadership in developing and providing innovative services for mentally retarded individuals. This fact has been reflected in the social work literature. Kelman,[3] for example, observed that social workers in many cases had failed to meet the challenge of offering appropriate services and understanding to parents of retarded children. Likewise, Adams[4] pointed out that historically only a small number of social workers, primarily in institutional settings, have been involved in addressing the needs of the retarded. During the past 10 years, social workers have chosen to concentrate their efforts in areas such as individual psychotherapy or family therapy, rather than exploring treatment approaches with the retarded.

Michael J. Monfils • Department of Psychiatry, Nebraska Psychiatric Institute, University of Nebraska Medical Center, Omaha, Nebraska 68105.

This trend is significant because the value base of social work practice (which stresses the dignity and uniqueness of the person) is particularly applicable to the retarded. The recent philosophical foundation in service delivery to the retarded, which stresses a developing model of the person, is consistent with social work's focus on the acceptance and the individuality of each client. However, social work is only beginning to shift its emphasis from programs in institutions for the retarded to the development of support systems and advocacy in the community.

Social workers need to cultivate a renewed acceptance of retarded citizens as growing, changing persons, as well as a commitment to serve them in both institutional and community contexts. Strider and Menolascino[5] have pointed out four attitudes and skills that are critical to success in working with retarded individuals: (1) positive attitudes toward mental retardation; (2) a thorough knowledge of the medical syndromes that are associated with retardation; (3) the ability to describe diagnostic and prognostic information, taking into account the emotional reaction of parents; and (4) an understanding of the dynamics and the interaction of each family. These skills can serve as a foundation for social workers in addressing social work challenges with the retarded.

The purpose of this chapter is to describe and examine some of the new challenges that social workers face in addressing the mental health needs of retarded citizens, in both institutional and community settings. Several emerging roles in social work practice with the retarded are discussed, with particular emphasis on the unique contributions that social workers can make as they serve the retarded and their families.

16.2. Institutional Challenges

16.2.1. Social Groupwork

In many instances, social workers in institutions for the retarded have routinely performed custodial or maintenance functions, rather than assuming an active treatment responsibility for their clients. This custodial focus is evident in tasks such as report writing, occasional contacts with parents or agencies, and long hours spent in team meetings discussing clients. These activities contribute little to any lasting change or development on the part of the client. Within the past 10 years, however, new techniques in social groupwork have been developed and refined, making it possible for social workers in institutions to become therapeutic group leaders. These techniques can be used to teach clients basic and advanced social skills, thereby preparing them for entrance back into the community. The absence of appropriate interpersonal skills is often a barrier to successful placement of the retarded in community settings.

Zisfein and Rosen,[6] for example, have developed a structured group-counseling program that can be used with mild to severely retarded individuals to prepare them for social and vocational functioning in the community. The program relies heavily on the use of behavioral approaches and techniques, such as modeling, behavior rehearsal, and transfer training. Lee[7] found that a similar approach, social adjustment training, was effective with a group of moderately retarded residents in an institutional setting. Lee's approach likewise is designed to teach clients specific social-interactional skills that can be put to use in the community. Group approaches such as assertiveness training,[8] which have proved popular with other populations, can also be applied by social workers to retarded citizens in teaching them appropriate assertive responses and behavior. Most recently, a study by Matson and Senatore[9] indicated that a social-skills-training format, aimed at changing specific target behaviors of retarded clients, was more effective than a traditional psychotherapy approach. Once again, heavy emphasis in this approach is placed on active learning via role-play demonstrations and social feedback.

After reviewing approaches such as these, social workers in institutional settings should recognize that they have a wealth of material on which to draw in structuring groupwork strategies. One group model that would have broad application to a variety of institutional settings is the "theme-centered" method.[10] The social worker utilizing this approach would develop a specific theme for each group session, which would then serve as the basis for group discussion and interaction.

An assortment of themes can be put to use in groups with institutionalized residents. For example, clients can be taught decision-making skills or appropriate heterosexual behaviors. They can learn basic conversational skills and appropriate methods for expressing positive and negative feelings. Areas of self-help skills, such as personal dress and grooming, as well as awareness of social rules and responsibility, also need to be stressed. By learning how to assert themselves appropriately in the group setting, clients are less likely to be exploited by others; therefore, assertiveness training serves as another important theme. Other possible goals in group sessions may include learning to express appreciation to others, giving and receiving compliments, asking for help, expressing opinions, and improving personal posture and manners. These are all areas of interpersonal functioning that are more easily acquired by most people, yet have not been mastered by many retarded individuals.

The social worker as a group leader introduces the goal or theme for each session and attempts to reduce anxiety and to keep the group focused on the theme. Following discussion of the theme and verbal instruction regarding the concepts involved, the group leader models the appropriate response or behavior. Group members are encouraged to participate in role-play situations as a way of rehearsing the behavior or skill. Social reinforcement is provided by means of praise and verbal feedback from the group leader and the members. By introducing homework assignments and a review of the material from each prior group, training can be transferred into real-life situations.

This type of structured group can be beneficial to mild through profoundly retarded clients and allows the social worker to function as both therapist and teacher. An active, directive style of leadership is called for, in which interaction is encouraged, yet allowing at the same time for spontaneity.

16.2.2. Sexuality and the Retarded

The whole field of human sexuality and the mentally retarded is a second challenging area of concern for social workers in institutional settings. Mentally retarded persons in institutions have the same needs and desires with respect to their psychosexual development as other individuals do. These needs include a hunger for relationships, physical affection, and love. Social workers have many opportunities in institutions to develop programs and resources on sexuality, both for clients and for other staff members.

The sexual behavior or misbehavior of institutional residents is at times the subject of humor and derisive comments on the part of staff members. Behaviors such as public nudity and masturbation, inappropriate touching or gestures, and vulgar language on the part of clients are thus held up to ridicule, rather than being handled in a constructive and supportive learning environment. This attitude leads to frustration, anxiety, and continued uncertainty on the part of clients regarding their sexual identity and acceptable ways of expressing their needs.

What do social workers have to offer clients and staff in such a setting as a means of promoting a healthier, more positive outlook on sexuality? In working with individual residents, the initial medical-social approach should include an assessment of the client's physical sexual development and sexual knowledge or attitudes. Many retarded citizens are delayed in the rate of their physical development, such as in the development of secondary sex characteristics.[11] They are also, in many cases, lacking in basic knowledge concerning physiology, reproduction, contraception, and so on.[12] An assessment of the client's development and sophistication in these areas will assist in ascertaining the type of intervention that is required.

Social workers in institutions need to become more assertive in developing programs and education in sexuality for clients. These programs can be offered in both individual and small-group formats. A number of excellent resource or curriculum guides have been developed for this purpose,[13] as well as a variety of films and tapes. Basic sex education thus becomes the foundation for clients in developing their knowledge concerning sexual adjustment. Small-group sessions can then be used to further expand the individual's repertoire of heterosexual behaviors. Role-play exercises, rehearsing various heterosexual experiences and social situations, are a powerful tool in this regard. Clients are able to observe and learn from one another, as well as from the group leader, in a safe and nonthreatening environment.

Because of a history of poorly developed social skills, many retarded individuals are unable to form relationships with members of both sexes, a lack leading to personal isolation and loneliness. They have few friends or social-recreational outlets. As social workers strive to educate clients in the institution, their efforts should also develop in residents the necessary attitudes and abilities to enter into relationships with others. These relationships, characterized by mutual warmth and affection, will enhance the client's capacity for intimacy with others. Thus, the whole spectrum of attitudes and relationships, as well as factual information on sexuality, must be included in this approach.

Along with their efforts in working directly with residents, social workers also have the opportunity to provide education and in-service training in this area for staff members and paraprofessionals, either in one-to-one encounters with other individuals or in small-group training sessions. Because paraprofessional and direct-care staff are responsible for much of the actual day-to-day care of the residents, they frequently handle sexual problems as they occur. Therefore, they need to cultivate positive attitudes toward sexuality and the handicapped, as well as knowledge of specific management techniques that may be used when problems arise.

Helping professionals who work with the mentally retarded are beginning to affirm the right of the client to access to information on sexuality. By providing leadership and direction in this effort, social workers in institutions will be able to better prepare clients to eventually cope in a world filled with confusing and contradictory sexual values and practices. This is an area of responsibility in which social workers have much to contribute.

16.2.3. Boundary Work

Social work practice in institutions for the retarded can easily become a process of preserving and perpetuating the institutionalization of the residents, rather than an active mechanism of preparing them for community placement. Historically, social workers in other settings, such as public welfare or settlement houses, have developed case management and coordination services that have assisted clients in obtaining necessary community services. Horejsi[14] has referred to this type of work as "boundary work," which is "intervention at the interface of social systems."

There is great potential for increased intervention by institutional social workers at the boundaries of social service systems. One example of such intervention is in the promotion and coordination of discharge-planning efforts. The orderly process of preparing for discharge constitutes an essential element in the treatment plan for each individual. Discharge planning involves the careful anticipation of the psychosocial needs of the retarded citizen as he or she returns to the community. The assessment of client needs is an ongoing process in which a variety of needs may be identified, including a new residential placement, referrals to educational or vocational programs, or the development of behavior management programs. It is crucial to develop a plan that is tailored to the unique needs of each person and that takes into account the environment in which the individual will be placed.

Opportunities abound for social workers to be creative and imaginative in coordinating discharge-planning efforts. These efforts involve tasks such as information and referral, formal and informal "networking" with agencies and resources, and advocacy. All of these tasks are necessary in order to build and solidify linkages and cooperation between agencies, families, and professionals. In the author's experience, a predischarge conference has been found to be useful in preparing family members and agencies for the discharge of clients from institutions. Social workers can serve as coordinators for these meetings, at which the findings and recommendations of the treatment team are communicated to the family or the agencies involved. In discussion of plans for follow-up care, emphasis is placed on constructing a network of community services that will meet the individual's needs. Family members and agency representatives are given the opportunity to express their fears and concerns regarding the discharge plans. The conference is a prime opportunity for social workers to educate others concerning the client's needs and to enlist the cooperation and the support of others.

As social workers in institutions begin to assume a leadership role in client coordination and management, the issue of advocacy becomes an important concern. A social work advocate, as Pincus and Minahan[15] have noted, assists individuals in obtaining a needed resource or service from a resistant or unresponsive system. Mentally retarded persons, many of whom lack highly refined verbal skills, are especially in need of advocacy services. However, the question has been raised as to whether social workers are really in an appropriate position to act as effective advocates for the retarded.

Wolfensberger[16] and Adams[17] have both expressed reservations about the effectiveness of advocacy by professionals and agencies. Wolfensberger noted that competent private citizens may be in a better position than professionals to advocate for the retarded, as they are not bound by agency regulations or conflicts of interest. Adams stated that social workers in particular are placed in the uncomfortable position of weighing the rights of the individual against the rights of society, thereby making advocacy a troublesome task. Perhaps the social-work advocacy role should best be conceptualized as that of a catalyst and a leader who enlists the cooperation of citizen and legal advocates on behalf of the retarded client. Social workers can provide the inspiration and the direction that these advocates will require as they assess the needs of each person. Social workers thus develop a partnership and a relationship, characterized by trust and acceptance, with other advocates, rather than attempting to serve solely as the advocate for each resident.

16.3. Community Challenges

16.3.1. Family Supportive Services

Social work intervention with families of the retarded is undergoing a striking transformation as the psychosocial focus shifts from institutional care to a decentralized, community-based approach. Social work assistance to families now encompasses the entire family unit, so as to enhance the development and coping abilities of all family members. The responsibility for coordinating efforts with the family continues to rest primarily with the social work profession, but it is now shared more than ever with other disciplines.

The presence of a retarded child within a family requires adjustments on the part of the parents. Initially, the parents must modify their expectations of having a normal, healthy child and adjust to the painful reality of having a handicapped child in the family. Parental reactions to retardation, such as shock and anger, and adaptive versus maladaptive responses have been well documented in the literature.[18,19] By the time a child enters a program of formal education, the parents may already have sought out several professional evaluations and made sacrifices of personal time and energy to meet the special needs of the child.

One important function that social workers in community settings can perform is to evaluate the actual amount of stress that parents are experiencing in raising a retarded child.[20] The daily responsibility of caring for a retarded child in the home can at times be overwhelming. The challenge for social workers thus becomes one of developing and making available to families concrete services and resources, such as child or respite care, homemakers, parent training and support groups, recreational opportunities, or vocational placements. These are the much-needed, valuable types of programs that will make it possible for parents to keep their children in the home for as long as possible.

In talking with family members, the social worker may also assist them in reevaluating their attitudes and values concerning the retarded individual. Our society often places a negative value on mentally retarded persons,[21] as they are viewed by some persons as being deviant or different. In opposition to this negativism, social workers must stress the individual's potential for continued learning, growth, and development, thereby inviting families to value their children positively. This posture will help the parents to formulate a realistic, yet hopeful, assessment of the child's potential and needs.

With increasing numbers of retarded children now remaining with their families or in community settings for extended periods of time, the social work task becomes one of supporting the family throughout various stages and crises of the person's life. This task is in contrast with earlier times, when community social-work intervention often terminated at the time that the child was placed in an institution. The current challenge for social workers is to be available throughout the retarded citizen's life to offer a continuum of services to the family. These services may include instruction-management functions, support, and information, as well as family therapy in selected cases. The overall objective should be to prevent individual and familial dysfunction by anticipating stresses that may occur during key periods of individual development.[22] Examples of such stressful events would include the delayed attainment of early-childhood developmental milestones, entry into school, or the transition into semi-independent adult living arrangements.

Social workers in various settings (e.g., public welfare, community-based mental retardation agency, and medical social work) need to cultivate a sharper awareness of how they might help individuals and families to cope at these times of transition. The young-adult years are particularly difficult, as the retarded citizen struggles to make the passage from home and family to community living and the world of work. Goodman[23] has shown that issues such as unresolved feelings concerning separation and anxiety about long-term residential and vocational plans are key questions that social workers need to address. These problems can be effectively handled only through individualized planning and open communication and cooperation between parents and professionals. The social worker thus becomes the gatekeeper or mediator who channels individuals and families into appropriate service systems and programs.

Within the past 20 years, a drastic shift has occurred in the manner in which the parents of the retarded relate to social workers and other mental-health professionals. Parents are no longer content to settle for charity or second-class services for their children.[24] They are instead demanding humane and appropriate services and programs and have recent court decisions to support their demands. The new social-work posture in working with parents must be that of a partnership, a shared responsibility for planning and decision making. This partnership also is the foundation for effective advocacy on the part of parents and professionals alike.

16.3.2. Consultation

Consultation is a method of practice that has received increased emphasis and importance in social work in recent years. Rapoport[25] defined it as "a time-limited, purposeful, contractual relationship between a knowledgeable expert, the consultant, and a less knowledgeable professional worker, the consultee" (p.156–157). In the context of community-based social work with retarded clients, consultation is directed at enhancing the ability of other mental-health professionals to solve problems that relate to the behavior and adjustment of the client. Consultation should also aim to instill positive attitudes and values in professionals regarding work with the retarded. the social work consultant also functions at times as an educator, in terms of conveying and applying modern concepts concerning the habilitation of retarded citizens.

There are many avenues available to social workers who are interested in doing consultation related to the needs of the mentally retarded. Possible settings for consultation efforts include group homes, schools, nursing homes, hospitals, and community mental-health centers. If social workers are to serve as "expert" consultants in these settings, they will first have to become thoroughly acquainted with the needs of the mentally retarded. The field of retardation needs to receive increased emphasis and commitment in social work education, so that social workers will be better prepared to serve as consultants.

Caplan[26] has delineated four different types of consultation and has noted that client-centered case consultation is the most familiar type of consultation used by mental health professionals. The initial task for social work consultants who are performing client-centered consultation is to build a solid helping relationship with their consultees. This relationship then becomes the springboard for future training and development activities. The consultant functions as an educator who leads the consultees to view the retarded citizen's presenting problem "not as an isolated entity but in light of his total adjustment and abilities."[27] The social worker thus attempts to provide a positive view of the client's potential for growth and development.

As social workers begin to demonstrate increased expertise in client-centered consultation concerning retarded individuals, they may also be called on to provide program or administrative consultation to administrators or boards of directors. In these instances, the social workers will have opportunities to provide administrators with information and impressions regarding the needs of the agency or program from a systems perspective. This function may include offering valuable assistance in developing mental health programs or training and development activities for agency personnel.

The use of consultation with groups is another dynamic technique that social workers can refine for use with agencies and programs that work with the retarded. Group consultation is not new to social work, having been used by Kevin[28] with classroom teachers in the early 1960s. Yet, social-work group consultation specifically directed toward the needs of the retarded is only in its infancy, having developed recently as a result of legislation such as PL 94–142. Group consultation can be used to educate other individuals, such as teachers or paraprofessionals, regarding the mental health needs of the retarded. The group format is also appropriate for discussions of problem-solving techniques and behavior management strategies, for example, in group homes or residential treatment centers. The social worker becomes essentially a resource person for other professionals in these settings and is able to model appropriate attitudes and commitment toward retarded citizens.

Social workers in community mental-health centers frequently function as consultants to various community agencies and programs. However, mentally retarded citizens are often overlooked and underserved in these efforts. A recent survey in one state[29] revealed that only a small number of retarded citizens were receiving services or treatment of any sort at mental health centers in the state. Likewise, consultation to mental retardation programs and group homes was rarely provided. As many new community-based mental-retardation programs continue to develop across the country, there will be a corresponding need for consultation services by social workers and other mental-health professionals. Consultation in many instances will focus on the development of behavior modification programs for clients, as maladaptive behaviors are frequently the primary cause of the return of clients to institutions. What is needed in many situations is an emphasis on constructing new behaviors and skills in the client through the use of positive reinforcements.

Social workers who can develop consultation skills and expertise in mental retardation have an exciting opportunity to engage in prevention efforts at all levels. Mental health consultation can be used not only to prevent mental disorders, but also to bring together community resources. Although social workers may claim that they have insufficient time and resources to do anything other than tertiary prevention, mental health–mental retardation consultation must be seen as an important tool in primary and secondary prevention efforts. Prevention also includes educational programs and active outreach to individuals at risk.

16.3.3. Community Development

Social workers have demonstrated a history of involvement and concern in many localities as community developers, coordinators, and activists. In doing so, they have successfully broadened the focus of their interventions beyond the confines of the office or the therapy session. Yet, many challenges remain in the community-at-large with respect to developing programs and services for retarded persons. Let us examine some of the ways in which one group of social workers, those in school settings, might pinpoint their efforts on bridging the gaps between home, school, and community in constructing comprehensive strategies that will meet the psychosocial needs of retarded children. School social workers should be in a position of leadership in initiating and coordinating these efforts.

Although retarded children and their parents can benefit in many instances from individual or family therapy, it is apparent that psychotherapy alone is not sufficient in meeting the complex needs of these persons. Costin[30] has advocated that school social workers bring an ecological perspective to bear on the problems of children, in which the goal is to improve the interaction between the school and the community. A broader, systems-oriented approach is thus called for in which effective cooperation and interaction between community resources and agencies is promoted.

The coordination of the multiple services that are often needed is an important principle in the management of the school-aged retarded child.[31] This coordination implies that social workers are aware of existing resources and are knowledgeable in community organization strategies. In the absence of resources, social workers can assume responsibility in developing coalitions of parents and concerned citizens who will move to create new programs and services. Alliances with organizations such as the Association for Retarded Citizens may be fruitful in establishing concrete services for families, such as recreational programs for children, respite care arrangements, and parent groups. The social worker as a community organizer establishes and solidifies linkages between a variety of resources on behalf of the child and the family.

Community education is another important tool and method that school social workers can utilize in bridging gaps between school and community. Individuals in the community need to know what types of programs are being offered in the schools for retarded children, in order to realize that these children can be served in a normal setting. Education can also focus on changing the negative attitudes, such as anger, fear, and indifference, that many persons feel toward the retarded. By speaking to civic and parent groups and presenting modern approaches to the retarded, school social workers will begin to change societal attitudes and promote acceptance of special-education efforts.

Costin[30] has identified two objectives of school social-work practice that are especially pertinent in working with the retarded child and the community: (1) influencing interactions between organizations and institutions and (2) influencing social and environmental policy. The first of these objectives provides the school social worker with an opportunity to function as a mediator who promotes effective interaction between the school and community agencies and organizations. With regard to the retarded child, this mediating function involves maintaining appropriate communication and teamwork between the school and those agencies that are involved with each child. It also includes tasks such as information and referral, the arrangement of placements, and client advocacy.

The second objective thrusts school social workers into the social policy arena, in terms of evaluating and influencing school policies and protecting student rights. Retarded children are at risk, for example, of being subjected to inappropriate forms of discipline or punishment. School social workers must take the initiative in becoming involved in the formulation of school policies and in enlisting the input of the community. This responsibility also extends to participation in the legislative process on the state and national levels.

As an illustration, the author has served as a legislative liaison during the past year on a regional developmental-disabilities council. The council has been active in identifying issues, problems, and needs that affect developmentally disabled persons, and in influencing legislation affecting the lives of these citizens. Council members have been tracking relevant bills in the state legislature, contacting senators concerning high-priority bills, and arranging for testimony at legislative hearings. This type of input ensures that the interests of retarded and handicapped children will be cultivated and protected.

16.4. Conclusion

Social workers in institutional and community settings are presented with a plethora of opportunities to be of service to retarded citizens and their families. If social workers will open their eyes to the challenges that confront them, they will see that they have a variety of habilitative approaches at their disposal. Social work knowledge, combined with positive attitudes toward the client's developmental potential and a sincere commitment to serving the retarded, will pave the way for skilled intervention with these clients. This chapter has presented an overview of some of the new and emerging roles that social workers may adopt in addressing the unmet psychosocial needs of the mentally retarded. These strategies will need to be incorporated into institutional and community programs as social work's contribution to treatment, prevention, and outreach efforts. By applying a variety of techniques in meeting the complex needs of retarded citizens, social workers can provide new direction and leadership in this field for other mental-health professionals and for concerned citizens as well.

References

1. Butterfield E: Some basic changes in residential facilities, in Kugel RB, Shearer A (eds): *Changing Patterns in Residential Services for the Mentally Retarded.* Washington, D.C., President's Committee on Mental Retardation, 1976.

2. Scheerenberger RC: Public residential facilities: Status and trends. *Ment Retard* 19;59–60, 1981.
3. Kelman HR: Social work and mental retardation: Challenge or failure? *Soc Work* 3;37–42, 1958.
4. Adams M: *Mental Retardation and Its Social Dimensions*. New York, Columbia University Press, 1971.
5. Strider FD, Menolascino, FJ: Counseling parents of the mentally retarded infants, in Howells JG (ed): *Modern Perspectives in the Psychiatry of Infancy*. New York, Brunner/Mazel, 1979.
6. Zisfein L, Rosen M: Effects of a personal adjustment training group counseling program. *Ment Retard* 12;50–53, 1974.
7. Lee DY: Evaluation of a group counseling program designed to enchance social adjustment of mentally retarded adults. *J Couns Psychol* 24;318–323, 1977.
8. Gentile C, Jenkins JO: Assertive training with mildly mentally retarded persons. *Ment Retard* 18;315–317, 1980.
9. Matson JL, Senatore V: A comparison of traditional psychotherapy and social skills training for improving interpersonal functioning of mentally retarded adults. *Behav Ther* 12;369–382, 1981.
10. Cohn RC: Style and spirit of the theme-centered-interactional method, in Sager CJ, Kaplan HS (eds): *Progress in Group and Family Therapy*. New York, Brunner/Mazel, 1972.
11. Mosier HD, Grossman HJ, Dingmann HF: Secondary sex development in mentally dificient individuals. *Child Dev* 33;273–286, 1962.
12. Hall J, Morris HL, Barker HR: Sexual knowledge and attitudes of mentally retarded adolescents. *Am J Ment Defic* 77;706–709, 1973.
13. Strauss A: *Teaching Sex Education to Adults Who Are Labelled Mentally Retarded*. (Privately published; Al Strauss, P.O. Box 2141, Oshkosh, WI 54903.)
14. Horejsi CR: Developmental disabilities: Opportunities for social workers. *Soc Work* 24;40–43, 1979.
15. Pincus A, Minahan A: *Social Work Practice: Model and Method*. Itasca, MI, F. E. Peacock, 1973.
16. Wolfensberger W: *Citizen Advocacy for the Handicapped, Impaired, and Disadvantaged: An Overview*. Washington, D.C., President's Committee on Mental Retardation, 1972.
17. Adams M: Science, technology, and some dilemmas of advocacy. *Science* 180;840–842, 1973.
18. Dobson JC, Koch R (eds): *The Mentally Retarded Child and His Family*. New York, Brunner/Mazel, 1976.
19. Baruth L, Burggraf M: *Counseling Parents of Exceptional Children*. New York, Guilford, Special Learning Corporation, 1979.
20. Menolascino FJ: *Challenges in Mental Retardation: Progressive Ideology and Services*. New York, Human Sciences Press, 1977.
21. Mandelbaum A, Wheeler ME: The meaning of a defective child to parents. *Soc Casework* 41;360–367, 1960.
22. Wikler L: Chronic stresses of families of mentally retarded children. *Fam Relations* 30;281–288, 1981.
23. Goodman DM: Parenting an adult mentally retarded offspring. *Smith College Studies in Social Work* 48;209–234, 1978.
24. Menolascino FJ, Eaton LF: Future trends in mental retardation. *Child Psychiatr Hum Dev* 10;156–168, 1980.
25. Rapoport L: Consultation in social work, in *Encyclopedia of Social Work*, vol I. Washington, D.C., National Association of Social Workers, 1977.
26. Caplan G: *The Theory and Practice of Mental Health Consultation*. New York, Basic Books, 1970
27. Szymanski LS, Leaverton DR: Mental health consultation to educational programs for retarded persons, in Szymanski LS, Tanguay PE (eds): *Emotional Disorders of Mentally Retarded Persons*. Baltimore, University Park Press, 1980.
28. Kevin D: Use of the group method in consultation, in Rapoport L (ed): *Consultation in Social Work Practice*. New York, National Association of Social Workers, 1963.

29. West MA, Richardson M: A statewide survey of CMHC programs for mentally retarded individuals. *Hosp Commun Psychiatr* 32;413–416, 1981.
30. Costin LB: School social work as specialized practice. *Soc Work* 26;36–43, 1981.
31. Donaldson JY, Menolascino FJ: Therapeutic and preventive interventions in mental retardation, in Sholevar GP (ed): *Emotional Disorders in Children and Adolescents*. New York, Spectrum Publications, 1980.

V

Research and Future Directions

Introduction

It is hoped that the reader now has an understanding and a background concerning this population, their service needs, and the training priorities and recommendations for carrying out these service needs. However, a comprehensive handbook would not be complete if it did not address the research on this particular population. Fortunately, we have been able to benefit from the contribution of two psychiatrists with outstanding credentials in this area of specialization. The focus of Chapter 17 is to review the current status and the future directions of research on the mentally ill-mentally retarded individual. Tanguay and Szymanski point out that the recent changes in the dually diagnosed population in terms of movement into the community presents a unique opportunity to conduct research with them, particularly as there is now a greater emphasis on the biological aspects of mental health research. As a result, these authors call for greater leadership and participation by child psychiatrists such as has been recommended by the American Academy of Child Psychiatry.

These authors also delineate the critical problems that face researchers in both clinical and basic research. First, in the clinical research area, we have been faced with a major problem in terms of a uniform diagnostic classification system. Using autism to illustrate a well-defined body of knowledge and research for the dually diagnosed population, the authors point out the numerous problems that must be dealt with. Diagnostic improvements via the DSM-III have helped, but there still remains a need for research into how useful and valid a nosological approach is in identifying the necessary ingredients for development and maturation. The authors further point out that epidemiological studies are perhaps somewhat deficient because research conducted on institutional populations tends to focus on those behaviors that are of major concern to the staff, whereas other problems (e.g., depression) perhaps remain unnoticed. They further recommend that double-blind studies be conducted in providing treatment and research, that prevention and research be encouraged for early intervention, and that cost analysis evaluations with the mildly retarded be investigated.

In basic research, the three major areas of prevention, early intervention, and the habilitation of those individuals who have been classified as autistic are presented. The authors summarize electrophysiological research, ranging from polygraphic sleep studies to auditory brain-stem responses, as being promising, particularly with the development of more sophisticated technology. Neuropharmacological research, ranging from serotonergic metabolism to endocrine functioning, is also encouraging, along with new breakthroughs in genetic research via computer technology.

The authors conclude the chapter by offering five excellent recommendations on research that medical schools and residency training programs will find useful, particularly in training child psychiatrists. These recommendations, they feel, will lead to the development of role models who actually deliver services, provide training, and conduct research in a multidisciplinary setting.

In Chapter 18, Dr. Menolascino addresses the challenge of attempting to transpose the modern mental-retardation system so that it directly serves the chronically mentally ill. Menolascino feels that it is possible to utilize a service model that he helped establish and has consulted with over the last 15 years in implementing this model with the "at-risk" elderly and the chronically mentally ill. Menolascino demonstrates that there are several commonalities among the retarded, the chronically mentally ill, and the elderly that make it possible to serve each of them in a comprehensive, community-based rehabilitation program.

It is obvious to those who have worked in this field that the residential component is often the critical basis of a comprehensive, community-based service system. Several distinct advantages are presented for providing a complete continuum of residential services for this population. Comparison of this model with other models that care for the chronically disabled person is reviewed for the reader. It is pointed out that the current service system has several huge gaps in it, most likely because of the fragmentation of the mental health professionals who treat this population. In agreement with the previous chapter, Menolascino also points out the importance of psychiatry and its role in the treatment of chronic patients, and he goes on to point out various medical models and problems in the delivery of human services. The chapter concludes by providing an overview of a community-based service model of mental retardation that offers specific techniques, recommendations, model components of a community-based system, and recommendations to mental health professionals in terms of their commitment if they hope to be successful with this population.

In closing, we hope that we have met the objectives of this book, to answer questions about who are the mentally ill-mentally retarded, what are their needs, why they need to be served, where they can best be served, and how to serve them.

We are optimistic about the future of this field because of the increased interest shown by professionals, despite the predicted shortage of child psychiatrists, and also because of the political, social, and financial reasons for serving this population. It is currently one of the hottest topics in both the mental health and the mental retardation fields. Yet, we have had very little research or demonstration and technical assistance projects that typically communicate knowledge to professionals and paraprofessionals in the field.

We are also optimistic because typically the scientific knowledge in a given area tends to double every 5–10 years, and it appears that we are on the threshold of major advances with the mentally ill-mentally retarded individual. Our ability to enhance the lives of these individuals via prevention, reversal, and habilitation is encouraging because of these biomedical and behavioral advances.

The biomedical field is advancing in knowledge thanks to diagnostic tools such as the PETT (positron emission transaxil tomograph) and the NMR (nuclear magnetic resonance) machines, which will allow us an open window to the brain's functioning, thereby allowing us to assessing the efficacy of our treatment via pharmacological, nutritional, and physiological approaches. In genetics, the use of the cell-sorter and gene-splicing recombinant DNA procedures also provide hope for the future elimination and prevention of the genetic disorders that cause or contribute to these mental health problems. These technological advances and hardward equipment are just now being made available across the country to major research and medical centers. With ongoing treatment via this technology, we should see even further advances of a rather dramatic nature in the next 20 years.

The behavioral research of the 1960s and 1970s of the hundreds of "techniques" involving analyzing, evaluating, and modifying behavior is now paying off in the *packaging* of these procedures into solid, individualized program plans that are capable, if properly implemented, of impressive improvement in the clients' behavior and productivity. Most impressive have been the early intervention and prevention studies, which indicate an excellent cost–benefit return. The editors of this book are also particularly optimistic about the combined potential of the biomedical and the behavioral specialists, who in working together can have an impact on those individuals with complex impairments of both emotional and cognitive functioning.

It has been recommended throughout this book that we now encourage the establishment of comprehensive interdisciplinary centers that engage in service to, training of, and research on the mentally ill-mentally retarded. Such centers are pivotal in providing in-service training and continuing education for professionals and paraprofessionals in both the mental health and the mental retardation fields.

In addition, role models will be necessary, particularly at the M.D. and Ph.D. level, from the child psychiatrist to the habilitation psychologist, if we are to meet the challenge of serving people with these combined impairments in community settings.

And last, we are just beginning, in this country, to understand the importance of providing greater assistance and support to the family if we are to effectively reverse and prevent the problems of this challenging population.

17

Psychiatric Research in Mental Retardation
Current Status and Future Directions

Peter E. Tanguay and Ludwik S. Szymanski

"Psychiatric" research in mental retardation may be defined from a number of viewpoints. *Psychiatric* might be taken to mean that the research has been performed by psychiatrists. Insofar as mental retardation is concerned, it could mean research performed by child psychiatrists, as they are much more likely (perhaps because they deal with development) to be concerned with mental retardation than is the general psychiatrist. Inasmuch as the child psychiatrist is broadly trained in biological issues, in child development, and in clinical assessment and treatment, it could be expected (even demanded of the profession as a whole) that child psychiatrists play a major role in research into the causes and treatment of serious psychopathology in childhood, including mental retardation.[1] Project Future,[2] an enterprise set in motion by the American Academy of Child Psychiatry, concluded in its final report (1983) that many more child psychiatrists must develop expertise in research, must become active in designing and carrying out research studies, and must provide leadership in child mental-health research. To this end, the report recommended that more training programs in child psychiatry provide research experience, and that postresidency research fellowships be made available to supplement such programs as the NIMH's Research Scientist Development Awards.

Implementation of the above recommendation is, in our viewpoint, long overdue. For, as Anders[3] has noted, the majority of child mental-health research projects are done by nonphysicians. Using figures provided by NIMH, which summarized funded projects for the past several years, Anders identified 14 projects involving children diagnosed as having early infantile autism, schizophrenia, or mental retardation. Nine of the projects were directed by Ph.D./M.A. professionals, whereas only five were carried out by physicians. And despite the American Psychiatric Association's call for increased participation by psychiatrists in the study and treatment of retarded persons, we have been able to find very few papers on mental retardation in the two leading American psychiatric journals (*Archives of General Psychiatry* and *American Journal of Psychiatry*) in the past 10 years. Those papers that can be found

Peter E. Tanguay • Department of Psychiatry, University of California at Los Angeles, Los Angeles, California 90049.   *Ludwik S. Szymanski* • Department of Psychiatry, Children's Hospital, 300 Longwood Avenue, Boston, Massachusetts 02115.

are mostly case reports. It would appear that psychiatrists have not yet seriously taken up the study of mental retardation. For these reasons, we conclude that if "psychiatric research" were limited to only those projects involving psychiatrists, our discussion of the subject would be limited indeed.

One could, on the other hand, interpret *psychiatric* as referring to a category of illness. Because there is no consensus on precisely what is "psychiatric illness," such an interpretation could be equally misleading.

We therefore opt for a relatively broad interpretation of the term *psychiatric research* and discuss here studies of the cause and treatment of retardation *per se* or of mental health issues in retarded persons. In the interests of brevity, we especially focus on current research needs, as engendered by the current state of our knowledge.

Within the past decade, the field of mental retardation has undergone profound changes, affecting both the type and the scope of possible research. For one, the increasing emphasis on the "normalization" of the environment of the retarded person has led to the entry of retarded citizens into the community outside of large state institutions. This entry has provided scientists[4,5] a unique opportunity to study the course of the personality and lifestyle development of retarded persons in the community, as well as to gain an understanding of the manner in which behavioral-emotional disorders arise in mentally retarded persons outside hospitals, how best these can be treated, and how often such disorders result in placement failure. Despite the important public-health issues involved, the research has most often been conducted by sociologists and psychologists. A review of the literature indicates that psychiatrists rarely study this subject.

Within the past decade, there has also been an explosion of interest in the biological aspects of mental illness. In part, this phenomenon has been a result of the availability of new methods of investigation and better instruments. Some of these methods have been used to study mentally retarded individuals as well as the mentally ill. The study of mentally retarded persons not only may be helpful in providing information useful in the prevention and treatment of retardation *per se* but may well prove helpful in elucidating normal brain–behavior relationships or in clarifying neurodevelopmental abnormalities in diverse neurological disorders.[6] The current state of this research, as well as its shortcomings, is described in Section 17.2.

In addition, a multimodal, interdisciplinary approach to the management and treatment of mental retardation has come to the fore. Such a model is equally important in research, inasmuch as emotional disorders in retarded as well as nonretarded persons are multidetermined.[7]

17.1. Clinical Research

Clinical research includes the study of diagnostic issues in mental retardation, the search for more effective treatment of psychopathology in retarded persons, and the investigation of preventive measures.

17.1.1. Diagnostic Issues

A problem common to many past studies of retarded persons has been an inconsistent and idiosyncratic use of diagnostic categories. Prior to 1980, the diagnostic systems in use did not provide specific enough diagnostic criteria and left much to the individual clinician's subjective judgment. Thus, it was difficult to compare the results of different studies, or even, sometimes, to accept them at face value. The publication of the American Psychiatric Association's new system of classification (DSM-III)[8] did much to improve the degree to which categories were defined with exactitude. Equally important in the DSM-III has been the inclusion of several commonly accepted categories (such as early infantile autism) that had hitherto been omitted from the system of classification. There are, however, certain serious shortcomings in the system as it now stands. For one, developmental issues are given relatively little consideration. The category of schizophrenia in children (an illness in which failures in certain aspects of cognitive development are paramount) can be diagnosed only by means of criteria more appropriate for adults. One such criterion is "thought disorder." But what is thought disorder in a child, who cannot be expected to show cognitive maturity? Because of this difficulty, it is well nigh impossible (unless one accepts certain physical traits as pathognomonic of schizophrenia, as Cantor[9] suggested) to diagnose schizophrenia in a child below 7 years of age or in a nonverbal retarded adult. On the other hand, recent research has clearly indicated that schizophrenia can be seen in children,[9,10] and that, with early stimulation and education, these children can be helped.

A more disturbing observation has been recently made in a series of papers[11-13]; some of the categories of developmental psychopathology (including early infantile autism, PDD childhood onset, specific language and reading disorders, and schizophrenia in children, all of which may coexist with retardation) may be invalid as specific nosological entities. What may be needed is a system of classification that deals not with such global "symptoms" as "inability to relate to others," "absent or deviant language," or "thought disorder," but with failure to develop certain elemental motor, affective, cognitive, and mnemonic skills necessary for psychological adaptation. Although our understanding of the development of such skills is rudimentary at present, recent neuropsychological studies have suggested, for example, that there may be two relatively separate lines of cognitive operations: holistic and sequential thought. Although it is beyond the scope of the present chapter to describe these operations, it is suggested [11-13] that, in terms of these two factors alone, the disparate features of the various syndromes listed above can be seen as an expression of varying profiles of deficit in holistic or sequential processing skills, as well as in motor or mnemonic skill. Such a new system of classification, based on "profiles of elemental handicaps," is not suggested as a replacement for Axis I of DSM-III, but as perhaps a new axis. We need research that will study whether such a nosological approach is useful and valid, and more important, we need studies designed to identify what autonomous ele-

mental skills may be integral to development, and how these unfold with maturation.

17.1.2. Epidemiological Issues

In the past, studies of mental illness in mentally retarded persons were
largely done with individuals in large institutions, or with retarded persons who
were specifically referred for mental health consultation. The extent to which
the findings of such studies are applicable to the general population of mentally
retarded persons is not known and should be studied. We suspect that the
incidence of certain types of mental illness (such as depression) may be largely
underestimated. Depressed persons may not be seen as a "trouble" by institutional staff who deal with them, and hence, they may not be referred. There
is a need for large-scale studies of random populations of retarded persons of
various ages, developmental levels, backgrounds, and socioeconomic status.

17.1.3. Treatment

Much of the research to date on the effects of medication has focused on
assessing response in terms of nonspecific symptoms such as aggression or
self-abuse. In one unpublished study that has come to our attention, poor eating
etiquette ("pigging") was among the symptoms rated to assess response. Such
an approach is akin to asking, in a group of patients with "fever" or "cough,"
whether antibiotics are useful. What we need are well-designed, double-blind,
controlled studies of the effects of various modalities of treatment on important
symptoms and handicaps of retarded persons. A number of such studies now
exist. The recent investigation of Rivinus and Harmatz[14] on the treatment of
manic-depressive disorder in retarded persons is one example.

17.1.4. Prevention

Despite our belief that mild mental retardation is largely a result of adverse
environmental factors, including inadequate prenatal care, maternal ill health,
prenatal substance abuse, poor postnatal nutrition, and lack of adequate language and social stimulation in infancy and early childhood, there is a need for
additional study of which factors are most important in etiology, and how cost-
effective programs of social intervention aimed at prevention may be developed. Perhaps the best example of such research is the research carried out
in relation to the implementation and assessment of the Head Start program.[15]
With the nation's decreasing interest in Great Society legislation, there is a
danger that such studies will lapse and that such programs will decrease.

17.1.5. Professional Attitudes

Although the reluctance of many psychiatrists and other mental-health
professionals to work with mentally retarded persons is well known,[1] and per-

haps attributable to ignorance and lack of experience, ways of reversing this unfortunate situation must be sought. It has been our experience in child psychiatry that the solution may require some type of bootstrap operation. As members of the Mental Retardation and Developmental Disabilities Committee of the American Academy of Child Psychiatry, we have sought to foster increased teaching of mental-retardation–related subjects in child-psychiatry training programs. But even when training directors wish to provide their trainees with in-depth experience in the evaluation and treatment of mentally retarded persons, they tell us that they are unable to do so because of the acute shortage of child psychiatrists and psychologists who are experts in these areas. Although books can be found on the subject, didactic experience alone is not at all sufficient for training purposes. There is a need for clinician role models for child psychiatrists, models who themselves are involved in the delivery of services to mentally retarded persons. Teaching must be through example, through communication of attitudes of confidence and hope. Perhaps the most effective solution at this time would be to establish model training programs in a few large centers, assisted by federal money specially earmarked for this purpose. A few such programs are already operational,[16] in which child psychiatrists, working in close affiliation with a university-affiliated facility (a specific federally funded program) have provided training in mental retardation to child psychiatrists. More such programs will be needed.

17.2. Basic Research

With few exceptions (most notably the discovery of PKU and other inborn errors of metabolism or of the specific chromosome abnormalities of Down's and other genetic syndromes), most major advances in the prevention and treatment of retarded persons have come from behavioral, educational, and socioanthropological research.

And yet, for moderate to severe forms of mental retardation (including those in which the children are autistic or otherwise psychotic), this is not enough. We are faced, in these individuals, with developmental failure, striking at the biological substrate of learning and humanity. Advances in the prevention and treatment of such disorders can come about only through a better understanding of the fundamental biological factors that go awry in such instances.

Scientists, of course, have not neglected such fields of inquiry. Nor has the National Institute of Mental Health been reluctant to fund such research. Witness the excellent work being done at the dozen federally funded mental-retardation research centers throughout the country. To the impatient clinician, however, it may not seem that much of practical import is resulting from this work, and to a certain extent, this assessment is correct. What we have is a large number of first-rate investigators addressing fundamental issues in neuroanatomy and neurophysiology, in developmental biology, in neurobiochemistry and neuropharmacology—attacking important questions whose answers must be found if the relationship between brain and behavior is to be keenly understood. And between these scientists and the clinicians who work with retarded persons, clinging like aerialists to the tenuous guy-wires that link the two groups, are the few clinician–basic-scientists who are attempting to use the techniques of basic science (the radioimmune assays, the mass-spectros-copy–gas-chromatography analysis, the event-related potentials of electrophy-siology, and such) to study the etiology, treatment, and prevention of devel-opmental psychopathology, including mental retardation. The degree to which they have been successful—and the manner in which this research may need to be conducted in the future—is the subject of the remainder of this chapter. To some extent, our narrative reflects the old adage that nature yields her secrets with the utmost reluctance. The major problem may be not how little we understand the neurobiology of human development, but how, even with the aid of computers and sophisticated electronic measuring devices, the tools with which we work are limited.

As stated in the title of the chapter, our goal is to assess the current status and the future directions of research. To do so as expeditiously as possible, we propose, in this section, to avoid a mere listing of the disparate, uncon-nected, and all-too-often unprepossessing basic research studies that have been done with retarded persons in general and to concentrate, instead, on what we believe to be the most cohesive body of research studies that have been carried out to date. Such an approach not only can provide a good sense of the historical development of the topic but can also give a clearer sense of what more can be done. The body of research to which we refer is the research that has been done with children who have been diagnosed as suffering from early infantile autism, a syndrome in which there is both serious psychopathology and mental retardation. A relatively large number of good, biologically oriented research investigators have been attracted to studying autistic children in the past two decades. As a result, biological studies of autistic children represent the best single body of basic research in the field of mental retardation today.

17.2.1. Electrophysiological Research

The history of electrophysiological research with autistic children did not begin until the middle 1960s. The specific techniques on which this research was based were largely a product of the electronic revolution of the 1950s. That we must, at each stage in our research endeavors, wait for the development of new research tools is typical of our current dilemma: basic biological re-search into the etiology and treatment of mental retardation is entirely depen-dent on new techniques, and each time a new technique is developed, there is a rush to exploit its applications, so that with perseveration and luck a few new ideas and answers are added to our knowledge base, but invariably, the work comes to a halt because the technique proves inadequate, and investi-gators await the development of the next level of technology to continue their work.

For this reason, electrophysiological studies of retarded and autistic chil-dren have been more often "technique-oriented" than based on profound biological hypotheses. A few investigators have postulated specific anatomical substrates or phenomena as defective (e.g., brain stem or vestibular system[17]) or, more recently, abnormalities in the development of hemispheric speciali- zation (see Tanguay *et al.*[18] for a review), or abnormalities in the limbic sys- tem,[19] but even in these instances, the manner in which particular hypotheses have been studied has been largely determined by the latest electrophysiol- ogical technique. As new techniques have appeared, individual investigators have eagerly seized the opportunity offered by the latest method, so that the history of electrophysiological research with autistic children reflects the de- velopment of the field of human electrophysiology itself.

The first electrophysiological studies were of the EEG. They yielded pos- itive results: 51% of autistic children were found[20] to have many EEG abnor- malities (e.g., focal slowing, focal spikes, paroxysmal spike and wave dis- charges), an observation that has since been confirmed by many others.[21-23] This finding certainly helped to reinforce the idea that autistic children had neurobiological abnormalities, but the lack of uniform findings between chil- dren, as well as the lack of a precise localization of the abnormalities in most instances, soon led to the realization that simple visual EEG analysis did not hold much promise in terms of understanding the precise nature of the neural abnormalities of the children. Other global measures, such as the galvanic skin response, have shared a similar fate: although under certain conditions autistic children had a lower GSR response,[24] it was not possible to link this observation with a specific neuropathological hypothesis.

Realizing the above, investigators attempted to quantify EEG character- istics in a more precise manner. Hermelin and O'Conner[25] compared the amount and patterning of alpha activity in the EEGs of normal, autistic, and retarded subjects and concluded that, although autistic children did not differ in terms of cortical arousal during the resting state, under visual stimulus con- ditions they tended to habituate more quickly than normals. Again, the finding did not lead to any fruitful line of research.

But simultaneously with the above, a popular new use of the EEG had made its appearance: sleep research. Following the discovery that EEG and eye-movement-activity phenomena varied over a fixed cycle during sleep,[26] there was an explosion of polygraphic sleep studies in the 1960s, including ones of autistic children. Immediately, it was found that autistic children had quite normal sleep cycles,[26,27] but that certain phasic events occurring during REM sleep might be abnormal. Specifically, Ornitz *et al.*[28] found that autistic children had markedly immature development of eye-movement burst activity (so that by ages 2–5 they continued to resemble 6- to 8-month old children), a finding subsequently confirmed by Tanguay *et al.*[29] At the same time, Ritvo *et al.*[30] were reporting that autistic children had markedly decreased vestibular res- ponsivity to whirling stimulation in the dark (though not in the light), an ob- servation subsequently confirmed by further studies.[31] Because the final com- mon pathways that mediate eye-movement activity during sleep involve the medial and descending vestibular nuclei, Ornitz concluded that the above find- ing demonstrated that autistic children have an abnormality in vestibular function at the level of the brain stem, which, in turn, led to a state of "perceptual inconstancy," which itself was responsible for the symptoms of the disorder.[17] Others[18] have argued that the syndrome is more likely to represent abnormalities in forebrain functioning than abnormalities in the brain stem. Although they had yielded interesting results, the eye-movement activity and vestibular studies were limited in the information that they could further provide in relation to brain stem function, and for this reason, this work was largely halted.

A third line of electrophysiological research that flourished in the 1960s and has continued (albeit with considerable refinement of technique) to the present has been the study of auditory "evoked responses" in autistic and mentally retarded persons. By means of computers, the EEG signal can be treated in such a way as to greatly increase the signal-to-noise ratio of the EEG response to a stimulus. Initially, it was noted that the gross morphology of the waveform of the auditory evoked response seemed normal in autistic children during sleep.[32] It was fortunate that the latter studies were done in sleep, for we now realize that most evoked-response research in waking subjects during the 1960s and the early 1970s was seriously flawed because the investigators had not known enough to control for certain "endogenous" responses. An example of an endogenous response is the so-called P300 potential, a positive potential occurring 300–400 msec after stimulus onset, which is emitted when a "rare" stimulus is perceived against a background of "frequent" stimuli of a different type. To date, there has been only one P300 study of a very small number of autistic persons,[33] in which it was found that the P300 of autistic persons was decreased in amplitude in comparison to normal subjects. Whether this finding is indicative of the autistics' reduced attention to the task, or whether it has a more specific physiological meaning is not known at present.

A final evoked-response technique that has been popularized within the past half-dozen years is *auditory brain-stem responses*. The technique has proved to be extremely reliable and robust. A series of 1,500 or more very brief click stimuli are given to subjects at a rate of 10 or 20 per second, and the resultant evoked response, amplified 200,000 times, is recorded. The response consists of a series of waves within the first 6 msec after stimulus onset, representing responses generated in the auditory nerve and in the brain-stem auditory system. Several investigators have studied these short-latency evoked responses in autistic children.[17] One common finding has been that some autistic children show unusually long transmission time of the response through the brain stem. Tanguay *et al.*[17] suggest three possible interpretations of this finding: They may have no causal relationship to the child's autistic handicaps; they may represent distortions in auditory input that impair the learning of language; or they may reflect events during an earlier period of development in which abnormal input directly caused maldevelopment of the forebrain systems necessary for language and cognitive function.

In summary, then, electrophysiological approaches to understanding early infantile autism and mental retardation are becoming increasingly sophisticated and are beginning to yield more interesting results. Whether existing techniques are sufficient to answer our questions remains to be seen, but one thing is certain: if we do not continue this work we are certain to find nothing, whereas the alternative has at least a hope of success.

17.2.2. Neuropharmacological Research

In a manner somewhat parallel to the situation in the field of electrophysiology, there has been a surge of interest in using the latest neuropharmacological techniques to study psychiatric impairment and mental handicaps in the past two decades. As with electrophysiology, advances in understanding the pathophysiology of early infantile autism or other mental retardation syndromes have been slow. A few isolated studies, with largely negative findings, have delved into such topics as hair amino acids[34] and serum copper or zinc levels[35] in autistic children. In general, however, biochemical research on the subject of infantile autism and mental retardation has focused on three topics: serotonergic metabolism, catecholaminergic metabolism, and endocrine function.

Insofar as infantile autism is concerned, the study of serotonergic metabolism has attracted the greatest number of investigators over the longest period of time (see DeMyer *et al.*[36] for a review of this work). In all of this research, one finding has been well established: blood serotonin levels are markedly elevated in some autistic and some nonautistic mentally retarded subjects. The results appear to be related inversely to IQ. Beyond this finding, it has not been possible to understand the manner in which serotonergic metabolism is distributed in some autistic and mentally retarded persons, or even if the peripheral elevations of serotonin in some individuals are related to abnormal serotonin metabolism in the brain. Most recently, Geller *et al.*[37] have reported promising results (in the form of increased IQ scores) in autistic children who were given fenfluramine, a drug that decreases blood serotonin levels. Only three children were studied, however. Much further investigation will be needed before this finding can be fully understood.

Studies of catecholamine metabolites in the urine and the cerebrospinal (CSF) fluid of autistic and mentally retarded children have been carried out by a number of investigators, but the research has been hampered by the realization that we are dealing with dynamic biochemical systems, and that study of a single enzyme or metabolite may yield little in the way of interpretable results. One series of studies by Cohen and his colleagues at Yale[38,39] examined CSF levels of various dopaminergic and serotonergic metabolites after the administration of probenacid. Autistic children were found to have decreased 5-HIAA levels in comparison to nonautistic psychotic children. Based on these findings, they postulated that autistic children may suffer from an overactivity of the dopaminergic system which could, in part, be associated with the various movement stereotypes seen in early infantile autism.

The endocrine investigations have included study of the stress response and the circadian rhythmicity of 11-hydroxicorticosteroids,[40] of free fatty acid metabolism,[41] and of hypothalamic-pituitary-thyroid axis function[42] in autistic children. All three approaches have found autistic children to be abnormal.

They have been reported as having disturbances in the development of circadian rhythmicity, greater variability in free fatty acid levels, and deficient effects of thyrotropin-releasing hormone compatible with, but not diagnostic of, hypothalamic disease. None of these results has led to further productive research, however.

17.2.3. Genetic Studies

As noted earlier, genetic studies of moderately to profoundly retarded children have been very successful in delineating many specific chromosome abnormalities. This has not been true of early infantile autism. Contrary to the prevailing beliefs of the 1960s, however, opinion has shifted strongly toward the belief that, for at least a subgroup of autistic children, genetic factors do play an important role[43–45] in the development of the syndrome. The genetic factors do not appear to be responsible for the specific symptoms of autism *per se* but appear to influence development of a variety of serious neurological, cognitive, and language disorders. More recently, Brown[46] and Meryash *et al.*[47] have reported genetic findings of a somewhat different nature: the occurrence of the fragile-X syndrome in a small number of autistic individuals.

17.3. Conclusions

Based on the directions taken by research in the past decade and on current results, we suggest that future research be guided by the following ideas:

1. Research aimed at understanding the causes and treatment of mental retardation must not be limited to studies of humans who are mentally retarded. We need neurobiological and neurodevelopmental research spanning the phylogenetic range from single-cell organisms to humans. Such basic studies are needed to reach an understanding of the principles of neural development and function and to develop new hypotheses on which future work in humans will be based.

2. At a clinical level, we must remain ready to exploit each new advance in methodology as it becomes available. Among the promising techniques for the immediate future are the newer methods of event-related potential study, including P300-type responses and auditory brain-stem responses, and the new computer-enhanced imaging techniques, especially the PET scan and nuclear magnetic resonance scanning. The latter methods hold promise of research into biochemical processes *in vivo*, an important addition to the analysis techniques of the 1970s.

3. It may not be effective to study groups solely on the basis of DSM-III diagnoses. It may be necessary to isolate fundamental developmental skills and attributes that contribute to the broad symptom clusters used to define syndromes in the DSM-III and to study individuals in terms of their levels of development within such clusters. Rather than confusing comparisons of "re-

tarded," "autistic," and "schizophrenic" groups of children, it may be more important to study children in terms of specific types of cognitive, language, motor, and attentional handicaps.[11-13] Handicaps in "fundamental lines of development" may cut across diagnostic categories and may be better indices of psychopathology than the global symptoms that serve to delineate diagnostic categories in the DSM-III.

4. Research must be carried out on an interdisciplinary basis. Major advances in knowledge often come not from within a single field of research, but at the intersection between fields. When this happens, a well-articulated hypothesis from one field may suddenly take on a new meaning as it is used to illuminate a process in the other field. As an example,[11-13] Piaget's stage model of cognitive development may take on a different (and more complete) meaning when viewed in the light of what we know about hemispheric specialization and its development.

5. Scientists who work with human subjects must understand that the traditional statistical approaches to research are not the sole *modus operandi*. There are times, especially when a field of research is new, when single-case studies and reports of subjective observations can be quite valuable in developing new hypotheses. Both the statistical double-blind method and the clinical observation method are valuable, and each must be brought to bear on important questions about human development.

References

1. Cushna B, Szymanski LS, Tanguay PE: Professional roles and unmet manpower needs, in Szymanski L, Tanguay P (eds): *Emotional Disorders of Mentally Retarded Persons*. Baltimore, University Park Press, 1980.
2. *Project Future*. Washington, D.C., American Academy of Child Psychiatry, 1983.
3. Anders T: The child psychiatrist and research. *J Am Acad Child Psychiatr* 2(16);570–571, 1982.
4. Edgerton RB: *Lives in Process: Mildly Retarded Adults in Community Settings*. Washington, D.C., AAMD Monograph #6, 1982.
5. Edgerton RB: Deinstitutionalizing the retarded: An example of values in conflict, in Johnson AW, Grusky O, Ravens BH (eds): *Contemporary Health Services: A Social Science Perspective*. Boston, Auburn House, 1982.
6. Winokur B: Subnormality and its relation to psychiatry. *Lancet* 2;270–273, 1974.
7. Tanguay PE: A field-theory approach to understanding developmental disabilities, in Szymanski L, Tanguay P (eds): *Mental Illness in Mental Retardation: Assessment, Treatment and Consultation*. Baltimore, University Park Press, 1980.
8. American Psychiatric Association: *Diagnostic and Statistical Manual*, ed 3 (DSM-III). Washington, D.C., Author, 1980.
9. Cantor S: *The Schizophrenic Children*. Toronto, Ontario, Canada, Eden Press, 1982.
10. Cantor S, Evans J, Pearce J, *et al*: Childhood schizophrenia: Present but not accounted for. *Am J Psychiatr* 139;758–762, 1982.
11. Tanguay PE: Toward a developmental classification of serious psychopathology in children, Part I: Shortcomings in a phenomenological system of classification, *Journal of American Academy of Child Psychiatry*, in press.
12. Tanguay PE: Toward a developmental classification of serious psychopathology in children, Part II: Elemental cognitive capacities: Development and relationship to psychopathology, *Journal of American Academy of Child Psychiatry*, in press.

13. Tanguay PE: Toward a developmental classification of serious psychopathology in children, Part III: Dissociations in development of elementary cognitive capacities in children. *Journal of American Academy of Child Psychology*, in press.

14. Rivinus TM, Harmatz JS: Diagnosis and lithium treatment of affective disorders in the retarded: Five case studies. *Am J Psychiatr* 12;109–114, 1982.

15. Miller LB, Dyer JL: Four preschool programs: Their dimensions and effects. *Soc Res Child Develop Monogr* 40 (5–6 Serial No.162);1–162, 1975.

16. Tanguay PE, Szymanski LS: Training of mental health professionals in mental retardation, in Tanguay PE, Szymanski LS (eds): *Emotional Disorders of Mentally Retarded Persons*. Baltimore, University Park Press, 1980.

17. Ornitz EM: The disorders of perception common to early infantile autism and schizophrenia. *Compr Psychiatr* 10;259–274, 1969.

18. Tanguay PE, Edwards RM, Buchwald J, et al: Auditory brain-stem responses in autistic children. *Arch Gen Psychiatr* 39;174–180, 1982.

19. Damasio AR, Maurer RG: A neurological model for childhood autism. *Arch Neurol* 35;777–786, 1978.

20. White PT, DeMyer W, DeMyer M: EEG abnormalities in early childhood schizophrenia: A double-blind study of psychiatrically disturbed and normal children during promazine sedation. *Am J Psychiat* 120;950–958, 1964.

21. Creak M, Pampiglione G: Clinical and EEG studies on a group of 35 psychotic children. *Dev Med Child Neurol* 11;218–227, 1969.

22. Gubbay SS, Lobascher M, Kingerlee P: A Neurological appraisal of autistic children: Results of a western Australian survey. *Dev Med Child Neurol* 12;422–429, 1970.

23. Taft LT, Cohen HJ: Hypsarrhythmia and infantile autism: A clinical report. *J Autism Child Schizophr* 1;327–336, 1971.

24. Bernal ME, Miller WH: Electrodermal and cardiac response of schizophrenic children to sensory stimuli. *Psychophysiology* 7;155–168, 1971.

25. Hermelin B, O'Conner, N: Measures of occipital alpha rhythm in normal, subnormal, and autistic children. *Br J Psychiatry* 114;603–610, 1968.

26. Dement W, Kleitman N: Cyclic variations in EEG during sleep and their relation to eye movements, body motility, and dreaming. *Electroencephalogr Clin Neurophysiol* 9;673–690, 1957.

27. Ornitz EM, Ritvo ER, Walter RD: Dreaming sleep in autistic and schizophrenic children. *Am J Psychiatr* 122;419–424, 1965.

28. Ornitz EM, Wechter V, Hartman D, et al: The EEG and rapid eye movements during REM sleep in babies. *Electroencephalogr Clin Neurophysiol* 30;350–353, 1971.

29. Tanguay PE, Ornitz EM, Forsythe AM, et al: Rapid eye movement (REM) activity in normal and autistic children during REM sleep. *J Autism Child Schizophr* 6;275–288, 1976.

30. Ritvo ER, Ornitz EM, Eriator A, et al: Decreased postrotatory nystagmus in early infantile autism. *Neurology* 19;653–658, 1969.

31. Ornitz EM, Forsythe AB, Tanguay PE, et al: The recovery cycle of the averaged auditory evoked response during sleep in autistic children. *Electroencephalogr Clin Neurophysiol* 37;173–174, 1974.

32. Ornitz EM, Ritvo ER, Panman LM, et al: The auditory evoked response in normal and autistic children during sleep. *Electroencephalogr Clin Neurophysiol* 25;221–230, 1968.

33. Novick B, Kurtzberg D, Vaughn HG: An electrophysiologic indication of defective information storage in childhood autism. *Psychiatr Res* 1;101–108, 1979.

34. Johnson RJ, Wiersema V, Kraft IA: High amino acids in childhood autism. *J Autism Child Schizophr* 4;177–178, 1974.

35. Jackson MJ, Garrod PJ: Plasma, zinc, copper and amino acid levels in the blood of autistic children. *J Autism Child Schizophr* 8;203–208, 1978.

36. DeMyer MK, Hingtgen NJ, Jackson RK: Infantile autism reviewed: A decade of research. *Schizophr Bull* 7;388–451, 1981.

37. Geller E, Ritvo ER, Freeman BJ, et al: Fenfluramine decreases blood serotonin and improves symptoms in three autistic boys. *N Engl J Med* 307;165–169, 1982.

38. Cohen D, Shaywitz A, Johnson W, *et al*: Biogenic amines in autistic and atypical children: Cerebrospinal fluid measures of monovanillic acid and 5-hydroxyindoleacetic acid. *Arch Gen Psychiatr* 31;845–853, 1974.
39. Cohen DJ, Young JG: Review article: Neurochemistry and child psychiatry. *J Am Acad Child Psychiatr* 34;353–411, 1977.
40. Yamazaki K, Saito Y, Okada F, *et al*: An application of neuroendocrinological studies in autistic children and Heller's syndrome. *J Autism Child Schizophr* 5;323–332, 1975.
41. DeMyer MK, Schwier H, Bryson CQ, *et al*: Free fatty acid response to insulin and glucose stimulation in schizophrenic, autistic, and emotionally disturbed children. *J Autism Child Schizophr* 1;436–452, 1971.
42. Campbell M, Hollander CS, Ferris S, *et al*: Response to thyrotrophin releasing hormone stimulation in young psychotic children: A pilot study. *Psychoneuroendocrinology* 3;195–201, 1978.
43. Bartak L, Rutter M, Cox A: A comparative study of infantile autism and specific developmental receptive language disorder, I. The children. *Br J Psychiatr* 126;127–145, 1975.
44. Folstein S, Rutter M: Infantile autism: A genetic study of 21 twin pairs. *J Child Psychol Psychiatr* 18;297–321, 1977.
45. Ritvo ER, Ritvo EC, Brothers AM: Genetic and immunohematologic factors in autism. *J Autism Devel Dis* 12;109–114, 1982.
46. Brown WT, Jenkins EC, Friedman EC, *et al*: Autism is associated with the fragile-X syndrome. *J Autism Develop Dis* 12;303–308, 1982.
47. Meryash DL, Szymanski LS, Gerald PS: Infantile autism associated with the fragile-X syndrome. *J Autism Devel Dis* 12;295–301, 1982.

A Broader Perspective

Applying Modern Mental-Retardation Service-System Principles to All Chronically Disabled Persons

Frank J. Menolascino

18.1. Introduction

This concluding chapter considers the broader applications of some of the diagnostic, treatment, research, and service innovations discussed in this book. Specifically, it addresses the challenge of attempting to transpose the modern mental-retardation systems model so as to directly serve chronically mentally ill citizens. The achievements of mental retardation professionals in the last 20 years have been of great importance in demonstrating effective programs and systems for helping chronically disabled persons who had previously been deemed beyond help. It is time to attempt to apply these innovations on a broader scale to meet the needs of other devalued individuals, who, although they are not mentally retarded, could well be served by programs and services previously thought applicable *only* to the retarded. Of specific concern are the chronically mentally ill and the "at-risk" elderly; it is obvious that, as human service professionals, we must hasten the development of more effective systems of care for promoting the healthy adaptation and societal integration of these individuals.

It has long been a temptation for professionals associated with community-based service systems for the mentally retarded to think of that configuration of services as a model for serving other groups of needy, chronically disabled citizens. The experiences of the author[1] with a regional community-based system for the mentally retarded (i.e., the Eastern Nebraska Community Office of Retardation—ENCOR) strongly suggests the possible utilization of this service model for the at-risk elderly and the chronically mentally ill. The fact that many of ENCOR's patients, during my last 15-year period of observation and active service involvements, had, in addition to being mentally retarded, allied indices of old age or chronic mental illness has spurred my professional interest in this challenge. True, there is the planning pitfall of the Procrustean bed:

Frank J. Menolascino • Departments of Psychiatry and Pediatrics, Nebraska Psychiatric Institute, University of Nebraska Medical Center, Omaha, Nebraska 68105.

Only by ignoring the clinical differences between the retarded, the elderly, and the chronical mentally ill can one conceive of serving them in similar ways. However, when the specific service needs of these groups are closely viewed, separately or as a group, one is not overly impressed by their distinctive needs (i.e., that the retarded need a "special" educational setting, the chronic mentally ill need "only" psychiatric facilities, the elderly need "extensive" medical care, and so on). It appears that undue focus on issues of exclusive service needs or professional turf problems mandates that these three groups be served only in segregated care programs or facilities. The result of these traditional approaches has been a failure to see beyond our current inadequate systems of care and support for such individuals. Although these apparently diverse groups of chronically handicapped citizens present different features and challenges to a service system, it has become increasingly apparent that their primary needs are neither exotic nor exclusively medical. For example, the primary and basically similar service needs of the retarded, the chronic mentally ill, and the handicapped elderly are programs and environments that will administer to, and mitigate, their social-adaptive disabilities through resocialization, rehabilitation, and structured activities to maintain or enlarge their current skills. These programmatic approaches are seldom provided in our current service offerings to the mentally ill and the elderly. Yet, these services could be provided for the elderly and the mentally ill in community-based rehabilitation systems that are based on the mental retardation model. Such a system does not deny the medical needs of the individuals, and it provides for these through the use of consultant physicians. Its value is the primary focus it gives to providing humane living environments and alternate support structure to persons whose disabilities are not answered by our current systems.

The concern for initiating community-based, noninstitutional modes of treatment for chronically disabled persons is not novel. Fifteen years ago, a benchmark study in psychiatry[2] drew this conclusion from a study of chronic schizophrenic citizens living in Louisville:

> It is hoped that this study and its findings will serve as a model for demonstration projects and programs for care and treatment of the aged, the retarded, and even the alcoholic and addicted, all of whom have been woefully neglected and shunted aside. The aged and the retarded, in particular, share many of the characteristics of the schizophrenic—chronicity, disabling character of the problem, poor functioning, limited productive or economic potential, and of course, the absence of specific treatment. Like the schizophrenic, too, the senile and retarded numerically constitute an inordinately large number of all those admitted and residing in state institutions. Home care and drug and other therapy would seem to be most applicable as a substitute for institutionalization and in reducing the hopelessness and stigma presently associated with these problems. (p. 255)

There are several key commonalities among the retarded, the chronic mentally ill, and the declining elderly that make it reasonable to serve them in a comprehensive, community-based rehabilitation program. The first, as the Louisville study points out, are the behavioral dimensions of their specific disabilities: deficiencies in self-care living skills, in social adaptive skills, and in work skills. Whatever the etiology of the underlying disability, these behavioral defects can be treated and managed within a modern rehabilitation system.[22] The second similarity is the extent to which these individuals are unconnected to family and community social supports. For a number of reasons—difficulty in managing them, the "burden" they represent, the stigma of their disability, or even the sometimes misguided encouragement of mental health systems to let them learn independence without guidance or support—the retarded, the elderly, and the chronically mentally ill frequently lose connections with their natural family. The third similarity—their frequently noted living conditions of poverty and drift—flows from the first two. Not all chronically disabled persons descend to the sorry state so vividly documented by recent books, articles, and television documentaries on the fate of previously institutionalized individuals or the unserved chronically ill who literally roam the streets.[23] Nevertheless, the impoverished elderly and the welfare-hotel–sequestered mentally ill singularly dramatize the impoverished nature of the service systems we have founded for these vulnerable groups.

18.2. The Current Modern Service Model for the Mentally Retarded

The service model for the mentally retarded that was evolved over the last decade in the United States has been based on similar experiences in Scandinavian countries. In the 1960s, the Scandinavian countries embarked on the development of alternatives to institutional care based on the concept that mentally retarded persons could be better treated—both physically and developmentally—in small, community-based, normalizing environments. Accordingly, these countries did not initiate a policy of deinstitutionalization; instead, they formulated a national social policy of developing an array of services around each of the following major life dimensions of the mentally retarded: residential, educational, vocational, and leisure-time. Over the last two decades, the international focus of community-based service systems for the retarded has been on developing programs in these four areas. This focus has produced programs that enable mentally retarded persons with all levels of disability to live in community settings and to actively participate in varying ways in normal activities of school, work, recreation, and family life.

For many retarded persons, especially children who were already living with their natural families, the development of community services offered finite targeted services for their developmental needs. It was understood that these individuals already possessed a primary factor that favored their development: a secure position within an interpersonal milieu that fostered adaptive behavior and growth. For these individuals, there was no need to create that most difficult service—the alternative residence—that supplies warmth and concern for the disabled person's needs and the involvement in the community that is usually supplied by the handicapped person's family.

It is no exaggeration to see the residential component as the crucial foundation of a comprehensive, community-based service system. Without a system of alternative residences to serve the most atypical or abnormal individuals, who are also bereft of family and interpersonal supports, a human service system can hardly claim to be an alternative to the traditional "home" for chronically disabled individuals, the congregate-care public institution. The efforts of advocates of community-based systems to create service alternatives to institutionalization forced them to grapple early with the problem of creating residential environments in the community. After a decade, the early enthusiasm for the group home as the "answer" has given way to a larger perspective. Group homes are now seen as one component of a continuum of residential environments, each of which is structured in a way to address the most compelling of the client's needs: medical, behavioral, social, and developmental.

In their essay on the optimal residential continuum to serve the mentally retarded, McGee and Hitzing[3] pointed out several distinct advantages to establishing services to complete the continuum model of residential services for the mentally retarded and, by implication, for all chronically disabled citizens: (1) the continuum fills the "gaps" in residential services so that all disabled persons have an appropriate setting matched to their needs and abilities; (2) the continuum permits the client movement to less restrictive and less supportive settings as his or her gains in skills and functioning permit; and (3) the continuum is cost-effective, as at every step chronically disabled citizens are supported only to the degree that they require it.

Compared to models of care for other chronically disabled persons, the mental retardation model is highly developed. The model is, first of all, highly responsive to the ideology of normalization[4]—the energy and sense of which have vitalized the entire field of mental retardation. Second, the community-based model of services is sufficiently complex and flexible to permit services to all retarded persons. Finally, the model is no mere theoretical construct; it is an operational system in over 20 states in our country at this time.

18.3. Current Services for Chronically Disabled Persons

In our national social policy toward chronically disabled persons, we currently provide a set of services with huge gaps in it. As previously noted, retarded persons are probably the best served, although comprehensive community systems for their care nationally are still in the early stages of development, and hence, many retarded persons—especially those with allied mental illness—are still underserved. For the elderly person with diminished capacities for self-sustenance, there have been few services established except the total-care model of the nursing home. For the chronic mentally ill patient, there are few examples of community-based programs or facilities that offer any focused rehabilitative care between periodic readmissions for acute care and outpatient–day-hospital mental-health care. Although the chronic mental patient may live in a variety of residential settings in the community (e.g., board and care homes, welfare hotels, and private residential facilities), these tend to represent sheltered facilities that offer little in the realm of definitive mental health or rehabilitative care.

In general, all of these chronically disabled persons are faced with all-or-nothing service alternatives: either live in the community with poorly focused or inadequate partial supports, or accept the alternative of long-term institutionalization in some form of congregate-care facility. If we look closely at the community, we see how tenuous are the supports provided for these persons with marginal psychosocial capacities for survival. Elderly persons tend to receive food, special transportation provisions, occasional forgiveness of utility bills, and only passing attention to their needs for leisure activities and companionship. If they have no friends or family to help them, their last years are apt to be lonely, stressful, and undignified.

Surveys of the elderly disclose how frequently the nonmedical problems of isolation, the need for in-home assistance, and financial need have been the primary determinants in their decisions to enter nursing homes.[5-7] It has been estimated that, in nearly 10% of the elderly population, the capability for self-sufficiency and independent living is fragile.[8] For the chronic mentally ill, the service situation may be worst of all: there are few rehabilitative or residential services available to integrate them into purposive living; and they receive the "best" current psychiatric treatment for the acute episodes of their chronic mental illness and, after short-term hospitalization, tend to be placed back in the interpersonal situations that exacerbated their mental illness in the first place. Even in the best of systems, psychiatric "aftercare" amounts to little more than case following. Typically, little effort is made to begin the arduous task of resocialization, or rebuilding the patient's support systems. In addition, the stigma of chronic mental illness tends to be more intense and more difficult to accept on the part of the community than either retardation or old age.

At the other end of the service spectrum is the institutional life. Although the deinstitutionalization movement has diminished the populations of state institutions for the retarded and the chronically ill, we should not be blind to the existence of congregate-care facilities that have sprung up to "reinstitutionalize" these persons. Many of the individuals who have left the state institutions to live "in the community" now live, instead, in nursing homes and private proprietary homes for adults that house as many as 100 persons. Perhaps there are habilitation advantages to being "in the community" in this dubious way, but it is difficult to see how the quality of living in these settings—congregate care, segregation from the challenges and richness of community life, institutional dependence, and the scant opportunities for the use of adaptive social, work, and living skills—can provide for the rehabilitation of disabled persons. On the contrary, such settings promote stigmatization, decline of function, unnecessary dependence, and feelings of uselessness,[9,10] all of which human service systems must find ways to reverse, not promote.

The last 20 years have been "liberal" decades in their concern for protecting devalued citizens from abuse at the hands of institutions. The rights of mental patients and retarded persons have been increasingly recognized and protected. Nevertheless, these legal protections are still largely definitions of what may *not* be done to and for individuals entrusted to the institution's care. Such needy individuals still await definition (and action) as to what they are entitled to in terms of service and rehabilitation. The mentally diabled and handicapped are entitled to the least restrictive setting for treatment, but these minimally restrictive settings often do not exist, and this is the most obvious defect of the policy of deinstitutionalization. Deinstitutionalized persons have been freed from conditions that abused their humanity and unnecessarily restricted them at the price of depriving them of their sense of place and daily community interactions with people and activities—none of which are usually forthcoming in many of the communities into which they have been dumped. Instead, during the 1960s and 1970s, we have seen the great boom in the nursing-house industry, as well as the rise of dubious shelter facilities that do little more than put a roof over their clientele's heads and feed them. Deinstitutionalization has taken place at a time when it was assumed that support systems were available in the community. *Community*, by definition, is a network of individuals, families, social groups, and services, whose interaction defines the activities, the health, and the sense of purpose and place of its members. It was assumed that deinstitutionalized persons would resume relationships, find purpose, and gain a sense of place, when, in fact, many had been institutionalized in the first place because of their failure or inability to accomplish these life goals.

A major conceptual failure in our current service offerings to chronically disabled persons is the assumption that their presenting problems are concrete or discrete entities; rather, they are more likely to be symptoms of unmet broader needs. Human service systems have taken little cognizance of the decline of those societal infrastructures that in the past may have protected and given purpose to these individuals: their primary and extended family, their neighborhoods, and the sense of shared human purpose we call *community*. The service system tends to try to meet these needs via focused, economical approaches—and frequently overlooks the causative factors of poverty, isolation, lack of personal support systems, and poor social-adaptive skills. The stopgap financial aids given the elderly, the periodic rehospitalizations of the chronic mentally ill—these are indeed necessary measures for the survival of such individuals, but they in no way provide remediation of skills, a resumption of purposeful living, or the connection to community life needed by these persons if they are to survive more than minimally.

A modern human-service-systems approach to recovering such individuals from useless lives will hinge on the continuing change of public and professional attitudes toward the retarded, the elderly, and the chronically mentally ill. Although these attitudes have become more accepting and tolerant since the 1960s, there remains, in both public and professional attitudes, the debris of these individuals' developmental potential that is untapped. The stereotypes of the retarded as "dangerous deviants," "vegetables," or "idiots who are unable to learn" have pretty much been conquered in the last 20 years. But the negative stereotypes of the chronically mentally ill (e.g., "crazy," "dangerously unstable," "hopeless") and the elderly live on. And they live on because the current professional posture of avoidance toward these two groups lends credence and support to the stereotypes. Robert Butler, in *Growing Old in America—Why Survive?*,[11] speaks of the "senile write-off": the marked tendency of physicians to view the decline of elderly persons as necessarily the permanent and irreversible signs of major brain impairments. In the NIMH report *New Views on Older Lives*,[12] the lack of psychiatric interest in the elderly is even more vigorously noted: "Although a high proportion of nursing home patients are mentally ill, psychiatrists were found to play a negligible role in their care" (p. 122). Although the chronically mentally ill do receive periodic psychiatric care at the time of relapse and rehospitalization, research indicates that this care is quite perfunctory, as priority is given to patients presenting a "favorable" prognosis: high motivation, an intact family, and illness of recent onset.[13] It would appear, to judge from their usual noninvolvement on behalf of elderly and chronically mentally ill patients, that professionals have written off these disabled persons as hopeless and untreatable. Given such attitudes on the part of professional caregivers, it should not be surprising if public opinion acquiesces to what seems to be the prevailing attitude of professionals.

18.4. Challenges in Establishing Modern Systems of Service

Perhaps the biggest roadblock to the establishment of a modern system of care to serve the chronically disabled is the fragmentation of the mental health professions. Because we tend to regard ourselves, first of all, as psychiatrists, psychologists, social workers, and mental retardation professionals, we find it extremely difficult to face and resolve problems whose resolution is interdisciplinary in nature. Care of the mentally ill retarded person is a case in point. The care of such individuals requires the close cooperation of mental-retardation, mental-health, special-education, social-work, and vocational-rehabilitation professionals in the synchronization of treatment–management efforts. Until we can "bridge the gap" between these professions, the person with complex or multiple diagnoses will fit into no coordinated system of care. So it is also with the chronically mentally ill and the handicapped elderly: their needs are medical and developmental and they require the support of physicians and behavioral specialists, as well as the less specialized attention of those who can provide warmth and care. To serve all these disabled persons, we need a very high level of interdisciplinary cooperation.

One of the professions that I believe is most crucial to the establishment of such interdisciplinary human-service systems is the medical profession— and more specifically, psychiatry. Accordingly, it is appropriate to discuss the potential role of psychiatry in this endeavor. Indeed, it is both appropriate and timely, as the current era is a time when psychiatry is at a crossroads, poised between more fully accepting the social-community problems of the chronically disabled, and retreating to the more limited, traditional biomedical approach. It may be helpful to highlight the aspects of the traditional medical model of treatment that continues to produce major professional blind spots in the care of the chronically disturbed. Conceptually, the model of a streptococcal inflamed throat in a person can be utilized to illustrate the key elements of the medical model. The key physical signs and symptoms are noted by the physician, and a throat swab for a laboratory culture is obtained. The specific symptoms, coupled with the specific identified agent (i.e., the streptococcal bacteria), lead to *specific* treatment and resolution. However, this clear-cut medical model of diagnosis and treatment can become quite obscure if the signs and symptoms are indistinct, the specific cause is unknown, and definitive treatments are not available. On another level, as diagnosis and/or treatment becomes less specific and cure is not possible, then the number of treaters involved becomes rapidly enlarged as the more complex and long-standing symptoms persist to handicap the patient and tax the strength of his or her family support system. Accordingly, the traditional medical model of treatment of a specific *physical illness* owes its success to the subordination of all factors external to the doctor–patient relationship. Within the private office or the hospital environment, the physician can marshal all his or her attention, the hospital's technical resources, and the necessary fellow treaters to one narrowly circumscribed goal: to cure or arrest the disease process in the patient. Within this configuration, the patient's family, the community, and the political climate are matters that are not permitted influence over the physician's expertise, precisely because these "externals" have no scientifically verifiable effect on the course of the disease and the recovery.

In a more specific sense, the "medical model" is not monolithic. There are in fact three medical models: (1) the acute infection model; (2) the surgical model; and (3) the chronic illness model. What distinguishes these models is the increasing dependence of the physician on individuals other than himself or herself, as well as his or her need to exert influence over an increasing number of nonmedical factors.

18.4.1. Acute Infection Model

In the acute infection model (as discussed previously), the patient presents the physician with a specific, circumscribed problem, which the physician resolves essentially in the one-to-one physican–patient relationship and within a relatively brief time period. Even if hospitalization is required, other medical personnel function essentially as agents of the diagnosing physician. Ideally, the patient's recovery leaves no residual symptoms or disabilities that are likely to remain and hence become chronic.

18.4.2. Surgical Model

In the surgical model (e.g., gall bladder removal for biliary stone impaction), the delivery of care is complicated by the increasing number of medical steps necessary to resolve the patient's complaint. Straightaway, the admission to the hospital prevents one-to-one treatment, and now, the model becomes professionally more complex as to control and communication. Preoperative care, surgery, and postoperative care require the cooperation and integration of the concerns of a number of medical professionals and paraprofessionals.

Smooth functioning is assured, however, by the operation of traditional hierarchies and their common definitions of the patient's problem. Thus, to contrast the surgical with the acute infection model, we see that the treater-to-patient ratio has expanded, the likelihood of residual problems or disabilities (e.g., postoperative complications) has expanded, and the possibility that the physician and his or her helpers will need to more actively take into account the patient's family has increased.

18.4.3. Chronic Illness Model

Lastly, in the chronic illness model (which is well illustrated by the diagnosis and management of mental retardation or chronic mental illness), the focus is no longer on cure, but on the amelioration of discomfort and the maintenance of as much intact residual functioning as possible. Within this model, the task of the treaters may range from monitoring by a few professionals to the creation of total alternative interpersonal and technical instrumentation environments to maintain the individual medically, socially, and psychologically. The ratio of treaters to individuals expands considerably, as do the problems of cooperation and integration of the viewpoints and treatment intentions of several professional disciplines. Plans for long-term care must be formulated—a dimension that demands active and ongoing family understanding and inputs as to further complications or expected residuals.

18.5. Psychiatry and the Chronic Patient

One major aspect of psychiatry's current identity crisis has to do with the long-term, apparently intractable problems of many types of mental illness. It is the long-term (i.e., chronic) patient who forcefully raises questions that probe at psychiatry's identity:

1. Is the problem perhaps biomedical after all (rather than psychosocial or interactional), and hence, should the psychiatrist turn full-face toward medical management and research to solve such problems?

2. What is the value of psychotherapy, anyway,—especially for these individuals, who, unlike our prime psychotherapy candidates, do not seem to make major improvements, no matter what we do?

3. Is there something we should be doing outside the hospital walls with communities, other professions, and nonprofessionals to more effectively *help* these long-term patients (even if we cannot "cure" them)?

A central problem in psychiatry's efforts to redirect itself and redefine its tasks remains the chronic mentally ill patient and his or her continuing need for human service supports.

A recent report of the Group for the Advancement of Psychiatry analyzed and synopsized recent research in the service situation for chronically mentally ill citizens and suggested appropriate modern programs of rehabilitation and support.[13] The report states that these patients' adaptation depends on five groups of factors, related to:

1. The patient, the seriousness of his or her illness, and his or her current level of intact personality functions.
2. The family, and the extent to which their attitudes, expectations, and demands are realistic.
3. The community, and the extent to which it fosters tolerance, integration, and active effort on the part of disabled persons, and insists on quality residential care with easy access to specialized treatment when necessary.
4. The political climate, and its receptivity to advocates for the chronic patients.
5. Mental-health-system factors, including the availability of community care, the capacities and priorities of community mental-health centers, third-party payment patterns, and the willingness of mental health systems to commit themselves to a coherent system of short- and long-term residential and rehabilitative care.

In short, because the chronic patient is so frequently bereft of supports from self, others, or systems, an appropriate modern approach to treatment must account for many variables and continually attempt to adjust them to the needs of each chronic patient. The best example of the ecological approach remains the Louisville Home Care Study by Pasamanick,[2] but as the Group for the Advancement of Psychiatry (GAP) Report authors noted, this successful family support model has had no observable impact on current community-mental-health practice.

The medical model of psychiatry implies a number of treatment–management features, all of which have at one time or another been called counter-therapeutic vis-à-vis the long-term patient:

1. Focus on the diagnostic problem, rather than on growth in adaptation.
2. Focus of treatment efforts primarily on acute episodes.
3. Failure to consult or fully utilize the significant other in the patient's life for ongoing support purposes.
4. The tendency of aftercare responsibility to remain with the patient.
5. Persistent uninvolvement with advocacy groups (because that would compromise medical impartiality).
6. Disinclination to become involved with nonpsychiatric therapeutic approaches.

One problem of the medical model has been the persistent reluctance of medical practitioners to incorporate other models of service delivery, despite the apparent current failure of the community-mental-health-center model to adequately resolve the problems of service delivery for chronic, long-term patients. Though deinstitutionalization has been accepted as an appropriate step for putting that fairly discredited model into the past, the mental health profession has developed no really workable alternatives to care for those individuals who formerly occupied state hospital wards.

Our human service systems have a paucity of residential settings that could even remotely be considered individualized, humanizing, or truly "in the community." Most of the current community settings for the chronically disabled (e.g., private proprietary homes for adults, nursing homes, large group homes, and boarding houses) merely perpetuate in the community the aimless drift of institutional life. A more striking lack is the absence of a comprehensive continuum of care in natural community settings for such persons. No system now exists for the chronically disabled that, like the residential model for the retarded person, provides ongoing training to spur the growth of adaptive behavior and increased self-sustenance on the part of the individual. Finally, though we have the knowledge and the models of care available, we need the determination to bring such systems of care into being. The Group for the Advancement of Psychiatry[13] emphasized this need to act on the basis of our current knowledge:

> The literature of the last two or three years is replete with positive descriptions of halfway houses, day hospital programs, day care centers, transitional care services, sheltered workshops, welfare hotels, apartment living projects, drug clinics, resocialization training groups, foster homes, structured homes, and patient advocates or ombudsmen. Characteristically each report ends with the statement that "evaluation of the program in progress." However, one gains the impression that much experimental work is going on, and that we possess a host of techniques for improving our present poor record in providing community care services—if we have the will. (p. 337)

18.6. The Community-Based Services Model in Mental Retardation

18.6.1. Overview

It is necessary, at this time, that the field of mental health and its leaders look seriously at the "mental retardation model" of services, particularly its now 10-year-old development of services and support systems at the community level, such as the Eastern Nebraska Community Office of Retardation[14] and Macomb-Oakland in Michigan. Although at both the services and the state administration level it has been difficult to separate mental health services from mental retardation services, there has been, in some states, an impressive development of community-based systems for managing citizens who present many of the same problems as the chronically mentally ill. Mental health professionals should ask: What are the main components of the community-based mental-retardation model and are these adaptable to the context of mental health approaches?

It is important first to glance briefly at the remarkable changes that have taken place in the field of mental retardation in the last 20 years. As recently as 1960, the care and treatment of the mentally retarded took place almost exclusively in large congregate-care institutions. Retarded individuals who were not institutionalized had extremely few services available at the community level. Intellectually, mental retardation was a stagnant pond, with no springs of new ideas. In this context, the personnel shortage, the low esteem of the field, and psychiatry's avoidance of mental retardation as static and uninteresting could be understood as effects of a mode and milieu of treatment that were unremittingly bleak. At the current time, mental retardation professionals can point to the following developments as evidence of the dynamism of change in mental retardation:

1. A 350,000-member national advocacy association (The Association for Retarded Citizens of the United States).
2. Widely accepted ideologies of treatment and management (e.g. normalization and the developmental model).
3. The rapid and extensive development of comprehensive service systems at the community level.
4. A series of legal decisions over the last decade that have expanded the human and civil rights of the mentally retarded.
5. A vastly renewed professional field, measurable by a number of indices: the number of professionals, the members in professional societies, publications, research, and the number of students.

Without asserting that this rejuvenation has reached an endpoint—for the task of converting care for the retarded from the large-scale institutional model to the community model is far from over—it is fair to say that the last 20 years have brought major change and help to the lives of many retarded persons and their families. In the process, there have been developed a number of characteristic methods, attitudes, and approaches that explain the success of mental retardation professionals (and concerned parents!) in turning the field around. These methods, attitudes, and approaches—and one should note the extent to which they *contrast* with those prevalent in psychiatry—are as follows:

1. Focus less on the retarded citizen's insight, the origins of the problems, or the prognosis; rather, concentrate more on their potential for behavioral change and adaptation.
2. Cultivate an attitude of cooperation and collaboration in the retarded citizen's rehabilitation, instead of adversary or blame-casting attitudes (especially with parents).
3. Accept the interdisciplinary approach to diagnosis, habilitation, and management—with the accompanying interdisciplinary-team approach.
4. Relate to the parents of the retarded (except in extreme cases) as potential educable resources in the treatment, the prevention of potential problems, the provision of support systems, advocacy, and service monitoring. In most instances, the parents are very willing "co-treaters" of their son or daughter. An amalgamation of the pilot parents' program in retardation[15] and the People First program[16] is the prototype here.
5. Accept that nonprofessionals can offer much in the rehabilitation of the retarded—a direct corollary of the principle of normalization.
6. Focus on residential treatment alternatives (i.e., group homes and monitored independent living) as the crux of community-based programming for persons with chronic problems in adaptation to the world around them.

7. Actively support the efforts of advocates for retarded citizens, whether they are parents, concerned citizens, or other professionals.

8. Actively utilize information and public-relations approaches to educate the general public about the needs of handicapped persons. Beyond the consultation and education model of community psychiatry, tough and energetic public-relations thrusts must be utilized on an ongoing basis.

18.6.2. The Residential Rehabilitation Model

Perhaps the most important heuristic achievement of the community-based mental-retardation service systems has been the development of a residential care system that, at least potentially, can provide the advantages of community placement to persons of all levels of handicaps and functioning. In the case of the mentally retarded, residential services have been crucial to the success of community-based systems because (1) such services maintain in the community those individuals whose families are unable to keep them at home; and (2) residences can be structured in specialized ways—in staffing, activities, and architecture—to fit the individual needs of even severely handicapped persons. The development of specialized and individualized residences is a crucial feature of the modern residential systems model; it answers very directly the current apologies for the large institutions that the community-based systems cannot service the severely handicapped.

A comprehensive residential system incorporates the following key concepts and programs:

1. *The developmental maximation unit.* This is a residential setting for up to 20 medically fragile individuals with severe developmental disorders. The setting provides a homelike, stimulating environment and developmental remediation until medical stabilization and the procurement of an appropriate community placement (e.g., original family, foster care, or a special group home that is barrier-free and specially staffed) permit the individual to move to a less restrictive residential alternative.

2. *The group home, or training residence.* In this setting, three to five retarded citizens live with the staff members while participating in the daily community activities appropriate to their age, either work or school. The best conceived group homes use the period of placement as a period of socialization, training in community living skills, and preparation for greater living independence.

3. *The crisis assistance unit.* Typically, this unit provides care for individuals who normally live with their families, but who, because of family difficulties (e.g., medical illness of the mother) or the parents' need for respite, need short-term residential placement. The overriding principle of care here is to match a short-term family crisis with a short-term residential stay. Too often, a short-term family crisis has led to the inappropriate long-term "solution" of institutionalization.

4. *The alternative living unit (ALU).* The ALU rubric may apply to a foster care setting, a staffed apartment setting, or an independent-living arrangement

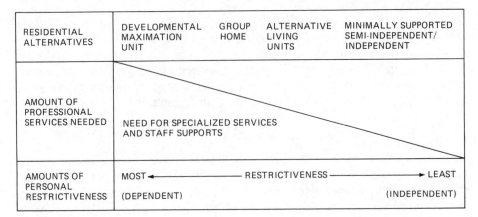

Figure 1. The modern residential system for the chronically handicapped.

for a retarded citizen. Flexible in structure, staffing, and intensity of specialized support, the ALU is maximally responsive to the retarded citizen's needs, whether he or she requires brief but intense long-term, or only periodic, support. Graphically these residential models are presented in Figures 1 and 2. The residential system model offers a continuum of units that provide specialized programming and staff support while permitting flexibility and potential

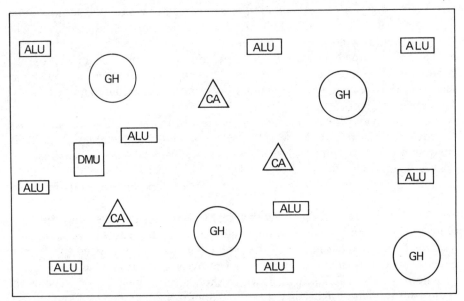

ALU = ALTERNATIVE LIVING UNIT   CA = CRISIS ASSISTANCE HOME
DMU = DEVELOPMENTAL MAXIMATION UNIT   GH = GROUP HOME (TRAINING RESIDENCE)

Figure 2. Comprehensive range of residential services.

movement into less restrictive physical and interpersonal settings. These specialized programs must also include the full range of educational intervention (e.g., from infant development programs to special preschools, special education in the primary school years), and then free vocational habilitation (sheltered workshops, job stations for the retarded in the midst of industrial plants, to semi-independent and independent work placements), and—most clearly: residential alternatives.

Figure 1 illustrates that even the most severely retarded can live in residential alternatives (e.g., outside of the primary family home) that are small and normalizing. Early in life, these complex children may need a medically and developmentally oriented setting such as the Developmental Maximation Unit that focuses on sustaining their life while maximizing their developmental growth. As they grow and develop, they graduate to a less restrictive physical setting such as a four to six person group home and, later, to a much smaller alternative residential setting (e.g., a staff department for two retarded citizens). If they developmentally progress further, they can graduate to semi-independent residential settings. Similarly, this needed array of residential services in a given demographic area must have <u>all</u> of these residential alternatives in order to serve the wide variety of levels and types of retarded individuals in a large city. This full system of residential services is depicted in Figure 2. The reader may obtain a more in-depth review of this topic by referring to Menolascino.[25]

This community-based system of services as exemplified by the ENCOR model can provide a comprehensive range of residential services for chronically handicapped citizens (i.e., in this instance for the mentally retarded, but it could readily be utilized for the chronic mentally ill, for handicapped or impaired elderly citizens). In Figure 3 are noted the combined elements, which need to be present, to provide the services required for many chronically handicapped populations.

Utilizing this basic framework of services ENCOR has been able to provide learning, work, and residential placements for retarded citizens at every level of functioning and allied handicaps, including allied major mental illness. Beyond the key program component of residential services, the reader should also note the other services (depicted in Figure 1). This is not an extensive list of services that are needed, and we are underscoring herein only one of the key service components: residential. The developmental maximation unit, the training residences, and the crisis assistance house can flexibly provide long-, medium-, and short-term care for clients with medical problems, lags in maturation, behavioral deficits, or temporary situational difficulties. It should be noted that the crisis assistance houses directly answer what repeated surveys of parents or other family members of the chronically handicapped request as their <u>most</u> pressing need: respite care. In brief, the developmental goal for all disabled individuals is the ready availability of alternative living units where their needs can be met in a variety of individualized ways in familylike environments.

Residential Alternatives	Chronic care units; group homes; clustered apartments; semi-independent and independent living alternatives
Vocational Alternatives	Sheltered workshops; job stations in industry; semi-independent and independent employment opportunities
Crisis Assistance	Supportive counseling; residential respite care; periodic help with physical activities
Assigned Counselors	Ongoing supportive, guidance, and crisis assistance
Health Care	Family practitioner; dental needs; general hospitals; and in-patient psychiatric care

Figure 3. Basic service components for populations of chronically impaired citizens (e.g., mentally retarded, mentally ill, and impaired elderly).

Before considering the types of residential placement that could be developed for the chronically mentally ill and the handicapped elderly by applying this model of residential care, we should consider the possible benefits that these persons could gain from specially supported living in the community. A primary gain is the maintenance of self-esteem and self-image that results from the person's being able to maintain her or his ties to family, friends, community, and familiar places. Such an individual, whether retarded, elderly, or chronically schizophrenic, could continue to own possessions, to be among persons of all ages, and to use his or her own volition (as the clinical condition permits) in regard to meals, recreation, and leisure-time activities. He or she would not be subject to the age segregation, the physical restrictions, the frequently demeaning and depressing medical atmosphere, or the choicelessness of institutional services such as state hospitals and nursing homes. Particularly for the handicapped elderly person, who is certainly at risk of further physical decline because of depressed mood, the maintenance of maximal health must be a major goal. Maintenance (in the case of the elderly) and even a sharpening (in the case of the chronically mentally ill) of personal and interpersonal living skills demand that these skills be frequently used.[24] Such maintenance and refinement are most easily and effectively accomplished in a real (not simulated) community, where work, household tasks, recreation, relations with others, and self-care require their continuing exercise. Community residential care supports and encourages a continued sense of self-responsibility, without which encouragement a person may give up and become totally dependent, as we frequently see in nursing homes and state hospitals.

Supported residential services (as in the Eastern Nebraska Community Office of Retardation) imply guidance on medical and psychological-behavioral assessment. Guidance here can include not only supervision to ensure, for example, that medications will be taken, dangerous undertakings will be avoided, and access will be gained to appropriate work and recreation; guidance connotes corrective and educational programming as well. A troubled individual may need psychotherapy; he or she may need a behavior change program that encourages adaptive behaviors and discourages those that are inappropriate. This modern service system provides access to the various generic agencies and service providers that can be used to meet these special needs. These mainstream services include the various therapies, work and leisure activities, educational opportunities (including career education for adults), and other services that help the chronically handicapped individual to attain or express optimal levels of functioning.

Lastly, another major benefit is the individualization of the residential environment to fit the particular needs of a chronically handicapped individual. With regard to staff support, this means providing as much or as little, as specialized or as general, staff aid as is necessary. For example, with many elderly and even chronically mentally ill persons, residential placement might require only minimal support staff, such as drop-in professional staff to check periodically on high-functioning persons. Alternatively, several staff persons would be needed with the more severely involved individual, so as to coordinate, administer, and conduct daily treatment, activity, and learning programs among a small group of like-functioning persons within a group-home residential model of care.

18.7. The Need for the Residential-Rehabilitation Model

The chronically disabled patient in the community—whether retarded, mentally ill, or elderly—remains one of the last outsiders in American life. In an era when social attitudes and societal policies were focused and broadened to provide acceptance and opportunities for various excluded social groups, these stigmatized disabled persons were neglected and ignored, and despite a genuine expansion of human services for persons with mental and physical problems, little has been done to aid them with their real needs.[25] In hundreds of cities across our country, the retarded and the mentally ill continue to shuffle aimlessly around the problem of survival, while the elderly decline quietly into poverty and helplessness or enter nursing homes, which are frequently institutional versions of that same condition. Neither the healing professions nor the human service systems have done much for these individuals except to treat partial ailments that result from the condition; it is as if helplessness and unconnectedness were not officially defined as a human problem. In their persistent attempts to bring about "care" and "recovery," the helping professions have often forgotten that there are extremes of the human condition, and that these extremes are neither "curable" nor subject to easy answers, although they are manageable. And the management and rehabilitation of the chronically disabled person remains one of the greatest challenges in the human services field at this time.

It is crucial that the challenge of serving the chronically handicapped be faced directly. The indirect method of general-hospital inpatient treatment or the community-mental-health-center approach has been shown to be inadequate, simply because the disabled person's problem is primarily in evidence when he or she is not in the hospital or the center. Proper treatment must focus on his or her extended life in the community.

It is necessary to face this challenge now in order not to squander the humanitarian concern of the last two decades, the current models adaptable to serving the long-term patient, and the fund of knowledge and techniques available for meeting the needs of chronically disabled persons. At the current time, now that we have achieved some degree of deinstitutionalization and the establishment of new community-based models of care, there is a real danger that the thrusts of community-based mental-retardation and community-psychiatry-service components will be blunted by overly stringent cost–service-benefit concerns and an inability to imagine service models of care for the chronically disabled other than long-term inpatient hospitalization.

Many are concerned that mental health professionals are turning back to the medical model of care precisely at a time when the field must go beyond it. In the words of Gurevitz,[17]

> Whether we like it or not, the mental health system increasingly will be identified with helping severely disturbed and chronic patients. We will gain sanction and credibility if we can deal with the problem constructively. Failing that, the mental health and other professions dealing with the chronic patient will be narrowed in scope and responsibility, and public support for developing and maintaining services for this population will be lost. If we choose not to bother with the chronic patient, we will have lost a major justification for all mental health services, not just those for the long-term or regressed patient. To ignore the problem would be to reaffirm the suspicions and stereotype of those who doubt the validity of accomplishments of mental health intervention. (p. 116)

It is necessary, then, to make a start, however imperfect, because the long-term patient will always be with us. Though prevention and treatment breakthroughs may reduce the number of retarded persons in need of residential services, the numbers of elderly disabled will grow as medical technology increases the average potential life span. The number of chronically mentally ill persons may increase as well, according to Dr. Morton Kramer,[18] recent Director of the Division of Biometry and Epidemiology of National Institute of Mental Health. He predicted that,

> the number of cases under treatment for schizophrenia will increase in the population during the coming decade. The chances of having at least one admission to a psychiatric facility for schizophrenia during a lifetime are now seven out of 100. Until there is a real breakthrough in our ability to prevent or cure this disorder, and unless we focus our energy on improving the long-term effectiveness of treatment and supportive care, the number of persons needing services is likely to further overwhelm the mental health system. (p. 12)

Because of the outcast status of the long-term disabled mentally ill or handicapped elderly persons in our society, we know very little about the prevention of their disabilities, the maintenance and growth of functions, and the long-range potential role of families in the treatment and rehabilitation of these individuals. With an effort to deal directly with these problems, we would learn more, much as the past decade of community-based services for the retarded has produced usable knowledge about their learning abilities, methods of training and teaching, and the maximization of their skills. At the present time, the lack of similar knowledge concerning the chronically mentally ill and the disabled elderly is a great impediment to the provision of effective services for individuals. As Harold Holder[19] wrote, "We do not understand personal support systems (why some work and some fail) and do not teach those who enter the treatment system much about developing healthy arrangements for themselves (p. 39). In using the community-based mental-retardation residential model as a template for developing genuinely supportive and rehabilitative systems for a variety of chronically disabled persons, we could learn a great deal that would remedy those specific areas of ignorance that so limit the applicability of community psychiatry and geriatric programs in the community.

Finally, we would take a large step toward buttressing and adapting those institutions—the family, the community, and neighborhood support systems— whose decline in modern America has much to do with the vulnerability and the unconnectedness of chronically disabled persons.

18.8. Conclusion and Summary

The history of community-based mental-retardation services in our country during the last two decades can point the way toward what is needed for serving *all* chronically disabled individuals, especially those with persistent mental illnesses and complex circumstances of aging. First, the crucial catalysts of change in mental retardation came from the interaction of several types of individuals:

1. The concerned professional who was willing to work with the mentally retarded and to actively advocate publicly on behalf of their rights to services and care.

2. Concerned parents who, beyond being activists for their sons or daughters, helped to initiate the early models of community-based treatment and management.

3. Concerned legislators who were open to the "cry for help" from organized professional and parent groups.

Similarly, mental health professionals can contribute to meaningful changes by actively working with chronic patients, by increasingly relating to parents of clients as potentially helpful resources, and by actively advocating for modern systems of treatment and management for chronic patients within their home communities.[20]

Second, we need to learn all we can about making initially small residential-rehabilitation services work on behalf of the chronically disabled. This would be a giant step away from the persisting traditional hospital-based medical model of mental-health service delivery. For many, it will mean learning the frustrations and difficulties of the rehabilitation team approach, and eventually seeing its direct and indirect benefits in the enhanced care of those they treat. The mental health professional must learn, too, the art of fully utilizing parents, generic community agencies, and the general public as supporters to be educated and worked with, instead of as adversaries. The effective education and attitude-changing of policy-making individuals and the general public are not the least of the tasks ahead, if the residential rehabilitation model is to succeed.

Because of the medical and psychiatric problems of the chronically disabled, practitioners of medicine and psychiatry must take a leading role in the establishment of this new model of services for these currently devalued and vulnerable individuals.[21] To succeed in this necessary endeavor, mental health professionals must continue to support several approaches that break with the traditional-professional postures of the past:

1. A sociobehavioral approach to assessment and treatment.
2. Willingness to utilize and integrate professionals from other disciplines who can actively contribute to the remediation model.
3. A posture of active and responsible advocacy, which implies, by definition, a strong positive belief in the possibility of the chronically mentally ill individual's potential for growth—and a willingness to act to gain public support for this potential.

This broader perspective—beyond the current challenges of serving the mentally retarded–mentally ill individual—will entail ongoing professional advocacy, work, and commitments. If this sounds difficult or naive, one should recall that it was this same posture of advocacy and activism that, in the 1970s, launched a new approach to mentally retarded citizens. The new approach has matured into a modern national model of residential and rehabilitation services for the retarded patient. It is my contention that the elements of this model are eminently useful in giving direction to programming our country's ongoing efforts to serve *all* of its chronically disabled citizens.

ACKNOWLEDGEMENT. The author is grateful for the efforts of Mr. Robert Coleman and for his help in compiling this chapter and herewith acknowledges both.

References

1. Menolascino FJ: *Eastern Nebraska Community Office of Retardation: 5-Year Plan.* Omaha, ENCOR, December 1979.
2. Pasamanick B, Scarpitto FR, Dinitz S: *Schizophrenics in the Community.* New York, Appleton-Century-Crofts, 1966.
3. McGee JJ, Hitzing W: *Current Residential Services: A Critical Analysis.* Lincoln, University of Nebraska Medical Center, Center for the Development of Community Alternative Service Systems (CASS), 1978.
4. Wolfensberger W: *Normalization.* Toronto, National Institute on Mental Retardation, 1972.
5. Downey GW: The view of old age: No deposit, no return. *Modern Nursing Home* 29;59–64, 1972.

6. Glasscote R: *Old Folks at Home*. Washington, D.C., American Psychiatric Association, 1976.
7. Butler R: New approach to problems of the elderly. *Psychiatric News*, March 1978.
8. Menolascino FJ: *Institutionalization: Issues and Challenges*. Unit 9 of Profiles of Aging Series. Omaha, University of Nebraska Medical Center, 1978.
9. Goffman E: *Asylums*. Garden City, NJ, Anchor Books, 1961.
10. Vail D: *Dehumanization and the Institutional Career*. Springfield, IL, C. C. Thomas, 1966.
11. Butler R: *Growing Old in America—Why Survive?* New York, Harper and Row, 1976.
12. Rosenfeld A: *New Views on Older Lives*. A Sample of NIMH Sponsored Research and Service Programs, USDHEW Publ. #(Adm) 78-687. Rockville, MD, NIMH, 1978.
13. Group for the Advancement of Psychiatry. *The Chronic Mental Patient in the Community*, vol 10, pub. #102, May 1978. New York, Group for the Advancement of Psychiatry, 1978.
14. Menolascino FJ: *Challenges in Mental Retardation: Progressive Ideology and Services*. New York, Human Sciences Press, 1977.
15. Menolascino FJ, Coleman R: The pilot parent program: Helping developmentally disabled children through their parents. *Child Psychiatr Hum Dev* 10(5);41–48, 1980.
16. President's Committee on Mental Retardation. *Islands of Excellence*. Washington, DC, Author, 1979.
17. Gurevitz H: Caring for chronic patients: Some cautions and concerns. *Hosp Comm Psychiatr* 21(2);42–44, 1978.
18. Lackner J: An overview of the issues. *Hosp Comm Psychiatr* 29(1);29–31, 1978.
19. Holder H: Building accountability into the service system. *Hosp Comm Psychiatr* 29(1);38–39, 1978.
20. Reiss S, Levitar G, McNally R: Emotionally disturbed mentally retarded people: An underserved population. *Am Psychol* 33(4);361–367, 1982.
21. Matson JL: *Psychopathology in the Mentally Retarded*. New York, Grune & Stratton, 1983.
22. Stein LI, Test MA (eds): *Alternatives to Mental Hospital Treatment*. New York, Plenum Press, 1978.
23. Talbot JA (ed): *The Chronic Mentally Ill: Treatment Programs and Services*. New York, Human Sciences Press, 1983.
24. Paul GL, Lentz RJ: *Psychosocial Treatments of Chronic Mental Patients*. Cambridge, Harvard University Press, 1977.
25. Talbot JA (ed): *The Chronic Mental Patient: Five Years Later*. New York, Grune & Stratton, 1983.

Author Index

Italic numbers indicate pages where complete reference citations are given.

Subject Index

Aberrant behavior, 278
Adjustment disorders in mental retardation, 254
Adrenergic activity, 173
Adult dual diagnosis patients, 274, 275
Affective Disorders, groups of, 18
Alcoholism, 25
Alpha activity, 409
Amenorrhea, 118
American Academy of Child Psychiatry, 403, 407
American Association on Mental Deficiency, 5, 47, 87, 349
American Dance Therapy Association, 300
American Hospital Association, 231
American Journal of Psychiatry, 403
American Psychiatric Association, 46, 50, 403, 405
Anorexia nervosa, 117–118
Antisocial personality, 24
Anxiety, 8
Anxiety reactions, 22
Archives of General Psychiatry, 403
Assertiveness training, 387
Association for Retarded Citizens, 385
Autism, 34–35, 52, 182
 differential diagnosis of, 35
Autosomal abnormalities, 31
Aversive consequences. See behavior therapy. 125, 133, 139, 267
 electrical stimulation, 123, 137, 143
 overcorrection, 123, 132, 136, 139, 143
 physical restraint, 132
 punishment procedures, 124, 137

Beacon House Program
 Independent Living Group
  arts and crafts therapy, 303
  clinical profile, 292
  community meeting, 9, 299
  cooking therapy, 298
  counselor role, 293
  daily program schedule, 294
  dance movement therapy, 299–301

Beacon House Program (*Cont.*)
 education, 302
 group psychotherapy, 294
 group therapist, 295
 horticulture therapy, 297
 music therapy, 301
 program organization, 293
 sensory integration, 296
 Subpopulation of, 291–292
Beacon House Research Study
 interpretation of results, 307
 methodology, 305
 randomization test for matched pairs, 305
Behavior, 45
 abnormal, 67–69
 atypical, 65
 client problem, 336
 developmental viewpoint, 102, 235
 disorders, 12
 functional explanation, 103
 maladaptive, in mentally ill-mentally retarded, 266
 misconceptions of, 290
 modification approach, 314
 primitive, 17, 62–64
Behavioral communication vs. volitional aggression, 205–206
Behavioral myopia, 207–208
Behavior disturbances, 3, 8, 404
 aggression, 118–125
 choice of medication, 175
 etiological factors, 9
 explanation of, 102–105
 management of, 279–281
 self-injurious, 133–137
 self-stimulatory, 137–139
 thought disorders, 405
Behavior modification. *See* Behavior therapy; Independent living
 impact of mental retardation-mental illness, 70–71
 paraprofessional staff involved with, 369
 success of programs, 369